Mathematical and Statistical Estimation Approaches in Epidemiology

Gerardo Chowell · James M. Hyman ·
Luís M. A. Bettencourt · Carlos Castillo-Chavez
Editors

Mathematical and Statistical Estimation Approaches in Epidemiology

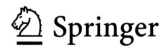 Springer

Editors

Dr. Gerardo Chowell
Arizona State University
School of Human Evolution & Social Change
Tempe AZ 85287-2402
USA
gchowell@asu.edu

Dr. James M. Hyman
Los Alamos National Laboratory
Los Alamos NM 87545
Mail Stop B284
USA
mac@t7.lanl.gov

Dr. Luís M. A. Bettencourt
Los Alamos National Laboratory
Los Alamos NM 87545
Mail Stop B284
USA
lmbett@lanl.gov

Dr. Carlos Castillo-Chavez
Arizona State University
Dept. Mathematics & Statistics
P.O.Box 871804
Tempe AZ 85287
USA
ccchavez@asu.edu

ISBN 978-90-481-2312-4   e-ISBN 978-90-481-2313-1
DOI 10.1007/978-90-481-2313-1
Springer Dordrecht Heidelberg London New York

Library of Congress Control Number: 2009926096

Printed on acid-free paper

Springer is part of Springer Science+Business Media (www.springer.com)

Preface

Mathematical and Statistical Estimation Approaches in Epidemiology compiles theoretical and practical contributions of experts in the analysis of infectious disease epidemics in a single volume. Recent collections have focused in the analyses and simulation of deterministic and stochastic models whose aim is to identify and rank epidemiological and social mechanisms responsible for disease transmission. The contributions in this volume focus on the connections between models and disease data with emphasis on the application of mathematical and statistical approaches that quantify model and data uncertainty.

The book is aimed at public health experts, applied mathematicians and scientists in the life and social sciences, particularly graduate or advanced undergraduate students, who are interested not only in building and connecting models to data but also in applying and developing methods that quantify uncertainty in the context of infectious diseases. Chowell and Brauer open this volume with an overview of the classical disease transmission models of Kermack-McKendrick including extensions that account for increased levels of epidemiological heterogeneity. Their theoretical tour is followed by the introduction of a simple methodology for the estimation of, the *basic reproduction number*, R_0. The use of this methodology is illustrated, using regional data for 1918–1919 and 1968 influenza pandemics. This chapter is followed by Greenwood and Gordillo's introduction to an analogous probabilistic framework. The emphasis is now on the computation of the distribution of the final epidemic size and the quantification of stochastically sustained oscillations. Next, the differences between *observable* and *unobservable* events in infectious disease epidemiology and their relationship to rigorous contact tracing and microbiological methodology are discussed in Chapter 3 by Nishiura et al. Furthermore, concepts like "dependent happening" and their role in identifying sources of infectious disease risk or in assessing vaccine efficacy are also discussed. In Chapter 4, Tennenbaum's engages us in a discussion of modeling perspectives and approaches through his discussion of the meaning of "contact". He challenges the reader to come up with novel approaches that bring together "ignored" biological and mechanistic aspects of the infection process.

Chapter 5 (Nishiura and Chowell) and Chapter 7 (Bettencourt) focus on real-time assessments of the reproduction number. The exposition is spiced with references to recent epidemic outbreaks. For example, Bettencourt uses his framework to estimate disease epidemiological parameters and to assess the effects of interventions in real time using data from the 2005 outbreak of Marburg hemorrhagic fever in Angola. In Chapter 8, Burr and colleagues review the theoretical and practical challenges associated with biosurveillance including the detection of disease outbreaks using traditional diagnosed case rates or syndromic surveillance data. In Chapter 6, Lloyd notes that parameter estimates are subject to uncertainty that arise not only from errors (noise) in the data but also from the structure of the model used in the fitting process. In other words, he argues that uncertainty must be evaluated at multiple levels to account for our ignorance or for the balance that each modeler must reach between biological detail and model complexity and objectives. Parameter estimation, Lloyd argues, must include structural sensitivity analyses. The use of historical data in epidemiological research is highlighted in Chapter 9 by Acuña-Soto's contribution. As he notes epidemiologists are reluctant to consider systematically the possibility of working with historical data albeit, as we have seen in the first Chapter, it is possible to extract valuable information from such data on influenza outbreaks. In fact, we acquired the kind of quantitative knowledge that let us quantify some of the differences between seasonal and pandemic influenza. Acuña-Soto's work[1], for example, on the epidemic of 1576 that killed 45% of the entire population of Mexico, highlights but a myriad of new possibilities for which the quantitative methods and approaches highlighted in this book can be put to good use.

Banks and colleagues in Chapter 11 provide a succinct overview of the statistical and computational aspects associated with inverse or parameter estimation problems for deterministic dynamical systems. Their results illustrate the impact that the marriage between statistical theory and applied mathematics is having in the study of infectious diseases while Chapter 10 (Arriola and Hyman) provides a general and thorough introduction to the field of sensitivity and uncertainty analyses, a central piece of any scientific work that is based on modeling.

The challenges and opportunities generated by studies of disease outbreak or disease dynamics in specific contexts are highlighted in the final chapters. Shim and Castillo-Chavez (Chapter 12) evaluate the potential impact that ongoing age-dependent vaccination strategies (in the United States and Mexico) are likely to have in reducing the prevalence of severe rotavirus infections. Rios-Doria et al. (Chapter 13) analyze the spatial and temporal dynamics of rubella in Peru, 1997–2006 via a wavelet time series analysis and other methods. The study is carried out in the context of changing policies that include the introduction of a vaccine and/or increases in vaccination rates. Cintron-Arias and colleagues (Chapter 15) model drinking as a "communicable" disease and, in the process, they highlight a new set of opportunities and possibilities for the applications of the mathematical and statistical approaches used in this volume. The focus here is on the evaluation of the role of relapse (ineffective treatment) on drinking dynamics but as a function of social network heterogeneity.

---

[1] R Acuna-Soto, LC Romero, and JH Maguire; Large epidemics of hemorrhagic fevers in Mexico 1545–1815; Am. J. Trop. Med. Hyg, 62(6), 2000, pp. 733–739.

The Editors would like to thank Melania Ruiz our associated Editor at Springer for her encouragement and infinite patience. We also thank the Springer publication staff for their support in helping us put this volume together. We also thank Carlos A. Torre for his technical support and sense of humor. Finally, we would like to thank all the authors for their timely and innovative contributions and their patience during the full process.

Tempe, AZ   Gerardo Chowell
Los Alamos, NM   James M. Hyman
Los Alamos, NM   Luís M.A. Bettencourt
Tempe, AZ   Carlos Castillo-Chavez

Contents

Contributors

Rodolfo Acuna-Soto Departamento de Microbiología y Parasitología, Facultad de Medicina, Universidad Nacional Autónoma de México, Delegación Coyoacán, México D.F. 04510, México, yvonne@ibt.unam.mx

Leon Arriola Department of Mathematiccal and Computer Sciences, University of WisconsinWhitewater, Whitewater, WI 53190, USA, arriolal@uww.edu

Luís M. A. Bettencourt Theoretical Division, MS B284, Los Alamos National Laboratory, Los Alamos NM 87545, USA; Santa Fe Institute, 1399 Hyde Park Road, Santa Fe, NM 87501, USA, lmbett@lanl.gov

Fred Brauer Department of Mathematics, The University of British Columbia, Vancouver, B.C., Canada V6T 1Z2, brauer@math.ubc.ca

Tom Burr Statistical Sciences Group, Los Alamos National Laboratory, Los Alamos NM 87545, USA, tburr@lanl.gov

Carlos Castillo-Chavez Mathematical, Computational, and Modeling Sciences Center, P.O. Box 871904, Arizona State University, Tempe, AZ 85287, USA; School of Human Evolution and Social Change, Arizona State University, Tempe, AZ 85287, USA; Department of Mathematics and Statistics, Arizona State University, Tempe, AZ, 85287, USA; Santa Fe Institute, 1399 Hyde Park Road, Santa Fe, NM 87501, USA, chavez@math.asu.edu

Gerardo Chowell School of Human Evolution and Social Change, Arizona State University, Box 872402, Tempe, AZ 85287, USA; Mathematical, Computational, Modeling Sciences Center, Arizona State University, Tempe, AZ 85287, USA; Division of Epidemiology and Population Studies, Fogarty International Center, National Institutes of Health, Bethesda, MD, USA, gchowell@asu.edu

Ariel Cintron-Arias Center for Research in Scientific Computation, Box 8205, North Carolina State University, Raleigh, NC 27695-8212, USA, acintro@unity.ncsu.edu

Marie Davidian Center for Research in Scientific Computation and Center for Quantitative Sciences in Biomedicine, North Carolina State University, Raleigh, NC 27695-8212, USA, davidian@eos.ncsu.edu

Luis F. Gordillo Department of Mathematics, University of Puerto Rico-RUM, Mayaguez, PR 00681-9018, USA, gordillo@math.uprm.edu

Dennis M. Gorman Department of Epidemiology and Biostatistics, School of Rural Public Health, Texas A&M Health Science Center, P.O. Box 1266, College Station, TX 77843-1266, USA, dennis-m-gorman@tamu.edu

Priscilla E. Greenwood Department of Mathematics and Statistics, Arizona State University, Tempe, AZ 85287-1804, USA, pgreenw@math.la.asu.edu

Paul J. Gruenewald Prevention Research Center, 1995 University Avenue, Suite 450, Berkeley, CA 94704, USA, paul@prev.org

James M. Hyman Theoretical Division, MS B284, Los Alamos National Laboratory, Los Alamos, NM 87545, USA, mac@t7.lanl.gov; hyman@lanl.gov

Hisashi Inaba Graduate School of Mathematical Sciences, University of Tokyo, 3-8-1 Komaba, Meguro-ku, Tokyo 153-8914, Japan, inaba@ms.u-tokyo.ac.jp

Masayuki Kakehashi Graduate School of Health Sciences, Hiroshima University, 1-2-3 Kasumi, Minami-ku, Hiroshima 734-8551, Japan, kakehashi@hiroshima-u.ac.jp

Alun L. Lloyd Biomathematics Graduate Program and Department of Mathematics, North Carolina State University, Raleigh, NC 27695, USA, alun_lloyd@ncsu.edu

Sarah Michalak Statistical Sciences Group, Los Alamos National Lab, Los Alamos NM 87545, USA, michalak@lanl.gov

Cesar Munayco-Escate Dirección General de Epidemiología, Ministerio de Salud, Perú, Jr. Camilo-Carrillo 402, Jesus Maria-Lima 11, Peru, cmunayco@dge.gob.pe

Hiroshi Nishiura Theoretical Epidemiology, University of Utrecht, Yalelaan 7, 3584 CL, Utrecht, The Netherlands, h.nishiura@uu.nl

Rick Picard Statistical Sciences Group, Los Alamos National Lab, Los Alamos NM 87545, USA, picard@lanl.gov

Daniel Rios-Doria School of Human Evolution and Social Change, Arizona State University, Box 872402 Tempe, AZ 85287, USA; Mathematical, Computational, Modeling Sciences Center, Arizona State University, Tempe, AZ 85287, USA, daniel@mathpost.asu.edu

John R. Samuels, Jr. Center for Research in Scientific Computation and Center for Quantitative Sciences in Biomedicine, North Carolina State University, Raleigh, NC 27695-8205, USA, jrsamue2@ncsu.edu

Fabio Sanchez Department of Biological Statistics and Computational Biology, Cornell University, Ithaca, NY 14853-7801, USA, fas9@cornell.edu

Eunha Shim Department of Epidemiology and Public Health, Yale School of Medicine, New Haven, CT, 06510, USA, eunha.shim@yale.edu

Karyn L. Sutton Center for Research in Scientific Computation and Center for Quantitative Sciences in Biomedicine, North Carolina State University, Raleigh, NC 27695-8212, USA, klsutton@unity.ncsu.edu

Stephen Tennenbaum Mathematical, Computational and Modeling Sciences Center, Arizona State University, Tempe, AZ 85287-1904, USA, set1@asu.edu

H. Thomas Banks Center for Research in Scientific Computation and Center for Quantitative Sciences in Biomedicine, North Carolina State University, Raleigh, NC 27695-8212; Department of Mathematics and Statistics, Arizona State University Tempe, AZ, 85287-1804, USA, htbanks@ncsu.edu

Xiaohong Wang Mathematical, Computational, and Modeling Sciences Center, P.O. Box 871904, Arizona State University, Tempe, AZ 85287, USA, Xiaohong.Wang@asu.edu

Alvaro Witthembury Dirección General de Epidemiología, Ministerio de Salud, Perú, Jr. Camilo-Carrillo 402, Jesus Maria-Lima 11, Perú, awhittembury@dge.gob.pe

The Basic Reproduction Number of Infectious Diseases: Computation and Estimation Using Compartmental Epidemic Models

Gerardo Chowell and Fred Brauer

Abstract The basic reproduction number (R_0) is a central quantity in epidemiology as it measures the transmission potential of infectious diseases. In this chapter we review the basic theory of the spread of infectious diseases using simple compartmental models based on ordinary differential equations including the simple Kermack-McKendrick epidemic model, SIR (susceptible-infectious-removed) models with demographics, the SIS (susceptible-infectious-susceptible) model, backward bifurcations, endemic equilibria, and the analytical derivation of R_0 using the next-generation approach. This theory is followed by simple methodology for the estimation of R_0 with its corresponding uncertainty from epidemic time series data. The 1918–1919 influenza pandemic in Winnipeg, Canada, and the 1968 influenza pandemic in US cities are used for illustration.

Keywords Influenza · Pandemic · Epidemiology · Basic reproduction number · Model

1 Thresholds in Disease Transmission Models

One of the fundamental results in mathematical epidemiology is that mathematical epidemic models, including those that include a high degree of heterogeneity exhibit a "threshold" behavior. In epidemiological terms, this can be stated as follows: *There is a difference in epidemic behavior when the average number of secondary infections caused by an average infective during his/her period of infectiousness, called the* basic reproduction number, *is less than one and when this quantity exceeds one.*

G. Chowell (✉)
School of Human Evolution and Social Change, Arizona State University, Tempe, AZ 85287, USA; Mathematical, Computational, Modeling Sciences Center, Arizona State University, Tempe, AZ 85287, USA; Division of Epidemiology and Population Studies, Fogarty International Center, National Institutes of Health, Bethesda, MD, USA
e-mail: gchowell@asu.edu

G. Chowell et al. (eds.), *Mathematical and Statistical Estimation Approaches in Epidemiology*, DOI 10.1007/978-90-481-2313-1_1,
© Springer Science+Business Media B.V. 2009

There are two different situations. If the course of the disease outbreak is rapid enough that there are no significant demographic effects (births, natural deaths, recruitment) on the population being studied, then the disease will die out if the basic reproduction number is less than one, and if it exceeds one there will be an epidemic.

If, on the other hand, there is a flow into the population of individuals who may become infected, through births, recruitment, or recovery of infected individuals with no immunity against reinfection, then there is a different alternative. If the basic reproduction number is less than one, the disease dies out in the population. Mathematically this is expressed by the fact that there is a disease-free equilibrium approached by solutions of the model describing the situation. If the basic reproduction number exceeds one, the disease-free equilibrium is unstable and solutions flow away from it. There is also an *endemic* equilibrium, with a positive number of infective individuals, indicating that the disease remains in the population.

However, the situation may be more complicated. We shall see later that in certain circumstances it is possible to have an endemic equilibrium with a reproduction number less than one.

We begin by describing the threshold phenomenon and the basic reproduction number in epidemic models.

2 The Simple Kermack-McKendrick Epidemic Model

An epidemic, which acts on a short temporal scale, may be described as a sudden outbreak of a disease that infects a substantial portion of the population in a region before it disappears. Epidemics usually leave many members untouched. Often these attacks recur with intervals of several years between outbreaks, possibly diminishing in severity as populations develop some immunity.

One of the questions that first attracted the attention of scientists interested in the study of the spread of communicable diseases was why diseases would suddenly develop in a community and then disappear just as suddenly without infecting the entire community. One of the early triumphs of mathematical epidemiology [54] was the formulation of a simple model that predicted behavior very similar to that observed in countless epidemics. The Kermack-McKendrick model is a compartmental model based on relatively simple assumptions on the rates of flow between different classes of members of the population.

We formulate our descriptions as *compartmental models*, with the population under study being divided into compartments and with assumptions about the nature and time rate of transfer from one compartment to another. Diseases that confer immunity have a different compartmental structure from diseases without immunity. We will use the terminology SIR to describe a disease which confers immunity against re-infection, to indicate that the passage of individuals is from the susceptible class S to the infective class I to the removed class R. On the other hand, we will use the terminology SIS to describe a disease with no immunity against re-infection, to indicate that the passage of individuals is from the susceptible class to the infective class and then back to the susceptible class. Other possibilities include $SEIR$ and $SEIS$ models, with an exposed period between being infected and becoming infective, and $SIRS$ models, with temporary immunity on recovery from infection.

In order to model such an epidemic we divide the population being studied into three classes labeled S, I, and R. We let $S(t)$ denote the number of individuals who are susceptible to the disease, that is, who are not (yet) infected at time t. $I(t)$ denotes the number of infected individuals, assumed infectious and able to spread the disease by contact with susceptibles. $R(t)$ denotes the number of individuals who have been infected and then removed from the possibility of being infected again or of spreading infection. Removal is carried out either through isolation from the rest of the population or through immunization against infection or through recovery from the disease with full immunity against reinfection or through death caused by the disease. These characterizations of removed members are different from an epidemiological perspective but are often equivalent from a modeling point of view which takes into account only the state of an individual with respect to the disease.

In formulating models in terms of the derivatives of the sizes of each compartment we are assuming that the number of members in a compartment is a differentiable function of time. This may be a reasonable approximation if there are many members in a compartment, but it is certainly suspect otherwise.

The basic compartmental models to describe the transmission of communicable diseases are contained in a sequence of three papers by W.O. Kermack and A.G. McKendrick in 1927, 1932, and 1933 [54–56]. The first of these papers described epidemic models. What is often called the Kermack-McKendrick epidemic model is actually a special case of the general model introduced in this paper. The general model included dependence on age of infection, that is, the time since becoming infected.

The special case of the model proposed by Kermack and McKendrick in 1927 which is the starting point for our study of epidemic models is

$$S' = -\beta S I$$
$$I' = \beta S I - \alpha I$$
$$R' = \alpha I .$$

It is based on the following assumptions:

(i) An average member of the population makes contact sufficient to transmit infection with βN others per unit time, where N represents total population size (mass action incidence).

(ii) Infectives leave the infective class at rate αI per unit time.

(iii) There is no entry into or departure from the population; in particular there are no deaths from the disease. Thus population size is a constant N_0.

The assumptions of a rate of contacts proportional to population size N_0 with constant of proportionality β, and of an exponentially distributed recovery rate are unrealistically simple. More general models can be constructed and analyzed, but our goal here is to show what may be deduced from extremely simple models. It will turn out that many more realistic models exhibit very similar qualitative behaviors. In our model R is determined once S and I are known, and we can drop the R equation from our model, leaving the system of two equations

$$S' = -\beta S I \qquad (1)$$
$$I' = (\beta S - \alpha)I \,,$$

together with initial conditions for $S(0)$, $I(0)$. We are unable to solve this system analytically but we learn a great deal about the behaviour of its solutions by a qualitative approach. We remark that the model makes sense only so long as $S(t)$ and $I(t)$ remain non-negative. Thus if either $S(t)$ or $I(t)$ reaches zero we consider the system to have terminated. We observe that $S' < 0$ for all t and $I' > 0$ if and only if $S > \alpha/\beta$. Thus I increases so long as $S > \alpha/\beta$ but since S decreases for all t, I ultimately decreases and approaches zero. If $S(0) < \alpha/\beta$, I decreases to zero (no epidemic), while if $S(0) > \alpha/\beta$, I first increases to a maximum attained when $S = \alpha/\beta$ and then decreases to zero (epidemic). We think of introducing a small number of infectives into a population of susceptibles and ask whether there will be an epidemic. It is not difficult to show that $I(t) \to 0$ and $S(t) \to S_\infty > 0$ as $t \to \infty$. The quantity $\beta S(0)/\alpha$ is a threshold quantity, called the *basic reproduction number* and denoted by $\mathcal{R}_0$, which determines whether there is an epidemic or not. If $\mathcal{R}_0 < 1$ the infection dies out, while if $\mathcal{R}_0 > 1$ there is an epidemic.

The definition of the basic reproduction number $\mathcal{R}_0$ is that the basic reproduction number is the number of secondary infections caused by a single infective introduced into a wholly susceptible population of size $N_0 \approx S(0)$ over the course of the infection of this single infective. In this situation, an infective makes βN_0 contacts in unit time, all of which are with susceptibles and thus produce new infections, and the mean infective period is $1/\alpha$; thus the basic reproduction number is actually $\beta N_0/\alpha$ rather than $\beta S(0)/\alpha$.

If we integrate the sum of the two equations of (1) from 0 to ∞ and let $t \to \infty$ we obtain

$$\alpha \int_0^\infty I(s)ds = S(0) + I(0) - S_\infty = N_0 - S_\infty.$$

The first equation of (1) may be written as

$$-\frac{S'(t)}{S(t)} = \beta I(t).$$

Integration from 0 to ∞ gives the *final size relation*

$$\log \frac{S(0)}{S_\infty} = \int_0^\infty \beta I(t) dt$$
$$= \frac{\beta(N_0 - S_\infty)}{\alpha} \tag{2}$$
$$= \mathcal{R}_0 \left[1 - \frac{S_\infty}{N_0} \right].$$

This final size relation shows that the size of the epidemic $N_0 - S_\infty$ is completely determined by the basic reproduction number.

3 More Elaborate Epidemic Models

There are many elaborations of the basic model (1). For example, one might assume an exposed period of mean duration κ following infection and preceding becoming fully infective, possibly with infectivity during the exposed period but reduced by a factor ε,

$$S' = -\beta S(I + \varepsilon E)$$
$$E' = \beta S(I + \varepsilon E) - \kappa E \tag{3}$$
$$I' = \kappa E - \alpha I.$$

In addition we have initial conditions

$$S(0) = S_0, \quad E(0) = E_0, \quad I(0) = I_0, \quad S(0) + E(0) + I(0) = N_0.$$

In order to calculate the basic reproduction number, we observe that an exposed member introduced into a susceptible population transmits $\varepsilon \beta N_0$ infections in unit time for a mean duration of $1/\kappa$ followed by βN_0 infections in unit time during the infective period of mean length $1/\alpha$. Thus

$$\mathcal{R}_0 = \beta N_0 \left(\frac{1}{\alpha} + \frac{\varepsilon}{\kappa} \right).$$

A calculation very similar to the derivation of the final size relation for (1) gives

$$\log \frac{S(0)}{S_\infty} = \int_0^\infty \beta [I(t) + \varepsilon E(t)] dt$$
$$= \mathcal{R}_0 \left[1 - \frac{S_\infty}{N_0} \right] - \frac{\varepsilon \beta I_0}{\kappa}.$$

If all initially infected members of the population are latent, this takes exactly the same form as (2), but if some have already completed the exposed stage there is a correction term in the final size relation.

Another extension of the model (1) is an SIR model in which a fraction γ of infected members in unit time are removed for treatment. The mean period for treated members before recovery is $1/\eta$ and treatment decreases infectivity by a factor σ. This leads to a model

$$
\begin{aligned}
S' &= -\beta S(I + \sigma T) \\
I' &= \beta S(I + \sigma T) - (\alpha + \gamma)I \\
T' &= \gamma I - \eta T.
\end{aligned}
\tag{4}
$$

Much as for the model (3) we calculate

$$
\mathcal{R}_0 = \beta N_0 \left[\frac{1}{\alpha + \gamma} + \frac{\gamma}{\alpha + \gamma} \frac{\sigma}{\eta} \right]
$$

and we obtain exactly the same final size relation (2).

These refinements of the simple Kermack-McKendrick epidemic model and models with more compartments are included in the general epidemic model of Kermack and McKendrick [54]. This model include a dependence of infectivity on the time since becoming infected (age of infection). In this model $\varphi(t)$ is the total infectivity at time t, defined as the sum of products of the number of infected members with each infection age and the mean infectivity for that infection age. We let $B(\tau)$ be the fraction of infected members remaining infected at infection age τ and let $\pi(\tau)$ with $0 \leq \pi(\tau) \leq 1$ be the mean infectivity at infection age τ. Then we let

$$
A(\tau) = \pi(\tau)B(\tau),
$$

the mean infectivity of members of the population with infection age τ.

The age of infection epidemic model is

$$
\begin{aligned}
S' &= -\beta S \varphi \\
\varphi(t) &= \varphi_0(t) + \int_0^t \beta S(t - \tau)\varphi(t - \tau)A(\tau)d\tau \\
&= \varphi_0(t) + \int_0^t [-S'(t - \tau)]A(\tau)d\tau.
\end{aligned}
\tag{5}
$$

The basic reproduction number is

$$
\mathcal{R}_0 = \beta N_0 \int_0^\infty A(\tau)d\tau,
$$

because an infective introduced into a susceptible population makes βN_0 contacts in unit time and the total infectivity over the duration of the infection is $\int_0^\infty A(\tau)d\tau$.

We write

$$-\frac{S'(t)}{S(t)} = \beta\varphi_0(t) + \beta\int_0^t [-S'(t-\tau)]A(\tau)d\tau.$$

Integration with respect to t from 0 to ∞ gives

$$\begin{aligned}
\ln\frac{S_0}{S_\infty} &= \beta\int_0^\infty \varphi_0(t)dt + \beta\int_0^\infty\int_0^t [-S'(t-\tau)]A(\tau)d\tau dt \\
&= \beta\int_0^\infty \varphi_0(t)dt + \beta\int_0^\infty A(\tau)\int_\tau^\infty [-S'(t-\tau)]dt d\tau \\
&= \beta\int_0^\infty \varphi_0(t)dt + \beta[S_0 - S_\infty]\int_0^\infty A(\tau)d\tau \qquad (6) \\
&= \beta[N_0 - S_\infty]\int_0^\infty A(\tau)d\tau + \beta\int_0^\infty [\varphi_0(t) - (N_0 - S_0)A(t)]dt \\
&= \mathcal{R}_0\left[1 - \frac{S_\infty}{N_0}\right] - \beta\int_0^\infty [(N_0 - S_0)A(t) - \varphi_0(t)]dt.
\end{aligned}$$

Here, $\varphi_0(t)$ is the total infectivity of the initial infectives when they reach age of infection t. If all initial infectives have infection age zero at $t = 0$, $\varphi_0(t) = [N_0 - S_0]A(t)$, and

$$\int_0^\infty [(N_0 - S_0)A(t) - \varphi_0(t)]dt = 0.$$

Then (6) takes the form

$$\ln\frac{S_0}{S_\infty} = \mathcal{R}_0\left(1 - \frac{S_\infty}{N_0}\right), \qquad (7)$$

and this is the general final size relation, exactly the same form as for the simple model (1).

If there are initial infectives with infection age greater than zero, let $u_0(\tau)$ be the average infectivity of these individuals. Then, since $u_0(\tau) \leq B(\tau)$,

$$\begin{aligned}
\varphi_0(t) &= (N_0 - S_0)u_0(\tau)\pi(t+\tau)\frac{B(t+\tau)}{B(\tau)} \\
&\leq (N_0 - S_0)A(t+\tau) \leq (N_0 - S_0)A(\tau).
\end{aligned}$$

Thus, the initial term satisfies

$$\int_0^\infty [(N_0 - S_0)A(t) - \varphi_0(t)]dt \geq 0.$$

The final size relation is sometimes presented in the slightly different form

$$\ln \frac{S_0}{S_\infty} = \mathcal{R}_0 \left(1 - \frac{S_\infty}{S_0} \right), \tag{8}$$

with an initial term which is assumed small and omitted, see for example [5, 30, 87].

Calculation of $\mathcal{R}_0$ for the model (5) requires calculation of the integral $\int_0^\infty A(\tau)d\tau$. In a model with multiple stages this calculation may be complicated but the approach given in [90] can simplify it.

The results we have developed assume mass action incidence, and this is not realistic. It is more plausible to assume that incidence is a saturating function of total population size. If there are no disease deaths, the total population size is constant and there is no loss of generality in assuming mass action incidence. If there are disease deaths, the total population size decreases with time. This does not affect the calculation of the reproduction number, but the final size relation becomes an inequality. If the disease death rate is small, the final size relation is an approximate equality and may still be used to estimate the epidemic size.

4 *SIR* Models with Demographics

Epidemics may sweep through a population and then disappear, but there are diseases which are endemic in many parts of the world and which cause millions of deaths each year. We have omitted births and deaths in our description of epidemic models because the time scale of an epidemic is generally much shorter than the demographic time scale. In effect, we have used a time scale on which the number of births and deaths in unit time is negligible. To model a disease which may be endemic we need to think on a longer time scale and include births and deaths.

The simplest *SIR* model with births and deaths is formulated by adding births and deaths to the epidemic model (1). We assume that the birth rate is a function $\Lambda(N)$ of total population size N and that there is a natural death rate in each compartment proportional to the size of the compartment; this corresponds to an assumption of an exponentially distributed life span. We assume also a density-dependent contact rate and that there are no disease deaths. This gives a model

$$\begin{aligned}
S' &= \Lambda(N) - \beta(N)SI - \mu S \\
I' &= \beta(N)SI - \mu I - \alpha I \\
N' &= \Lambda(N) - \mu N.
\end{aligned} \tag{9}$$

The total population size N uncouples in this model and satisfies the differential equation

$$N' = \Lambda(N) - \mu N .$$

The *carrying capacity* of population size is the limiting population size K, satisfying

$$\Lambda(K) = \mu K, \qquad \Lambda'(K) < \mu .$$

The condition $\Lambda'(K) < \mu$ assures the asymptotic stability of the equilibrium population size K. It is reasonable to assume that K is the only positive equilibrium, so that

$$\Lambda(N) > \mu N$$

for $0 \le N \le K$. For most population models,

$$\Lambda(0) = 0, \qquad \Lambda''(N) \le 0 .$$

However, if $\Lambda(N)$ represents recruitment into a behavioral class, as would be natural for models of sexually transmitted diseases, it would be plausible to have $\Lambda(0) > 0$, or even to consider $\Lambda(N)$ to be a constant function. If $\Lambda(0) = 0$, we require $\Lambda'(0) > \mu$ because if this requirement is not satisfied there is no positive equilibrium and the population would die out even in the absence of disease.

The theory of *asymptotically autonomous systems* [15, 64, 80, 81] implies that if N has a constant limit then the system is equivalent to the system in which N is replaced by this limit. Then the system (9) is equivalent to the system

$$
\begin{aligned}
S' &= \Lambda - \beta S I - \mu S \\
I' &= \beta S I - \mu I - \alpha I
\end{aligned}
\tag{10}
$$

in which β stands for the constant $\beta(K)$ and Λ for the constant $\Lambda(K) = \mu K$.

We shall analyze the model (10) qualitatively; our analysis will also apply to the more general model (9) if there are no disease deaths.

Just as for the epidemic models considered earlier, the basic reproduction number is the number of secondary infections caused by a single infective introduced into a wholly susceptible population. Because the number of contacts per infective in unit time is βN_0, and the mean infective period (corrected for natural mortality) is $1/(\mu + \alpha)$, the basic reproduction number is

$$\mathcal{R}_0 = \frac{\beta N_0}{\mu + \alpha}.$$

Our approach will be to identify equilibria (constant solutions) and then to determine the asymptotic stability of each equilibrium. Asymptotic stability of an equilibrium means that a solution starting sufficiently close to the equilibrium remains close to the equilibrium and approaches the equilibrium as $t \to \infty$, while instability of the equilibrium means that there are solutions starting arbitrarily close to the equilibrium which do not approach it. To find equilibria (S_∞, I_∞) we set the right side of each of the two equations equal to zero. The second of the resulting algebraic equations factors, giving two alternatives. The first alternative is $I_\infty = 0$, which will give a disease-free equilibrium, and the second alternative is $\beta S_\infty = \mu + \alpha$, which will give an endemic equilibrium, provided $\beta S_\infty = \mu + \alpha < \beta N_0$. If $I_\infty = 0$ the other equation gives $S_\infty = N_0 = \Lambda/\mu$. For the endemic equilibrium the first equation gives

$$I_\infty = \frac{\Lambda}{\mu + \alpha} - \frac{\mu}{\beta} . \tag{11}$$

We linearize about an equilibrium (S_∞, I_∞) by letting $y = S - S_\infty$, $z = I - I_\infty$, writing the system in terms of the new variables y and z and retaining only the linear terms in a Taylor expansion. We obtain a system of two linear differential equations,

$$y' = -(\beta I_\infty + \mu)y - \beta S_\infty z$$
$$z' = \beta I_\infty y + (\beta S_\infty - \mu - \alpha)z .$$

The coefficient matrix of this linear system is

$$\begin{bmatrix} -\beta I_\infty - \mu & -\beta S_\infty \\ \beta I_\infty & \beta S_\infty - \mu - \alpha \end{bmatrix}$$

We then look for solutions whose components are constant multiples of $e^{\lambda t}$; this means that λ must be an eigenvalue of the coefficient matrix. The condition that all solutions of the linearization at an equilibrium tend to zero as $t \to \infty$ is that the real part of every eigenvalue of this coefficient matrix is negative. At the disease-free equilibrium the matrix is

$$\begin{bmatrix} -\mu & -\beta N_0 \\ 0 & \beta K - \mu - \alpha \end{bmatrix},$$

which has eigenvalues $-\mu$ and $\beta N_0 - \mu - \alpha$. Thus, the disease-free equilibrium is asymptotically stable if $\beta N_0 < \mu + \alpha$ and unstable if $\beta N_0 > \mu + \alpha$. Note that this condition for instability of the disease-free equilibrium is the same as the condition for the existence of an endemic equilibrium.

In general, the condition that the eigenvalues of a 2×2 matrix have negative real part is that the determinant be positive and the trace (the sum of the diagonal elements) be negative. Since $\beta S_\infty = \mu + \alpha$ at an endemic equilibrium, the matrix of the linearization at an endemic equilibrium is

$$\begin{bmatrix} -\beta I_\infty - \mu & -\beta S_\infty \\ \beta I_\infty & 0 \end{bmatrix} \tag{12}$$

and this matrix has positive determinant and negative trace. Thus, the endemic equilibrium, if there is one, is always asymptotically stable. If the quantity

$$R_0 = \frac{\beta N_0}{\mu + \alpha} = \frac{N_0}{S_\infty} \tag{13}$$

is less than one, the system has only the disease-free equilibrium and this equilibrium is asymptotically stable. In fact, it is not difficult to prove that this asymptotic stability is global, that is, that every solution approaches the disease-free equilibrium. If the quantity $\mathcal{R}_0$ is greater than one then the disease-free equilibrium is unstable, but there is an endemic equilibrium that is asymptotically stable. The disease model exhibits a *threshold* behavior: If the basic reproduction number is less than one the disease will die out, but if the basic reproduction number is greater than one the disease will be endemic. The asymptotic stability of the endemic equilibrium means that the compartment sizes approach a steady state. If the equilibrium had been unstable, there would have been a possibility of sustained oscillations. Oscillations in a disease model mean fluctuations in the number of cases to be expected, and if the oscillations have long period could also mean that experimental data for a short period would be quite unreliable as a predictor of the future. Epidemiological models which incorporate additional factors may exhibit oscillations. A variety of such situations is described in [45, 46]. In general, a reproduction number greater than one signifies persistence of the infection.

Like epidemic models, disease transmission models including births and deaths can be put into an age of infection framework as in [13]. This allows the calculation of the reproduction number for models with multiple infective or treatment compartments.

If there are disease deaths in an SIR model with births and deaths, the analysis is more complicated. Because the total population size is not constant, the dimension of the model can not be reduced to two, and the stability analysis of a system of higher dimension is more complicated. However, the fundamental threshold property continues to hold [13]. This also extends to more complicated models with more compartments.

Epidemic models also exhibit a threshold behavior but of a different kind. For these models, SIR models without births or natural deaths, the threshold distinguishes between a dying out of the disease and an epidemic, or short term spread of disease.

5 The SIS Model

In order to describe a model for a disease from which infectives recover with no immunity against reinfection and that includes births and natural deaths but no disease deaths as in the model (9), we may modify the model (9) by removing the equation for R and moving the term αI describing the rate of recovery from infection to the equation for S. This gives the model

$$S' = \Lambda(N) - \beta(N)SI - \mu S + \alpha I \qquad (14)$$
$$I' = \beta(N)SI - \alpha I - \mu I$$

describing a population with a density-dependent birth rate $\Lambda(N)$ per unit time, a proportional death rate μ in each class, and with a rate α of departure from the infective class through recovery with no immunity against reinfection.

As for the SIR model, since the system (14) is asymptotically autonomous and since $S + I$ is a constant N_0, it is equivalent to the single equation

$$I' = \beta I(N_0 - I) - (\alpha + \mu)I, \qquad (15)$$

where S has been replaced by $N_0 - I$. But (15) is a logistic equation which is easily solved by an equilibrium analysis. We find that $I \to 0$ if

$$\mathcal{R}_0 = \frac{\beta N_0}{\mu + \alpha} < 1$$

and $I \to I_\infty > 0$ with

$$I_\infty = N_0 - \frac{\mu + \alpha}{\beta} = N_0 \left(1 - \frac{1}{\mathcal{R}_0} \right)$$

if $\mathcal{R}_0 > 1$. Thus the SIS model exhibits the same threshold behavior as the SIR model. In fact, this holds even without births and natural deaths; the flow of new susceptibles coming from recovery from infection maintains the disease.

If there are disease deaths in the SIS model, the analysis is more complicated but the result is the same.

6 Backward Bifurcations

In compartmental models for the transmission of communicable diseases there is usually a basic reproduction number $\mathcal{R}_0$, representing the mean number of secondary infections caused by a single infective introduced into a susceptible population. If $\mathcal{R}_0 < 1$ there is a disease-free equilibrium which is asymptotically stable, and the infection dies out. If $\mathcal{R}_0 > 1$ the usual situation is that there is an endemic equilibrium which is asymptotically stable, and the infection persists. Even if the endemic equilibrium is unstable, the instability commonly arises from a Hopf bifurcation and the infection still persists but in an oscillatory manner. More precisely, as $\mathcal{R}_0$ increases through 1 there is an exchange of stability between the disease-free equilibrium and the endemic equilibrium (which is negative as well as unstable and thus biologically meaningless if $\mathcal{R}_0 < 1$). There is a bifurcation, or change in equilibrium behavior, at $\mathcal{R}_0 = 1$ but the equilibrium infective population size depends continuously on $\mathcal{R}_0$. Such a transition is called a forward, or transcritical, bifurcation.

It has been noted [33, 39, 40, 57] that in epidemic models with multiple groups and asymmetry between groups or multiple interaction mechanisms it is possible to have a very different bifurcation behavior at $\mathcal{R}_0 = 1$. There may be multiple positive endemic equilibria for values of $\mathcal{R}_0 < 1$ and a backward bifurcation at $\mathcal{R}_0 = 1$.

The qualitative behavior of an epidemic system with a backward bifurcation differs from that of a system with a forward bifurcation in at least three important ways. If there is a forward bifurcation at $\mathcal{R}_0 = 1$ it is not possible for a disease to invade a population if $\mathcal{R}_0 < 1$ because the system will return to the disease-free equilibrium $I = 0$ if some infectives are introduced into the population. On the other hand, if there is a backward bifurcation at $\mathcal{R}_0 = 1$ and enough infectives are introduced into the population to put the initial state of the system above the unstable endemic equilibrium with $\mathcal{R}_0 < 1$, the system will approach the asymptotically stable endemic equilibrium.

Other differences are observed if the parameters of the system change to produce a change in $\mathcal{R}_0$. With a forward bifurcation at $\mathcal{R}_0 = 1$ the equilibrium infective population remains zero so long as $\mathcal{R}_0 < 1$ and then increases continuously as $\mathcal{R}_0$ increases. With a backward bifurcation at $\mathcal{R}_0 = 1$, the equilibrium infective population size also remains zero so long as $\mathcal{R}_0 < 1$ but then jumps to the positive endemic equilibrium as $\mathcal{R}_0$ increases through 1. In the other direction, if a disease is being controlled by means which decrease $\mathcal{R}_0$ it is sufficient to decrease $\mathcal{R}_0$ to 1 if there is a forward bifurcation at $\mathcal{R}_0 = 1$ but it is necessary to bring $\mathcal{R}_0$ below 1 if there is a backward bifurcation.

These behavior differences are important in planning how to control a disease; a backward bifurcation at $\mathcal{R}_0 = 1$ makes control more difficult. One control measure often used is the reduction of susceptibility to infection produced by vaccination. By vaccination we mean either an inoculation which reduces susceptibility to infection or an education program such as encouragement of better hygiene or avoidance of risky behavior for sexually transmitted diseases. Whether vaccination is inoculation or education, typically it reaches only a fraction of the susceptible population and is not perfectly effective. In an apparent paradox, models with vaccination may exhibit backward bifurcations, making the behavior of the model more complicated than the corresponding model without vaccination. It has been argued [9] that a partially effective vaccination program applied to only part of the population at risk may increase the severity of outbreaks of such diseases as HIV/AIDS.

We give a simple example of a backward bifurcation by incorporating vaccination into a simple SIS model, following the elementary approach of [11].

The model we will study adds vaccination to the simple SIS model (15) described in the preceding section. We add the assumption that in unit time a fraction φ of the susceptible class is vaccinated. The vaccination may reduce but not completely eliminate susceptibility to infection. We model this by including a factor σ, $0 \le \sigma \le 1$, in the infection rate of vaccinated members with $\sigma = 0$ meaning that the vaccine is perfectly effective and $\sigma = 1$ meaning that the vaccine has no effect. We assume also that the vaccination loses effect at a proportional rate θ. We describe the new model by including a vaccinated class V, with

$$I' = \beta [N_0 - I - (1 - \sigma)V] I - (\mu + \gamma)I \qquad (16)$$
$$V' = \varphi[N_0 - I] - \sigma\beta V I - (\mu + \theta + \phi)V.$$

The system (16) is the basic vaccination model which we will analyze. We remark that if the vaccine is completely ineffective ($\sigma = 1$), then (16) is equivalent to the SIS model (15). If there is no loss of effectiveness of vaccine, $\theta = 0$, and if all susceptibles are vaccinated immediately (formally, $\varphi \to \infty$), the model (16) is equivalent to (15) with β replaced by $\sigma\beta$ and has basic reproduction number

$$\mathcal{R}_0^* = \frac{\sigma\beta K}{\mu + \gamma} = \sigma\mathcal{R}_0 \leq \mathcal{R}_0.$$

We will think of the parameters μ, γ, θ, φ and σ as fixed and will view β as variable. In practice, the parameter φ is the one most easily controlled, and with this interpretation in mind, we will use $R(\varphi)$ to denote the basic reproduction number of the model (16), and we will see that

$$\mathcal{R}_0^* \leq \mathcal{R}(\varphi) \leq \mathcal{R}_0.$$

Equilibria of the model (16) are solutions of

$$\beta I [N_0 - I - (1 - \sigma)V] = (\mu + \gamma)I \qquad (17)$$
$$\varphi[N_0 - I] = \sigma\beta V I + (\mu + \theta + \varphi)V.$$

If $I = 0$ then the first equation of (17) is satisfied and the second equation leads to

$$S = \frac{\mu + \theta}{\mu + \theta + \varphi} N_0, \quad V = \frac{\varphi}{\mu + \theta + \varphi} N_0.$$

This is the disease-free equilibrium.

The matrix of the linearization of (16) at an equilibrium (I, V) is

$$\begin{bmatrix} -2\beta I - (1 - \sigma)\beta V - (\mu + \alpha) + \beta N_0 & -(1 - \sigma)\beta I \\ -(\varphi + \sigma\beta V) & -(\mu + \theta + \varphi + \sigma\beta I) \end{bmatrix}$$

At the disease-free equilibrium this matrix is

$$\begin{bmatrix} -(1 - \sigma)\beta V - (\mu + \alpha) + \beta N_0 & 0 \\ -(\phi + \sigma\beta V) & -(\mu + \theta + \varphi) \end{bmatrix}$$

which has negative eigenvalues, implying the asymptotic stability of the disease-free equilibrium, if and only if

$$-(1 - \sigma)\beta V - (\mu + \alpha) + \beta N_0 < 0.$$

Using the value of V at the disease-free equilibrium this condition is equivalent to

$$\mathcal{R}(\varphi) = \frac{\beta N_0}{\mu + \alpha} \cdot \frac{\mu + \theta + \sigma\phi}{\mu + \theta + \varphi} = R_0 \frac{\mu + \theta + \sigma\varphi}{\mu + \theta + \varphi} < 1.$$

The case $\varphi = 0$ is that of no vaccination with $\mathcal{R}(\varphi) = \mathcal{R}_0$, and $\mathcal{R}(\varphi) < \mathcal{R}_0$ if $\varphi > 0$. In fact, it is not difficult to show, using a standard a priori bound argument, that if $\mathcal{R}_0 < 1$ the disease-free equilibrium is globally asymptotically stable [57]. We note that $\mathcal{R}_0^* = \sigma \mathcal{R}_0 = \lim_{\varphi \to \infty} \mathcal{R}(\phi) < \mathcal{R}_0$.

6.1 Endemic Equilibria

If $0 \le \sigma < 1$ endemic equilibria are solutions of the pair of equations

$$\beta [N_0 - I - (1 - \sigma)V] = \mu + \gamma \tag{18}$$
$$\varphi[N_0 - I] = \sigma\beta V I + (\mu + \theta + \varphi)V.$$

We eliminate V using the first equation of (18) and substitute into the second equation to give an equation of the form

$$AI^2 + BI + C = 0 \tag{19}$$

with

$$
\begin{aligned}
A &= \sigma\beta \\
B &= (\mu + \theta + \sigma\varphi) + \sigma(\mu + \gamma) - \sigma\beta N_0 \\
C &= \frac{(\mu + \gamma)(\mu + \theta + \varphi)}{\beta} - (\mu + \theta + \sigma\varphi)N_0.
\end{aligned}
\tag{20}
$$

If $\sigma = 0$ (19) is a linear equation with unique solution.

$$I = N_0 - \frac{(\mu + \gamma)(\mu + \theta + \varphi)}{\beta(\mu + \theta)} = N_0 \left[1 - \frac{1}{\mathcal{R}(\varphi)} \right]$$

which is positive if and only if $\mathcal{R}(\varphi) > 1$. Thus if $\sigma = 0$ there is a unique endemic equilibrium if $\mathcal{R}(\varphi) > 1$ which approaches zero as $\mathcal{R}(\phi) \to 1+$ and there can not be an endemic equilibrium if $\mathcal{R}(\varphi) < 1$. In this case it is not possible to have a backward bifurcation at $\mathcal{R}(\varphi) = 1$.

We note that $C < 0$ if $\mathcal{R}(\varphi) > 1$, $C = 0$ if $\mathcal{R}(\varphi) = 1$, and $C > 0$ if $\mathcal{R}(\varphi) < 1$. If $\sigma > 0$, so that (19) is quadratic and if $\mathcal{R}(\varphi) > 1$ then there is a unique positive root of (19) and thus there is a unique endemic equilibrium. If $\mathcal{R}(\varphi) = 1$, then $C = 0$ and there is a unique non-zero solution of (19) $I = -B/A$ which is positive if and only if $B < 0$. If $B < 0$ when $C = 0$ there is a positive endemic equilibrium for $\mathcal{R}(\varphi) = 1$. Since equilibria depend continuously on φ there must then be an interval to the left of $\mathcal{R}(\varphi) = 1$ on which there are two positive equilibria. This establishes that the system (16) has a backward bifurcation at $\mathcal{R}(\varphi) = 1$ if and only if $B < 0$ when β is chosen to make $C = 0$.

We can give an explicit criterion in terms of the parameters $\mu, \alpha, \theta, \varphi, \sigma$ for the existence of a backward bifurcation at $\mathcal{R}(\varphi) = 1$. When $\mathcal{R}(\varphi) = 1$, $C = 0$ so that

$$(\mu + \theta + \sigma\varphi)\beta N_0 = (\mu + \alpha)(\mu + \theta + \varphi) \tag{21}$$

The condition $B < 0$ is

$$(\mu + \theta + \sigma\varphi) + \sigma(\mu + \alpha) < \sigma\beta N_0$$

with βN_0 determined by (21), or

$$\sigma(\mu + \alpha)(\mu + \theta + \varphi) > (\mu + \theta + \sigma\varphi)[(\mu + \theta + \sigma\varphi) + \sigma(\mu + \alpha)]$$

which reduces to

$$\sigma(1 - \sigma)(\mu + \gamma)\varphi > (\mu + \theta + \sigma\varphi)^2. \tag{22}$$

A backward bifurcation occurs at $\mathcal{R}(\varphi) = 1$ if and only if (22) is satisfied. We point out that there can not be a backward bifurcation if the vaccine is perfectly effective, $\sigma = 0$. Also, it is possible to prove that for the corresponding SIR model with vaccination a backward bifurcation is not possible.

If (22) is satisfied, so that there is a backward bifurcation at $\mathcal{R}(\varphi) = 1$, there are two endemic equilibria for an interval of values of β from

$$\beta N_0 = \frac{(\mu + \alpha)(\mu + \theta + \varphi)}{\mu + \theta + \sigma\varphi}$$

corresponding to $\mathcal{R}(\varphi) = 1$ to a value β_c defined by $B = -2\sqrt{AC}$. Thus there are two endemic equilibria if β is chosen so that

$$-2\sqrt{AC} < B < 0.$$

It is possible to prove that the larger one is asymptotically stable while the lower one is unstable and separates the regions of attraction of the disease-free equilibrium and the asymptotically stable endemic equilibrium.

7 Calculation of Reproduction Numbers

We have calculated reproduction numbers directly by following the course of a disease through a population from an initial infective. This is possible because we have examined only situations in which all new infections are in a single compartment. If new infections may be in multiple compartments, it is necessary to use a next generation operator approach [29, 30]. If the model is a system of ordinary differential equations, the next generation approach may be formulated in matrix-theoretic terms [82]. In this section we outline this approach, referring the reader to [82] for details.

A compartment is called a disease compartment if its members are infected. Note that exposed and asymptomatic compartments are disease compartments in this sense. Suppose that there are n disease compartments and m non-disease compartments, and let $x \in R^n$ and $y \in R^m$ be the subpopulations in these compartments respectively. We denote by $\mathcal{F}_i$ the rate at which secondary infections increase the ith disease compartment. We define the $n \times n$ matrix V describing the transitions between infected states as well as removals from infected states through death and recovery. For any non-negative vector x, the components of the vector Vx represent the net rate of decrease of each infected compartment. Since this rate cannot be positive if the compartment is empty, it follows that the off-diagonal entries of V must be negative or zero. Similarly, the sum of the components of the vector Vx, which represents the net rate of decrease in infected individuals due to death and recovery, must be non-negative for every non-negative vector x.

The compartmental model can then be written in the form

$$x' = \mathcal{F}(x, y) - Vx \tag{23}$$
$$y' = g(x, y),$$

with non-negative initial conditions such that at least one component of $x(0)$ is positive.

The disease-free set $\{(x, y) | x = 0, y \geq 0\}$ is invariant. Suppose that a point $(0, y_0)$ is a locally asymptotically stable equilibrium of the system without disease

$$y' = g(0, y)$$

in the sense that solutions that start close to $(0, y_0)$ remain close to $(0, y_0)$. Such a point is referred to as a disease-free equilibrium. The community matrix of the system without disease at this equilibrium is

$$g_y(0, y_0),$$

and this assumption implies that all the eigenvalues of $g_y(0, y_0)$ have negative or zero real parts.

The point $(0, y_0)$ is also an equilibrium of the system (23). We define

$$F = \mathcal{F}_x(0, y_0).$$

If all eigenvalues of $F - V$ have negative real parts, then this equilibrium is also asymptotically stable for (23).

The number of secondary infections produced by a single infected individual can be expressed as the product of the expected duration of the infectious period and the rate at which secondary infections occur. For the general model with n disease compartments, these are computed for each compartment for a hypothetical index case. The expected time the index case spends in each compartment is given by the integral $\int_0^\infty \varphi(t, x_0)\, dt$, where $\varphi(t, x_0)$ is the solution of (23) with $F = 0$ (no secondary infections) and nonnegative initial conditions, x_0, representing an infected index case:

$$x' = -Vx, \quad x(0) = x_0. \tag{24}$$

In effect, this solution shows the path of the index case through the disease compartments from the initial exposure through to death or recovery with the ith component of $\varphi(t, x_0)$ interpreted as the probability that the index case (introduced at time $t = 0$) is in disease state i at time t. The solution to (24) is $\varphi(t, x_0) = e^{-Vt}x_0$, where the exponential of a matrix is defined by the Taylor series

$$e^A = I + A + \frac{A^2}{2!} + \frac{A^3}{3!} + \cdots + \frac{A^k}{k!} + \cdots$$

This series converges for all t. Thus

$$\int_0^\infty \varphi(t, x_0)\, dt = \int_0^\infty e^{-Vt} x_0\, dt = V^{-1} x_0.$$

The (i, j) entry of the matrix V^{-1} can be interpreted as the expected time an individual initially introduced into disease compartment j spends in disease compartment i. The (i, j) entry of the matrix F is the at which rate secondary infections are produced in compartment i by an index case in compartment j. Hence, the expected number of secondary infections produced by the index case is given by

$$\int_0^\infty F e^{-Vt} x_0\, dt = F V^{-1} x_0.$$

The matrix $K = FV^{-1}$ is called the next generation matrix [29, 30] for the system at the disease-free equilibrium. The (i, j) entry of K is the expected number of secondary infections in compartment i produced by individuals initially in compartment j, assuming, of course, that the environment seen by the individual remains homogeneous for the duration of its infection.

It is shown in [82] that V is a non-singular M-matrix. This implies that the eigenvalues of V all have positive real part, and V^{-1} is a matrix with non-negative entries [7]. The next generation matrix, $K = FV^{-1}$, is nonnegative and the properties of matrices imply that K has a nonnegative eigenvalue, $\rho(FV^{-1})$, such that there are no other eigenvalues of K with modulus greater than $\mathcal{R}_0$ and there is a nonnegative eigenvector ω associated with $\mathcal{R}_0$. This eigenvector is in some sense the distribution of infected individuals that produces the greatest number, $\mathcal{R}_0$, of secondary infections per generation. Thus, $\mathcal{R}_0$ and the associated eigenvector ω suitably define a "typical" infective and the basic reproduction number can be defined rigorously as the spectral radius of the next generation matrix, K.

It is possible to show that the spectral radius of $K = FV^{-1}$ has absolute value less than 1 if and only if all eigenvalues of the matrix $F - V$ have negative real part [82]. Thus the disease-free equilibrium $(0, y_0)$ of (23) is (locally) asymptotically stable if and only if $\mathcal{R}_0 < 1$.

If all new infections are in one compartment, the matrix F has rank 1 and thus the matrix $K = FV^{-1}$ also has rank 1. Then all but one of the eigenvalues of K are zero, and since the sum of the eigenvalues of K is equal to the trace of K, the spectral radius is the remaining eigenvalue,

$$\rho(K) = tr(K).$$

8 Estimating R_0 Using a Compartmental Epidemic Model

In practice, the reproduction number denoted simply by R and defined as the number of secondary cases generated by a primary infectious cases in a partially protected population might be useful. R can also be estimated from the initial growth phase of an epidemic in such a partially immunized population. In a randomly mixing population, the relationship between the basic reproduction number (R_0) and the reproduction number (R) is given by $R = (1 - p)R_0$ where p is the proportion of the population that is effectively protected against infection (in the beginning of an epidemic). Besides, for many recurrent infectious diseases including seasonal influenza, estimating the background immunity p in the population is extremely difficult due to cross-immunity of antigenically-related influenza strains and vaccination campaigns.

Statistical methods to quantitatively estimate R_0 have been reviewed by Klaus Dietz [32]. Depending on the characteristics of data and underlying assumptions of the models, R_0 can be estimated using various different approaches [28]. Here we focus on the estimation of R_0 from an inverse problem perspective using compartmental epidemic models based on systems of ordinary differential equations. While in previous sections the focus is on mass action incidence, here we model epidemics assuming standard incidence. A recent review on methods for the estimation of the basic reproduction number in the context of the 1918–1919 influenza pandemic has been given by Chowell and Nishiura (2008) [25].

The simple SEIR model classifies individuals as susceptible (S), exposed (E), infectious (I), recovered (R), and dead (D) [3]. Susceptible individuals in contact with the virus enter the exposed class at the rate $\beta I(t)/N$, where β is the transmission rate, $I(t)$ is the number of infectious individuals at time t and $N = S(t) + E(t) + I(t) + R(t)$ is the total population for any t. The entire population is assumed to be susceptible at the beginning of the epidemic. Individuals in latent period (E) progress to the infectious class at the rate k (where $1/k$ suggests the mean latent period). We assume homogeneous mixing (*i.e.* random mixing) between individuals and, therefore, the fraction $I(t)/N$ is the probability of a random contact with an infectious individual in a population of size N. Since we assume that the time-scale of the epidemic is much faster than characteristic times for demographic processes (natural birth and death), background demographic processes are not included in the model. Infectious individuals either recover or die from influenza at the mean rates γ and δ, respectively. Recovered individuals are assumed protected for the duration of the outbreak. The mortality rate is given by $\delta = \gamma$ [CFP/(1-CFP)], where CFP is the mean case fatality proportion. The transmission process can be modeled using the system of nonlinear differential equations:

$$
\begin{cases}
\dfrac{dS(t)}{dt} = -\dfrac{\beta S(t)I(t)}{N} \\[2ex]
\dfrac{dE(t)}{dt} = \dfrac{\beta S(t)I(t)}{N(t)} - kE(t) \\[2ex]
\dfrac{dI(t)}{dt} = kE(t) - (\gamma + \delta)I(t) \\[2ex]
\dfrac{dR(t)}{dt} = \gamma I(t) \\[2ex]
\dfrac{dD(t)}{dt} = \delta I(t) \\[2ex]
\dfrac{dC(t)}{dt} = kE(t)
\end{cases}
\tag{25}
$$

where $C(t)$ is the cumulative number of infectious individuals. The basic reproduction number of the above system (25) is given by the product of the mean transmission rate and the mean infectious period, $R_0 = \beta/(\gamma + \delta)$.

8.1 Parameter Estimation

In the simplest manner, model parameters can be estimated via least-square fitting of the model solution to the observed data. That is, one looks for the set of parameters $\hat{\Theta}$ whose model solution best fits the epidemic data by minimizing the sum of the squared differences between the observed data y_t and the model solution $C(t, \Theta)$. That is, we minimize:

$$
X(\Theta) = \sum_{t=1}^{n} (\mathbf{y_t} - \mathbf{C(t, \Theta)})^2
\tag{26}
$$

The standard deviation of the parameters can be estimated by computing the asymptotic variance-covariance $AV(\hat{\Theta})$ matrix of the least-squares estimate by [27]:

$$\mathbf{AV}(\hat{\Theta}) = \sigma^2(\nabla_\Theta \mathbf{C}(\Theta_0) \, \nabla_\Theta \mathbf{C}(\Theta_0)^{\mathbf{T}})^{-1} \tag{27}$$

which can be estimated by

$$\hat{\sigma}^2(\hat{\nabla}_\Theta \mathbf{C}(\hat{\Theta})\hat{\nabla}_\Theta \mathbf{C}(\hat{\Theta})^{\mathbf{T}})^{-1} \tag{28}$$

where n is the total number of observations, $\hat{\sigma}^2$ is the estimated variance, and $\hat{\nabla}C$ are numerical derivatives of C. Estimates of $\hat{R}_0$ can be obtained by substituting the corresponding individual parameter estimates into an analytical formula of R_0. Further, using the delta method [8], we can derive an expression for the variance of the estimated basic reproduction number $\hat{R}_0$. An expression for the variance of R_0 for the simple SEIR model (Equations (25)) is given by:

$$V(\hat{R}_0) \approx \hat{R}_0^{\ 2} \left\{ \frac{V(\hat{\beta})}{\hat{\beta}^2} + \frac{V(\hat{\gamma})}{(\hat{\gamma} + \hat{\delta})^2} + \frac{V(\hat{\delta})}{(\hat{\gamma} + \hat{\delta})^2} \right.$$

$$\left. - \left(\frac{2}{\hat{\beta}(\hat{\gamma} + \hat{\delta})} \right) \left(Cov(\hat{\gamma}, \hat{\beta}) - \frac{\hat{\beta}Cov(\hat{\delta}, \hat{\gamma})}{\hat{\gamma} + \hat{\delta}} + Cov(\hat{\delta}, \hat{\beta}) \right) \right\}. \tag{29}$$

This expression depends on the variance (denoted by V) of the individual parameter estimates as well as their covariance (denoted by Cov).

8.2 Bootstrap Confidence Intervals

Another method to generate uncertainty bounds on the reproduction number is computing bootstrap confidence intervals by generating sets of realizations of the best-fit curve $C(t)$ [34]. Each realization of the cumulative number of case notifications $C_i(t)$ ($i = 1, 2, \ldots, m$) is generated as follows: for each observation $C(t)$ for $t = 2, 3, \ldots, n$ days generate a new observation $C_i'(t)$ for $t \geq 2$ ($C_i'(1) = C(1)$) that is sampled from a *Poisson* distribution with mean: $C(t) - C(t-1)$ (the daily increment in $C(t)$ from day $t-1$ to day t). The corresponding realization of the cumulative number of influenza notifications is given by $C_i(t) = \sum_{j=1}^{t} C_i'(t)$ where $t = 1, 2, 3, \ldots, n$. The reproduction number was then estimated from each of 1000 simulated epidemic curves to generate a distribution of R estimates from which simple statistics can be computed including 95% confidence intervals. These statistics need to be interpreted with caution. For example, 95% confidence intervals for R derived from our bootstrap sample of R should be interpreted as containing 95% of future estimates when the same assumptions are made and the only noise source is observation error. It is tempting but incorrect to interpret these confidence intervals as containing the *true* parameters with probability 0.95.

8.3 Example: The Transmissibility of the 1918 Influenza Pandemic in Winnipeg, Canada

The 1918–1919 influenza pandemic known as the Spanish influenza has been the most devastating in recent history with estimated worldwide mortality ranging from 20 to 100 million deaths [26, 67] with a case fatality of 2–6% [63, 79]. The first pandemic wave arrived to Winnipeg at the end of September 1918 probably brought by returning soldiers at the end of war (Fig. 1). The pandemic appears to have moved from the south of the city into the north (from the wealthy to the poor populations) [50]. The influenza mortality rate of influenza was 90 deaths per thousand in the north end, and 46 per thousand in the south.

Because influenza pandemics such as the Spanish flu from 1918 to 1919 are associated to the emergence of novel influenza strains to which most of the population is susceptible, it might be reasonable to assume that the reproduction number $R \approx R_0$. Previous studies have estimated that R_0 of the 1918–1919 influenza pandemic ranged between 1.5 and 5.4 [4, 19, 20, 22, 38, 65, 66, 70, 77, 83, 84] depending on the specific location and pandemic wave considered, type of data, estimation method, and level of spatial aggregation, which has ranged from small towns to entire nations with several million inhabitants. The variability of R_0 estimates suggests that local factors, including geographic and demographic conditions, could play an important role in disease spread [24, 76].

We estimated the reproduction number of the 1918 influenza pandemic in Winnipeg, Canada by fitting the simple SEIR model (25) to the initial phase of the cumulative number of reported cases. Figures 2 and 3 show the model fit to the epidemic data and the corresponding distributions of the reproduction number obtained

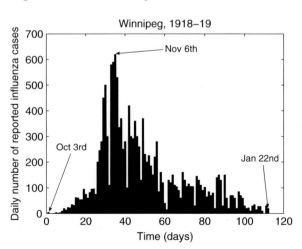

Fig. 1 Temporal distribution of Spanish influenza in Winnipeg, Canada in 1918. A total of 14868 cases were reported from October 3rd to January 22nd. Data source: [14]

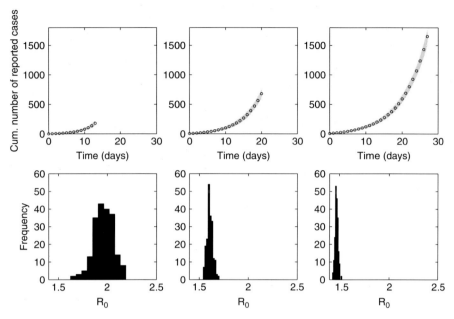

Fig. 2 Model fits (*top panels*) and the resulting distributions of the reproduction number (*bottom panels*) obtained assuming a generation interval of 3 days after fitting the simple SEIR epidemic model to the initial phase of the Fall influenza wave using 14, 21 and 28 epidemic days of the Spanish Flu Pandemic in Winnipeg, Canada. In the *top panel*, the epidemic data of the cumulative number of reported influenza cases are the *circles* and the *solid blue lines* are 200 realizations of the model fit to the data obtained through parametric bootstrapping as explained in the text

from parametric bootstrap of the model best fit using 14, 21 and 28 epidemic days of data and a generation interval of 3 and 6 days, respectively. Following a generation interval of 3 days [17, 88], the reproduction number was estimated to be ~2 (SD 0.1) using the first 14 days and ~1.6 (SD 0.03) using the first 21 epidemic days.

9 Estimation of the Reproduction Number Using the Intrinsic Growth Rate *r*

It is possible to relate the basic reproduction number (R_0) with the intrinsic growth rate (r). Moving forward from the compartmental epidemic models presented in the previous sections, the intrinsic growth rate is essentially the dominant eigenvalue of the characteristic equation obtained after linearizing the system of differential equations of the epidemic model around the disease free equilibrium. For the classical SIR model, the basic reproduction number as a function of the early-time and per-capita free growth rate r is given by $R_0 = 1 + r/\gamma$ [3] where $1/\gamma$ is the mean

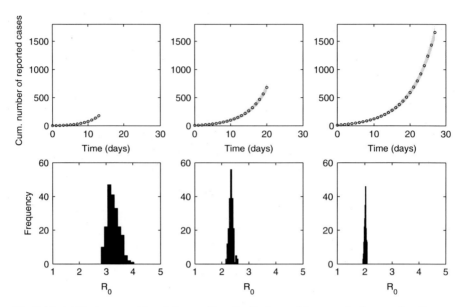

Fig. 3 Model fits (*top panels*) and the resulting distributions of the reproduction number (*bottom panels*) obtained assuming a generation interval of 6 days after fitting the simple SEIR epidemic model to the initial phase of the Fall influenza wave using 14, 21 and 28 epidemic days of the Spanish Flu Pandemic in Winnipeg, Canada. In the *top panel*, the epidemic data of the cumulative number of reported influenza cases are the *circles* and the *solid blue lines* are 200 realizations of the model fit to the data obtained through parametric bootstrapping as explained in the text

infectious period. When a latency period $(1/k)$ is included in the model, the relationship between R_0 and r becomes $R_0 = 1 + \frac{r^2 + (k+\gamma)}{k\gamma}$. It is important to highlight that these relationships are obtained under the assumption of exponential waiting times for the latent and infectious periods, and the impact of this assumption on estimates of R_0 has been highlighted in several publications (e.g., [59, 60, 73, 87, 89]). Wallinga and Lipsitch (2008) [86] have recently elucidated a general relationship between the generation time and R_0 and derived the following estimator for R_0 using the intrinsic growth rate:

$$\hat{R}_0 = \frac{1}{M(-r)}, \qquad (30)$$

where $M(-r)$ is the moment generating function of the generation time distribution $w(\tau)$, given the intrinsic growth rate r [86]. For example, when the generation time of the disease in question is considered to be fixed (no variance), an upper bound for the basic reproduction number can be easily obtained through the formula $R_0 = e^{rT}$ where T is the mean generation time. Similarly for generation intervals that are approximately normally distributed with mean T and variance σ^2 the reproduction number can be approximated by $R \approx e^{rT - \frac{1}{2}r^2\sigma^2}$.

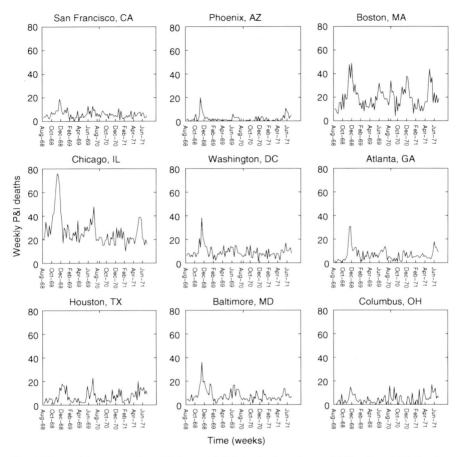

Fig. 4 The weekly pneumonia and influenza (P&I) deaths from August 1968 to June 1971 for nine representative US cities

9.1 Example: The Transmissibility of the 1968 Influenza Pandemic in US Cities

Following the devastating 1918–1919 influenza pandemic caused by the influenza virus A (H1N1), subsequent pandemics during the 20th century are attributed to subtypes A (H2N2) from 1957 to 1958 (Asian influenza) and A (H3N2) in 1968 (Hong Kong influenza) [62].

We estimated the reproduction number of the 1968 influenza pandemic for 85 US cities using weekly pneumonia and influenza (P&I) mortality [1]. The weekly series of P&I deaths for 9 representative US cties are shown for illustration in Fig. 4. We assumed an influenza generation interval of 3 days [17, 88]. We used the median P&I mortality during the 1970–1971 season as a constant baseline to extract influenza-related deaths during the 1968 influenza pandemic (e.g., excess

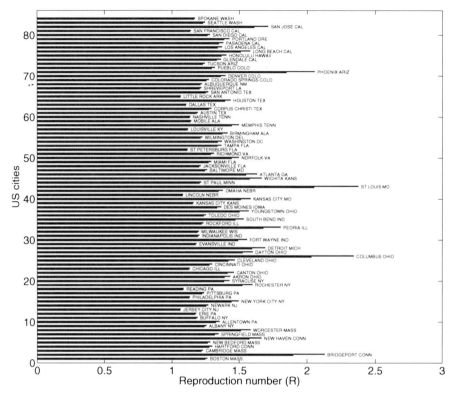

Fig. 5 Estimates of the reproduction number of the 1968 influenza pandemic for 85 US cities assuming an exponentially distributed (*blue*) or a fixed generation interval (*red*) with a mean of 3 days

P&I deaths above that median were considered to be influenza-related deaths). We estimated the intrinsic growth rate "r" for all those cities for which the initial epidemic phase comprised at least three epidemic weeks of data. We estimated "r" assuming an exponential growth phase $y = Ce^{rt}$. The longest epidemic period that is consistent with exponential growth and used to estimate "r" is determined via the goodness-of-fit test statistic.

We estimated a mean R for all the 85 US cities of 1.33 (95% CI: 1.29, 1.38) assuming exponentially distributed latent and infectious periods of 1.5 days each (3-day generation interval) while assuming a fixed generation interval of 3 days (zero variance) yielded an upper bound with mean $R = 1.37$ (95% CI: 1.32, 1.43). The city level R estimates assuming an exponentially distributed or a fixed generation interval are given in Fig. 5. For comparison, Rvachev and Longini (1985) [75] estimated $R = 1.89$ from influenza case incidence data for the pandemic wave starting in July 1968 in Hong Kong.

Acknowledgments We thank Ping Yan for kindly providing the time series data of the 1918 influenza pandemic in Winnipeg, Canada. The mortality data of the 1968 influenza pandemic in US cities was kindly facilitated by CDC.

References

1. Morbidity and Mortality Weekly Reports (MMWR). 121 US cities mortality surveillance (1968–1971) [http://www.cdc.gov/mmwr/].
2. Anderson RM and May RM (1982) Directly transmitted infectious diseases: Control by vaccination. *Science* 215:1053–1060.
3. Anderson RM and May RM (1991) Infectious Diseases of Humans: Dynamics and Control. Oxford University Press, Oxford.
4. Andreasen V, Viboud C and Simonsen L (2008) Epidemiologic characterization of the summer wave of the 1918 influenza pandemic in Copenhagen: Implications for pandemic control strategies. *J. Infect. Dis.* 197:270–278.
5. Arino J, Brauer F, van den Driessche P, Watmough J and Wu J (2007) A final size relation for epidemic models. *Math. Biosc. Eng.* 4:159–176.
6. Becker NG (1989) Analysis of Infectious Disease Data. Chapman and Hall, New York.
7. Berman A and Plemmons RJ (1994) Nonnegative Matrices in the Mathematical Sciences, Classics in Applied Mathematics 9, SIAM, Philadelphia.
8. Bickel P and Doksum KA (1977) Mathematical Statistics. Holden-Day, Oakland, California.
9. Blower SM and Mclean AR (1994) Prophylactic vaccines, risk behavior change, and the probability of eradicating HIV in San Francisco. *Science* 265: 1451.
10. Brauer F and Castillo-Chavez C (2000) Mathematical Models in Population Biology and Epidemiology. Springer-Verlag, New York.
11. Brauer F (2004) Backward bifurcations in simple vaccination models. *J. Math. Anal. Appl.* 298:418–431.
12. Brauer F (2005) The Kermack-McKendrick model revisited. *Math. Biosc.* 198: 119–131.
13. Brauer F (2008) Compartmental models in epidemiology. In: Brauer F, van den Driessche P, and Wu J (eds) Mathematical Epidemiology, Lecture Notes in Mathematics, Mathematical Biosciences Subseries 1945 Springer-Verlag, Berlin-Heidelberg: 19–79.
14. Cadham MFT (1919) The use of a vaccine in the recent epidemic of influenza. *Can. Med. Assoc. J.* 9:519–527.
15. Castillo-Chavez C and Thieme HR (1993) Asymptotically autonomous epidemic models. In: Arino O, Axelrod D, Kimmel M, Langlais M (eds) Mathematical Population Dynamics: Analysis of Heterogeneity, Vol. 1, Theory of Epidemics,, Wuerz, Winnipeg: 33–50.
16. Castillo-Chavez C, Feng Z and Huang W (2002) On the computation of R_0 and its role on global stability, in: Mathematical Approaches for Emerging and Reemerging Infectious Diseases: An Introduction, IMA Volume 125. Springer-Veralg, Berlin pp. 229-250.
17. Carrat F, Vergu E, Ferguson NM, et al. (2008) Time lines of infection and disease in human influenza: A review of volunteer challenge studies. *Am. J. Epidemiol.* 167(7): 775–785.
18. Cauchemez S, Boelle PY, Thomas G and Valleron AJ (2006) Estimating in real time the efficacy of measures to control emerging communicable diseases. *Am. J. Epidemiol.* 164:591–597.
19. Chowell G, Ammon CE, Hengartner NW and Hyman JM (2006) Transmission dynamics of the great influenza pandemic of 1918 in Geneva, Switzerland: Assessing the effects of hypothetical interventions. *J. Theor. Biol.* 241:193–204.
20. Chowell G, Nishiura H and Bettencourt LM (2007) Comparative estimation of the reproduction number for pandemic influenza from daily case notification data. *J. R. Soc. Interface* 4:155–166.
21. Chowell G, Miller MA and Viboud C (2008) Seasonal influenza in the United States, France, and Australia: Transmission and prospects for control. *Epidemiol. Infect.* 136:852–64.
22. Chowell G, Ammon CE, Hengartner NW and Hyman JM (2007) Estimating the reproduction number from the initial phase of the Spanish flu pandemic waves in Geneva, Switzerland. *Math. Biosci. Eng.* 4:457–470.
23. Chowell G, Bettencourt LMA, Johnson N, Alonso WJ and Viboud C (2008) The 1918–1919 influenza pandemic in England and Wales: Spatial patterns in transmissibility and mortality impact. *Proc. R. Soc. B* 275:501–509.

24. Chowell G, Bettencourt LMA, Johnson NPAS, Alonso WJ and Viboud C (2008) The 1918–1919 influenza pandemic in England and Wales: Spatial patterns in transmissibility and mortality impact. *Proc. Biol. Sci.* 275:501–9.
25. Chowell G and Nishiura H (2008) Quantifying the transmission potential of pandemic influenza. *Phys. Life Rev.* 5, 50–77.
26. Cunha BA (2004) Influenza: Historical aspects of epidemics and pandemics. *Infect. Dis. Clin. North Am.* 18:141–155.
27. Davidian M and Giltinan DM (1995) Nonlinear Models for Repeated Measurement data. Monographs on Statistics and Applied Probability 62. Chapman and Hall, New York.
28. De Jong MC, Diekmann O and Heesterbeek JA (1994) The computation of R_0 for discrete-time epidemic models with dynamic heterogeneity. *Math. Biosci.* 119:97–114.
29. Diekmann O, Heesterbeek JAP and Metz JAJ (1990) On the definition and the computation of the basic reproductive ratio $\mathcal{R}_0$ in models for infectious diseases in heterogeneous populations. *J. Math. Biol.* 28:365–382.
30. Diekmann O and Heesterbeek JAP (2000) Mathematical Epidemiology of Infectious Diseases: Model Building, Analysis and Interpretation. John Wiley and Sons, New York.
31. Dietz K (1988) Mathematical models for transmission and control of malaria. in: Malaria, Principles and Practice of Malariology, eds W.H. Wernsdorfer and I. McGregor. Churchill Livingstone, Edinburgh. pp.1091–1133.
32. Dietz K (1993) The estimation of the basic reproduction number for infectious diseases. *Stat. Methods Med. Res.* 2:23–41.
33. Dushoff J, Huang W and Castillo-Chavez C (1998) Backwards bifurcations and catastrophe in simple models of total diseases. *J. Math. Biol.* 36:227–248.
34. Efron B and Tibshirani RJ (1986) Bootstrap methods for standard errors, confidence intervals, and other measures of statistical accuracy. *Stat. Sci.* 1:54–75.
35. Ferguson NM, Donnelly CA and Anderson RM (2001) Transmission intensity and impact of control policies on the foot and mouth epidemc in Great Britain. *Nature* 413:542–548.
36. Ferguson NM, Cummings DAT, Cauchemez S, Fraser C, Riley S, Meeyai A, Iamsirithaworn S and Burke DS (2005) Strategies for containing an emerging influenza pandemic in Southeast Asia. *Nature* 437:209–214.
37. Fine PE (1993) Herd immunity: History, theory, practice. *Epidemiol. Rev.* 15:265–302.
38. Gani R, Hughes H, Fleming DM, Griffin T, Medlock J and Leach S (2005) Potential impact of antiviral drug use during influenza pandemic. *Emerg. Infect. Dis.* 11:1355–1362.
39. Hadeler KP and Castillo-Chavez C (1995) A core group model for disease transmission. *Math Biosc.* 128:41–55.
40. Hadeler KP and van den Driessche P (1997) Backward bifurcation in epidemic control. *Math. Biosc.* 146:15–35.
41. Halloran ME, Haber M, Longini IM and Struchiner CJ (1991) Direct and indirect effects in vaccine efficacy and effectiveness. *Am. J. Epidemiol.* 133:323–331.
42. Heesterbeek JAP (2002) A brief history of R_0 and a recipe for its calculation. *Acta Biotheor.* 50:189–204.
43. Heffernan JM, Smith RJ and Wahl LM (2005) Perspectives on the basic reproductive ratio. *J. R. Soc. Interface* 2:281–293.
44. Heffernan JM and Wahl LM (2006) Improving estimates of the basic reproductive ratio: using both the mean and the dispersal of transition times. *Theor. Popul. Biol.* 70:135–145.
45. Hethcote HW, Stech HW and van den Driessche P (1981) Periodicity and stability in epidemic models: a survey. In: Busenberg S and Cooke KL (eds.) Differential Equations and Applications in Ecology, Epidemics and Population Problems, Springer-Verlag, Berlin-Heidelberg: 65–82.
46. Hethcote HW and Levin SA (1989) Periodicity in epidemic models. In : Levin SA, Hallam TG, Gross LG (eds) Applied Mathematical Ecology. Biomathematics 18, Springer-Verlag, Berlin-Heidelberg-New York: 193–211.
47. Hethcote HW (2000) The mathematics of infectious diseases. *SIAM Rev.* 42:599–653.

48. Hyman JM and Li J (2000) An intuitive formulation for the reproductive number for the spread of diseases in heterogeneous populations. *Math. Biosci.* 167:65–86.
49. Johnson NP and Mueller J (2002) Updating the accounts: global mortality of the 1918–1920 "Spanish" influenza pandemic. *Bull. Hist. Med.* 76:105–115.
50. Jones EW (2005) Co-operarion in all human endeavour: Quarantine and immigrant disease vectors in the 1918–1919 influenza pandemic in winnipeg. *Can. Bull. Med. Hist.* 22:57–82.
51. Keeling MJ and Grenfell BT (2000) Individual-based perspectives on R(0). *J. Theor. Biol.* 203:51–61.
52. Keeling MJ and Eames KT (2005) Networks and epidemic models. *J. R. Soc. Interface* 2:295–307.
53. Kendall DG (1956) Deterministic and stochastic epidemics in closed populations. in: Third Berkeley Symposium on Mathematical Statistics and Probability 4, ed P. Newman. University of California Press, New York. pp. 149–165.
54. Kermack WO and McKendrick AG (1927) Contributions to the mathematical theory of epidemics – I. *Proc. R. Soc. A* 115:700–721 (reprinted in *Bulletin of Mathematical Biology* 53 (1991) 33–55).
55. Kermack WO and McKendrick AG (1932) Contributions to the mathematical theory of epidemics, part. II. *Proc. Roy. Soc. London* 138:55–83.
56. Kermack WO and McKendrick AG (1933) Contributions to the mathematical theory of epidemics, part. III. *Proc. Roy. Soc. London* 141:94–112.
57. Kribs-Zaleta CM and Velasco-Hernandez JX (2000) A simple vaccination model with multiple endemic states. *Math Biosc.* 164:183–201.
58. Lipsitch M, Cohen T, Cooper B, Robins JM, Ma S, James L, Gopalakrishna G, Chew SK, Tan CC, Samore MH, Fisman D and Murray M (2003) Transmission dynamics and control of severe acute respiratory syndrome. *Science* 300:1966–1970
59. Lloyd AL (2001) Destabilization of epidemic models with the inclusion of realistic distributions of infectious periods. *Proc. R. Soc. London B* 268:985–993.
60. Lloyd AL (2001) Realistic distributions of infectious periods in epidemic models: Changing patterns of persistence and dynamics. *Theor. Popul. Biol.* 60:59–71.
61. Ma J and Earn DJ (2006) Generality of the final size formula for an epidemic of a newly invading infectious disease. *Bull. Math. Biol.* 68:679–702.
62. MacKellar L (2007) Pandemic influenza: A review. *Popul. Dev. Rev.* 33:429–451.
63. Markel H, Lipman HB, Navarro JA, Sloan A, Michalsen JR, Stern AM and Cetron MS (2007) Nonpharmaceutical interventions implemented by US cities during the 1918–1919 influenza pandemic. *JAMA* 298:644–654.
64. Markus L (1956) Asymptotically autonomous differential systems. In: Lefschetz S (ed) Contributions to the Theory of Nonlinear Oscillations III. Annals of Mathematics Studies **36**, Princeton University Press, Princeton, N.J.: 17–29.
65. Massad E, Burattini MN, Coutinho FA and Lopez LF (2007) The 1918 influenza A epidemic in the city of Sao Paulo, Brazil. *Med. Hypotheses* 68:442–445.
66. Mills CE, Robins JM and Lipsitch M (2004) Transmissibility of 1918 pandemic influenza. *Nature* 432:904–906.
67. Murray CJ, Lopez AD, Chin B, Feehan D and Hill KH (2006) Estimation of potential global pandemic influenza mortality on the basis of vital registry data from the 1918–1920 pandemic: A quantitative analysis. *Lancet* 368:2211–2218.
68. Nishiura H, Dietz K and Eichner M (2006) The earliest notes on the reproduction number in relation to herd immunity: Theophil Lotz and smallpox vaccination. *J. Theor. Biol.* 241:964–967.
69. Nishiura H (2006) Mathematical and statistical analyses of the spread of dengue. *Dengue Bull.* 30:51–67.
70. Nishiura H (2007) Time variations in the transmissibility of pandemic influenza in Prussia, Germany, from 1918 to 1919. *Theor. Biol. Med. Model.* 4:20.

71. Nishiura H and Inaba H (2007) Discussion: Emergence of the concept of the basic reproduction number from mathematical demography. *J. Theor. Biol.* 244:357–364.
72. Patterson KD and Pyle GF (1991) The geography and mortality of the 1918 influenza pandemic. *Bull. Hist. Med.* 65:4–21.
73. Roberts MG and Heesterbeek JA (2007) Model-consistent estimation of the basic reproduction number from the incidence of an emerging infection. *J. Math. Biol.* 55:803–816.
74. Ross R (1911) The Prevention of Malaria. John Murray, London.
75. Rvachev LA, Longini IM (1985) A mathematical model for the global spread of influenza. *Math. Biosci.* 75:322.
76. Sattenspiel L and Herring DA (2003) Simulating the effect of quarantine on the spread of the 1918–1919 flu in central Canada. *Bull. Math. Biol.* 65:1–26.
77. Sertsou G, Wilson N, Baker M, Nelson P and Roberts MG (2006) Key transmission parameters of an institutional outbreak during the 1918 influenza pandemic estimated by mathematical modelling. *Theor. Biol. Med. Model.* 3:38.
78. Smith CE (1964) Factors in the transmission of virus infections from animal to man. *Sci. Basis Med. Annu. Rev.* 125–150.
79. Sydenstricker E (1921) Variations in case fatality during the influenza epidemic of 1918. *Public Health Rep.* 36:2201–2211.
80. Thieme HR and Castillo-Chavez C (1989) How may infection-age dependent infectivity affect the dynamics of HIV/AIDS? *SIAM J. Appl. Math.* 53:1447–1479.
81. Thieme HR (1994) Asymptotically autonomous differential equations in the plane. *Rocky Mountain J. Math.* 24:351–380.
82. van den Driessche P and Watmough J (2002) Reproduction numbers and subthreshold endemic equilibria for compartmental models of disease transmission. *Math. Biosc.* 180:29–48.
83. Viboud C, Tam T, Fleming D, Handel A, Miller MA and Simonsen L (2006) Transmissibility and mortality impact of epidemic and pandemic influenza, with emphasis on the unusually deadly 1951 epidemic. *Vaccine* 24:6701–6707.
84. Vynnycky E, Trindall A and Mangtani P (2007) Estimates of the reproduction numbers of Spanish influenza using morbidity data. *Int. J. Epidemiol.* 36:881–889.
85. Wallinga J and Teunis P (2004) Different epidemic curves for severe acute respiratory syndrome reveal similar impacts of control measures. *Am. J. Epidemiol.* 160:509–516.
86. Wallinga J, Lipsitch M (2007) How generation intervals shape the relationship between growth rates and reproductive numbers. *Proc. Roy. Soc. B* 274:599–604.
87. Wearing HJ, Rohani P, and Keeling MJ (2005) Appropriate models for the management of infectious diseases. *PLOS Med.* 2:621–627.
88. White LC and Pagano MA (2007) likelihood-based method for real-time estimation of the serial interval and reproductive number of an epidemic. *Stat. Med.* in press (doi: 10.1002/sim.3136).
89. Yan P (2008) Separate roles of the latent and infectious periods in shaping the relation between the basic reproduction number and the intrinsic growth rate of infectious disease outbreaks. *J. Theor. Biol.* 251:238–252.
90. Yang CK and Brauer F (2008) Calculation of $\mathcal{R}_0$ for age-of-infection models. *Math. Biosci. Eng.* 5:585–599.

Stochastic Epidemic Modeling

Priscilla E. Greenwood and Luis F. Gordillo

Abstract We review the topic of stochastic epidemic modeling with emphasis on compartmental stochastic models. A main theme is the usefulness of the correspondence between these and their large population deterministic limits, which describe dynamical systems. The dynamics of an ODE system informs us of the deterministic skeleton upon which the behavior of corresponding stochastic systems are built. In this chapter we present a number of examples, mostly in the context of susceptible-infected-removed (SIR) models, and point out how this way of thinking may be useful in understanding other stochastic models. In particular we discuss the distribution of final epidemic size, the effect of different patterns of infectiousness, and the quantification of stochastically sustained oscillations.

Keywords Epidemic modeling · Stochastic SIR · Final size distribution · Vaccination · Stochastically sustained oscillations · Variable infectiousness

1 Introduction

The topic of stochastic epidemic modeling is huge. There are many possible types of stochastic epidemic model. The decision of which type of model to choose, or to invent a new one, depends on the specific question to be explored and the data which is at hand or can be obtained. This chapter is a brief guide for newcomers, to the literature and to the construction of compartmental stochastic models. We will indicate some of the history of the subject in the next section. The one class of stochastic models which we will describe in some detail, compartmental models, is introduced in Section 3. Their natural form is multivariate Markov jump processes. When populations are large, they correspond, in the sense of non-limit approximation, to systems of stochastic differential equations. Their large population limits are systems of ordinary differential equations.

P.E. Greenwood (✉)
Department of Mathematics and Statistics, Arizona State University, Tempe, AZ 85287-1804, USA
e-mail: pgreenw@math.asu.edu

G. Chowell et al. (eds.), *Mathematical and Statistical Estimation Approaches in Epidemiology*, DOI 10.1007/978-90-481-2313-1_2,
© Springer Science+Business Media B.V. 2009

Following the section on stochastic compartmental models we will describe three stochastic phenomena that illustrate some of the questions to which these models can yield answers. They happen to be questions to which we have recently contributed. The first, in Section 4, concerns the form of the distribution of the final size of an epidemic. In the context of a susceptible-infected-removed (SIR) epidemic, the final size distribution is bimodal, quite strikingly if the reproduction number is just slightly larger than one. Hence a prediction of epidemic size based on deterministic modeling may be meaningless.

Section 5 concerns stochastically sustained oscillations, which occur if the corresponding dynamical system has damped oscillations. Such sustained oscillations may help to explain the semi-regular recurrence of infectious disease outbreaks. Multiscale analysis has allowed the phenomenon to be interpreted in terms of stochastic process behavior, so that the role it plays in oscillatory disease phenomena can be quantified.

Another interesting stochastic effect, in Section 6, concerns a class of stochastic models in which nearly all homogeneity is abandoned. Still it is possible to say something about the distribution of epidemic size. It depends on the infectiousness of infected participants only through their total, or integrated, infectiousness.

A concluding section contains general observations about the essential role of dynamical systems analysis in the understanding of stochastic dynamic effects in epidemic models and additional examples.

2 History

An early stochastic epidemic model was proposed by A.G. McKendrick in 1926, [38], which precedes his work with Kermack on deterministic models, [28]. An account of McKendrick's paper can be found in [25]. In 1928 and 1931, Reed and Frost, and Greenwood proposed discrete time stochastic models, which proceeded by generations of infectives, [18]. The Reed-Frost model was not published at the time, but was presented in lectures in 1928. Bartlett, [14], studied a continuous time stochastic SIR model, and this began a large literature of which we mention only a few highlights. The book of Bailey [6] (first printed in 1957) is about both deterministic and stochastic epidemic models and the estimation of their parameters. In 1993 the Isaac Newton Institute in Cambridge held a semester-long workshop on stochastic epidemic modeling. Three collections of papers edited by Mollison [40], by Isham and Medley [26], and by Grenfell and Dobson [21] resulted. The monograph of Daley and Gani [18] is probably the best general source on this subject. In particular their Chapter 1 is a fine account of the early history of epidemic modeling in general. In fact Daley and Gani are two of the outstanding figures on this area. Another authoritative survey, including maximum likelihood estimation and Monte Carlo Markov Chain (MCMC) methods is by Anderson and Britton, [3]. A revised edition is currently under preparation. Among further prominent contributors to the area are Frank Ball [7–9, 11] Andrew Barbour [12, 13], Niels Becker [15, 16],

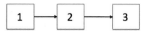

Fig. 1 A schematic compartmental representation. Particles "move" between different categories

David Kendall [27], Donald Ludwig [36], Anders Martin-Löf [39], Ingemar Nåsell [41, 42], Gian Paulo Scalia-Tomba [11, 46, 47], Tom Sellke [48].

3 Stochastic Compartmental Models

Before looking at particular epidemic models, let us become familiar with some notation and ideas about stochastic compartmental models. Later the compartments will become disease states and their members, which we refer to here as particles, will be individuals. We will represent compartments, or classes of individuals by boxes, for example three of them as in Fig. 1, and define a vector-valued process which describes the movement of particles into, and out of each box. Time is continuous. For each time, $t \geq 0$, $(X_1(t), X_2(t), X_3(t))$ is the number of particles in boxes 1, 2, and 3 respectively, where these three numbers sum up to $N(t)$, the total number of particles at that time.

An underlying structure, basic to the class of stochastic compartmental models, and indeed to all Markov jump processes, is the Poisson process. Suppose there is just one compartment, and just one process, $X(t)$, representing the number of particles in the box at time t. Particles enter the box at random times. The initial value, $X(0)$, is fixed and for some $\lambda > 0$,

$$P(X(t + \Delta t) - X(t) = 1) = \lambda \Delta t + o(\Delta t), \tag{1}$$

$$P(X(t + \Delta t) - X(t) = 0) = 1 - \lambda \Delta t + o(\Delta t). \tag{2}$$

The increments of $X(t)$ in disjoint time intervals are independent. Then $X(t), t \geq 0$ is called a Poisson process. The number λ is called the *intensity* or the *stochastic rate* of the process. The times between successive jumps of the process are exponentially distributed with parameter λ. Instead of being constant, $\lambda = \lambda(t)$ may depend on t and may also depend on the value of the process at time t. For example, if

$$P(X(t + \Delta t) - X(t) = 1) = aX(t)\Delta t + o(\Delta t), \tag{3}$$

then we say $aX(t)$ is the *conditional instantaneous stochastic rate* of the process at time t, where the conditioning is on the value of $X(t)$, or, once this is understood, we shorten this to : $aX(t)$ is the stochastic rate, or simply the rate. The rate per particle is a. This process is a *pure birth process*. If our model has several compartments, so that our stochastic process of counts has several components, then the conditional instantaneous stochastic rates of particles entering or leaving each compartment at time t may depend on the sizes of any of the components.

A Markov jump process necessarily has exponentially distributed times between the jumps. We saw this above in the description of the pure birth process, which involves just one component process and one type of jump. A compartmental epidemic model is a vector-valued process with a vector component for each compartment. There are several types of jumps, one type of jump for each arrow in the diagram. If the resulting multi-component process is Markov, each type of jump will occur according to a *locally Poisson* probability as in (1) above, and the times between jumps of any one type, given that nothing occurs in the interim to alter the rate, will be exponentially distributed with parameter given in terms of the states of the component processes at the beginning of the interval. Each component of the Markov jump process can be regarded as a birth and death process, with instantaneous stochastic rates depending on all the components.

The requirement that the inter-jump times be exponentially distributed is not essentially restrictive. There are ways to generalize without losing the advantages of Markov modeling. For example, additional stages can be introduced so that, for instance, one infective step occurs in a sum of independent exponential times, and the result will be a gamma-distributed time. What is important to the resulting stochastic process is how the conditional mean of each increment, each change between t and $t + \Delta t$, relates to the conditional variance of the increment. In the case of conditionally Poisson increments, which are often used in this type of modeling, and yield a Markov structure, the mean and variance are equal. The paper of Lloyd in this volume discusses this point further.

Example 1. A simple stochastic epidemic. In this example we will consider two compartments corresponding to susceptible and infective individuals. We will use the letters S and I respectively to refer to the compartments and also, without confusion we hope, to the number of individuals in each class. We will assume that the total number of individuals is constant and equal to N, that is, $S + I = N$. An individual who belongs to the class S may be contacted by an individual in I, who can transfer the infection. If that is the case, the susceptible individual changes his classification and belongs now to the class I, where he will remain indefinitely. Assume that individuals in each compartment are interchangeable, that the classes are homogeneously mixed, and that contacts between susceptible and infective individuals, or equivalently the movement of individuals from the class S to the class I, occur at random times. If β is the average number of contacts made by an average infective per unit of time that leads to an infection, the probability of a susceptible individual moving from class S to class I in the time interval $[t, t + \Delta t]$, that is, $S \to S - 1$ and $I \to I + 1$, is $\beta \frac{SI}{N} \Delta t + o(\Delta t)$.

This stochastic infection rate has come to be widely used, with various possible interpretations of the N in the denominator. One can think of each susceptible contacting everyone in the population with a rate β and encountering a proportion I/N of infectives. Or one may think of each infective contacting everyone in the population with a rate β and encountering a proportion S/N of susceptibles. Or one may think of the N in the denominator as a reduction of the infection rate due to incomplete mixing in population. From this last point of view, the denominator might be a different power of N or some other function of N. This point is discussed in [49].

The process (S_t, I_t), will represent the number of susceptible and infective individuals at time t. The probability of an infection during the time interval $[t, t+\Delta t]$ is

$$P((S_{t+\Delta t}, I_{t+\Delta t}) - (S_t, I_t) = (-1, 1)) = \beta \frac{S_t I_t}{N} \Delta t + o(\Delta t), \tag{4}$$

with the complementary probability

$$P((S_{t+\Delta t}, I_{t+\Delta t}) - (S_t, I_t) = (0, 0)) = 1 - \beta \frac{S_t I_t}{N} \Delta t + o(\Delta t). \tag{5}$$

Example 2. The stochastic SIR model. Consider three classes of individuals: susceptible, infected, and removed (by recovery or death). As in the previous example, we will use S, I and R to represent the compartments themselves, as well as the numbers of individuals in each compartment, and assume $S + I + R = N$, a constant. Thus, in the time interval $[t, t + \Delta t]$, the probability of an infection, that is, the simultaneous transitions $S \to S - 1$ and $I \to I + 1$ occur, is $\beta \frac{SI}{N} \Delta t + o(\Delta t)$, as in Example 1. If it is assumed that infected individuals recover with rate γ, the probability for a recovery, $I \to I - 1$ and $R \to R + 1$, in the interval $[t, t + \Delta t]$, is $\gamma I \Delta t + o(\Delta t)$. Because $R = N - S - I$, it is enough to consider the process (S_t, I_t). Thus, the probabilities of an infection and of a recovery during the time interval $[t, t + \Delta t]$ are

$$P((S_{t+\Delta t}, I_{t+\Delta t}) - (S_t, I_t) = (-1, 1)) = \beta \frac{S_t I_t}{N} \Delta t + o(\Delta t), \tag{6}$$

$$P((S_{t+\Delta t}, I_{t+\Delta t}) - (S_t, I_t) = (0, -1)) = \gamma I_t \Delta t + o(\Delta t), \tag{7}$$

with the complementary probability

$$P((S_{t+\Delta t}, I_{t+\Delta t}) - (S_t, I_t) = (0, 0)) = 1 - \left(\beta \frac{S_t}{N} + \gamma \right) I_t \Delta t + o(\Delta t). \tag{8}$$

This model, widely known as the *general stochastic epidemic*, was introduced by Barlett in 1949, [14]. An extensive study can be found, for instance, in [3, 18]. The *stochastic equations* describing this process, which are going to be used in Section 4, are obtained by adding and subtracting, to each increment of S_t and I_t, the conditional expectations, given the value of the process at the beginning of the corresponding time increment, say, of length Δt, [6]. Each increment of the process can be expressed as the expected value of the increment plus a sum of centered increments. In our example, the expected values of the increments $\Delta S = S_{t+\Delta t} - S_t$ and $\Delta I = I_{t+\Delta t} - I_t$ are $(-\beta \frac{S_t I_t}{N}) \Delta t$ and $(\beta \frac{S_t I_t}{N} - \gamma I_t) \Delta t$ respectively, so the increments can be written as

$$\Delta S = \left(-\beta \frac{S_t I_t}{N} \right) \Delta t + \Delta Z_1 \tag{9}$$

$$\Delta I = \left(\beta \frac{S_t I_t}{N} - \gamma I_t \right) \Delta t - \Delta Z_1 + \Delta Z_2, \tag{10}$$

where ΔZ_1 and ΔZ_2 are conditionally centered Poisson increments with mean zero and conditional variances $\beta(S_t I_t / N)\Delta t$ and $\gamma I_t \Delta t$.

Now let us consider what happens if we drop the terms ΔZ_i from Equations (9) and (10), and let Δt go to zero. The resulting ordinary differential equations,

$$\frac{dS}{dt} = -\beta \frac{S_t I_t}{N},$$
$$\frac{dI}{dt} = \beta \frac{S_t I_t}{N} - \gamma I_t,$$

define a deterministic model. If $\hat{\beta} S_t I_t$ is used instead of $\beta S_t I_t / N$, with $\hat{\beta} = \beta / N$, we have, after dropping the hats, the so called Kermack and McKendrick ODE model, [19],

$$\frac{dS}{dt} = -\beta S_t I_t, \tag{11}$$

$$\frac{dI}{dt} = \beta S_t I_t - \gamma I_t. \tag{12}$$

In these first two examples, many aspects of a real contagion process have been put aside, for instance latent periods, varying infection and recovery rates, partial immunity, behavioral changes. The inclusion of such features would make the model more realistic, but would complicate the analysis. The strategy in modeling a particular system is first to consider the simplest model, even though some of the aspects one might eventually wish to include are absent. One looks at the analysis and then one may add, one step at a time, additional features. Adding compartments rapidly complicates the analysis. It may be necessary to evaluate the effect of an additional feature by numerical methods or simulation. In the next example, to which we return in Section 5, the effect of births and deaths is taken into account.

Example 3. Stochastic SIR with demography. The stochastic SIR presented in Example 2 might be appropriate when the rates of movement between compartments, and hence the evolution of the disease, are fast enough so that the life span of an individual does not need to be taken into account. This is often acceptable as an idealization when one is interested in looking at functionals of a particular epidemic outbreak such as epidemic size, which we discuss in the next section. However, we may be interested in the longer term recurrent or endemic aspects of a disease, such as the childhood diseases mumps, measles, smallpox, chickenpox, polio or rubella. In this case, demography, meaning births and deaths of individuals, is often included in the model. A scheme including demography is shown in Fig. 2, where

Fig. 2 Schematic compartmental representation of SIR including "demography"

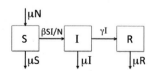

births occur only in the susceptible class and deaths occur, at the same rate per individual, in the three compartments. The transition rates for this model are shown in Table 1 below.

Table 1 Transition rates for the stochastic SIR model with demography

Transition	Rate
$S \rightarrow S + 1$	μN
$S \rightarrow S - 1$	$\beta \frac{SI}{N} \Delta t + \mu S$
$I \rightarrow I + 1$	$\beta \frac{SI}{N} \Delta t$
$I \rightarrow I - 1$	$(\gamma + \mu)I$
$R \rightarrow R + 1$	γI
$R \rightarrow R - 1$	μI

The stochastic rates of birth and death of individuals are assumed constant and equal to μ. This makes the expected value of the total population constant and equal to N. The corresponding probabilities of the events are

$$P((S_{t+\Delta t}, I_{t+\Delta t}) - (S_t, I_t) = (1, 0)) = P((S_{t+\Delta t}, I_{t+\Delta t}) - (S_t, I_t) = (-1, 0))$$

$$= \mu N \Delta t + o(\Delta t), \tag{13}$$

$$P((S_{t+\Delta t}, I_{t+\Delta t}) - (S_t, I_t) = (-1, 1)) = \beta \frac{S_t I_t}{N} \Delta t + o(\Delta t), \tag{14}$$

$$P((S_{t+\Delta t}, I_{t+\Delta t}) - (S_t, I_t) = (0, -1)) = (\gamma + \mu) I_t \Delta t + o(\Delta t). \tag{15}$$

As in Example 2, it is enough to consider the process (S_t, I_t), even though the total population at time t has become a stochastic process. The equations for (S_t, I_t) form a closed system if we take N to be the constant EN, the expected value of N_t. The stochastic equations describing this process, which will be used in Section 5, are obtained similarly, by adding and subtracting to each increment of S_t and I_t, the conditional expectations, given the value of the process at the beginning of the corresponding time increment. For this example, the expected values of the increments $\Delta S = S_{t+\Delta t} - S_t$ and $\Delta I = I_{t+\Delta t} - I_t$ are $(\mu(N - S_t) - \beta \frac{S_t I_t}{N}) \Delta t$ and $(\beta \frac{S_t I_t}{N} - (\gamma + \mu) I_t) \Delta t$ respectively, so the increments can be written as

$$\Delta S = \left(\mu(N - S_t) - \beta \frac{S_t I_t}{N} \right) \Delta t + \Delta Z_1 + \Delta Z_2, \tag{16}$$

$$\Delta I = \left(\beta \frac{S_t I_t}{N} - (\gamma + \mu) I_t \right) \Delta t - \Delta Z_2 + \Delta Z_3, \tag{17}$$

where ΔZ_1 is the difference of the centered Poisson increments corresponding to births and deaths in the susceptible class with mean zero and variance $\mu(N + S_t) \Delta t$. Similarly the centered Poisson increments corresponding to the infections and removals are ΔZ_2 and ΔZ_3 respectively, both with conditional mean zero and with conditional variances $\beta(S_t I_t / N) \Delta t$ and $(\gamma + \mu) \Delta t$. If we drop the terms ΔZ_i from

Equations (16) and (17), and let Δt go to zero. The resulting ordinary differential equations,

$$\frac{dS}{dt} = \mu(N - S_t) - \beta\frac{S_t I_t}{N},$$

$$\frac{dI}{dt} = \beta\frac{S_t I_t}{N} - (\gamma + \mu)I_t,$$

define a deterministic model, namely the deterministic SIR with demography, which has deterministic rates the same as the stochastic rates which yield the stochastic model defined by Equations (16) and (17).

When N is large, there is often a diffusion approximation to a stochastic compartmental model. We illustrate this in the case of Example 3. Let us normalize by dividing each of the stochastic processes in our model by N so that the state variables are the proportions of the total expected population in the susceptible and infective classes at each time, t and their jumps are of size $1/N$. Suppose we replace the conditionally centered Poisson increments, $\Delta Z_i/N$, by increments of Brownian motion, appropriate multiples of ΔW_i, with the same standard deviations as the Poisson increments they replace. We obtain a diffusion approximation to our Markov jump process model which can be written as

$$ds = (\mu(1 - s) - \beta si)\, dt + G_1 dW_1(t) - G_2 dW_2(t),$$

$$di = (\beta si - (\gamma + \mu)i)\, dt + G_2 dW_2(t) - G_3 dW_3(t), \qquad (18)$$

$$G_1 = \sqrt{\mu(1 + s)}, \quad G_2 = \sqrt{\beta si}, \quad G_3 = \sqrt{(\gamma + \mu)i},$$

where $s = S/N$ and $i = I/N$. Kurtz, [29, 30], showed that the normalized Markov jump process and the approximating diffusion (18) can be constructed on the same probability space in such a way that the maximum pointwise distance between their sample paths on a fixed finite interval of time is of order $\log N/N$. It is important to note that the diffusion approximation is good for N large but becomes less useful if N is too large. The limit of the solution of the stochastic system, as N goes to infinity, is in fact the solution of the deterministic model, where the states are the fractions of the total population in each class (18).

For epidemic models, a main concern is to find conditions under which a disease introduced into a community will develop into a large outbreak, and if it does, conditions under which the disease may become endemic. For stochastic models, all such questions are in terms of probabilities. A useful parameter in this regard, called the *basic reproductive number*, R_0, is defined as the expected number of secondary infective cases per primary case in a completely susceptible population, [19]. In Examples 2 and 3 above, the basic reproductive number is β/γ and $\beta/(\gamma + \mu)$, respectively. If the basic reproductive number is smaller than or equal to one, with a high probability the disease outbreak is relatively small. For this reason most studies of these examples concentrate on the complementary case. Arguably, the most important and interesting case is where R_0 is near one, as we shall see.

If the basic reproductive number is greater than one, the stochastic behavior of Examples 2 and 3 are very different. In Example 2, with no demography, the number of infected individuals generally increases, reaches a maximum and then generally decreases to zero. In Example 3, with demography, the solutions of the corresponding deterministic equations (see Section 5 below), will approach a non-trivial equilibrium as t increases, called the endemic equilibrium. Simulations of the stochastic model show almost periodic oscillations of the process around this equilibrium. We return to this striking phenomenon in Section 5.

Other stochastic epidemic models can be defined along lines similar to these three examples. Compartments may be added corresponding to latent, asymptomatic, quarantined, or other disease-associated states. In this chapter we will confine ourselves mostly to questions pertaining to Examples 2 and 3. It will be clear that these and similar questions about other compartmental stochastic models might be pursued using, in part, similar methods. The relation of stochastic compartmental models to limiting deterministic models, and their approximations by diffusions, are illustrated for the SIR model in this section. Essentially all stochastic compartmental models have deterministic limits and diffusion approximations which can be obtained by the arguments analogous to those indicated here and given in detail and in great generality by Kurtz [30]. Often it is useful, and justified, to work with the diffusion approximation to the jump Markov chain model. The deterministic large-N limit is also often of value for understanding the behavior of the stochastic dynamical system defined by the Markov chain model. One example is the information contained in the basic reproductive number, R_0, which can be regarded as a property of the deterministic limit. We see another example in Section 5 and discuss this point more generally in Section 7.

4 Distribution of the Final Epidemic Size

Public health policy may be influenced by predictions of how large an epidemic might be, that is, how many individuals ultimately become infected during the entire time an epidemic lasts. This involves the assumption that the disease in question does not become endemic and persist at a positive level indefinitely. In view of the nature of the dynamics of Examples 2 and 3 in Section 3, the assumption that there is a finite epidemic size pushes us in the direction of assuming that the population is fixed and finite, with no *demography*. In this case, the number of infectives will eventually reach zero, with probability one, so that the total number of individuals that are infected during the infectious process is almost surely finite, and the distribution of the final size of the epidemic can, in principle, be computed.

It was first observed by Bailey in 1953, [5], that the final size distribution for the stochastic SIR is bimodal, that is, there are two maxima. He provided formuli that allow the computation of the distribution of the final size if the population is rather small. Since then, the final size distribution has been investigated for various models, by Lefèvre and Picard [34, 35, 44], Ball [8, 9], Ball and Nåsell [10], Scalia-Tomba [46, 47], Martin-Löf [39], Ludwig [36] among others. For large populations, the computer storage needed for computation of the final size distribution, together with numerical precision, have been important issues.

For the SIR, if the basic reproductive number is greater than one, the general shape of the epidemic size distribution can be deduced intuitively as follows. With a large enough population, during the first stages of an epidemic, the number of infectives evolves approximately like a branching process. If the probability of zero offspring in any family is positive, then the branching process goes extinct with positive probability. The event of zero offspring corresponds to the event that an infective infects no-one else, and this has positive probability. If extinction does occur, it is likely to occur early. Correspondingly there are several sample paths of the process of infectives, I_t, which reach zero relatively soon. On the other hand, if early extinction does not happen then the finite number of susceptible individuals begins to be depleted, so that the process no longer behaves as a branching process. In this case the size of the epidemic may be approximately normally distributed.

There have been attempts to produce a rigorous argument for bimodality of the epidemic size distribution along these lines, but apparently without success. On the other hand, careful observation of simulations shows that some degree of bimodality of this distribution is present for any combination of parameters. The most striking biomodality occurs when the basic reproductive number is just slightly larger than one, as in Fig. 3.

Martin Löf, [39], found a normalization and relative rates, under which the process of infectives has a diffusion limit when, simultaneously, the total population, N, and the basic reproductive number approach infinity and one, respectively. Also, the distribution of the time until the epidemic stops converges to the time it takes a Brownian motion to hit a parabolic boundary. Martin Löf used an elegant approximation, using Airy functions, to produce the shape of the limiting epidemic size distribution by computation. Marion and Greenwood [37] found a way of computing the final size distribution for very large N, from which one can see the degree of agreement between Martin-Löf's limiting distributions and the pre-limit for large N. In this section we describe these results and others found in [22]. We look at the questions:

- How does the epidemic size distribution depend on the parameters of the model?
- Is there a way to incorporate a process of vaccination in the stochastic SIR that depends on the activity of the disease?
- How does the final epidemic size distribution change in the presence of vaccination?

In order to simplify notation we will re-scale the time to γt, and define $\lambda = \beta/\gamma$, which is the basic reproductive number. Then, in the notation of Example 2, $\beta = \lambda$, and $\gamma = 1$. We observe how the shape of the final size distribution depends on the parameters of the model by accurately computing the distribution in a memory-efficient fashion, which we indicate here. For this we need to look only at the

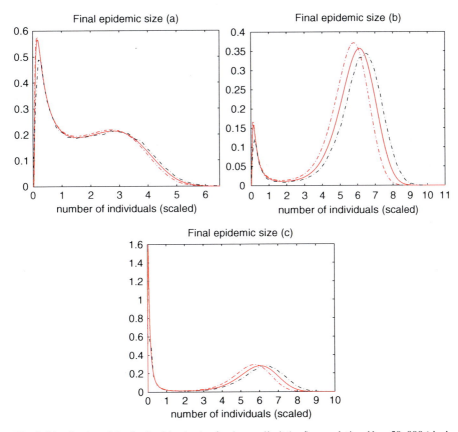

Fig. 3 Distribution of the final epidemic size for the pre-limit (*red*): population $N = 50,000$ (*dash-dots*) and $N = 500,000$ (*solid*). The limit distribution (*black*) is in *dash-dots*. The parameters are (a) $a = 1, b = 1$, (b) $a = 3, b = 1$ (c) $a = 3, b = 0.5$. For all the figures $\theta = 0$. Notice that the three figures have different scales. Epidemic size is about $N^{2/3}$ times the scaled value

times at which transitions occur, that is, points in time where an event, contagion or removal, happens. Ignoring the waiting times between events, we obtain a discrete-time Markovian structure from the continuous time SIR that has the same epidemic size as the SIR process. This is called the *discrete time embedded Markov chain of jumps*. Let us number the consecutive jumps of the continuous time Markov chain by j, so that j becomes the time parameter of the discrete time embedded Markov chain. The transition probabilities of this discrete time chain are given by

$$(\Delta S_j, \Delta I_j) = \begin{cases} (-1, 1) & \text{with probability } \frac{\lambda S_j I_j / N}{\lambda S_j I_j / N + I_j} = \frac{\lambda S_j}{\lambda S_j + N}, \\ (0, -1) & \text{with probability } \frac{I_j}{\lambda S_j I_j / N + I_j} = \frac{N}{\lambda S_j + N}. \end{cases} \tag{19}$$

We introduce the possibility of immunization through an additional type of jump, of the form $(-1, 0)$. An individual is removed from the susceptible class through immunization, which may occur at each time step of the embedded chain. We denote by θ the average ratio of the number of vaccinations to the number of jumps. Thus, for instance, if $\theta = 0.5$, there is one vaccination every two steps, on the average; if $\theta = 2$, there are two vaccinations per step, on the average. This entry into the model of the vaccination procedure can be modified in various ways. For example, immunization can be considered only at the times when someone is infected, or only when a recovery occurs. The parameter θ can also depend on time or it may even be random with its distribution being time-dependent, and/or dependent on the current state of the process. Partial effectiveness can be modeled by multiplying θ by the probability of successful vaccination. Note that in this model the number of vaccinated persons is not directly related to the number of susceptibles, but is tied to the intensity of the epidemic as it evolves.

Let U_j count the total number of infections which occur up to, and including, time j, disregarding the initial number of infected individuals. The probability that an individual gets infected in the time step from $j - 1$ to j, given the value U_{j-1}, and if there were initially n and m susceptible and infected individuals, is

$$p_{k,j} \equiv P(U_j = k + 1 | U_{j-1} = k) = \frac{\lambda(n - k - \theta(j - 1))}{\lambda(n - k - \theta(j - 1)) + (n + m)}, \qquad (20)$$

with the complementary probability

$$q_{k,j} \equiv P(U_j = k | U_{j-1} = k) = 1 - p_{k,j}. \qquad (21)$$

Although it does not appear in the notation, this probability is conditional on S_t being positive.

Let T denote the time at which the epidemic stops. Then U_T is the number of individuals ultimately infected, in addition to the original m infectives. At each time step an infection or a recovery happens. The process U_j is a random walk starting at 0, with a positive step when there is an infection and a zero step when there is a recovery. The epidemic stops when

$$U_t + m - (\text{number of recoveries}) = 0,$$

and

$$T = U_T + (\text{number of recoveries}).$$

Therefore, $U_T = (T - m)/2$. To obtain the distribution of U_T, it is enough to compute the distribution of the hitting time T. To compute this distribution we will use the following recursion. First define $W_j(k) = P(U_j = k, T > j)$ for non-negative integers, j. Notice that $W_0(k) = \delta_{k,0}$, $P(T = 0) = 0$ and, if $j - m$ is even,

$$P(T = j) = W_{j-1}\left(\frac{j - m}{2}\right) q_{\frac{j-m}{2}, j}. \qquad (22)$$

If $j - m$ is odd, then $P(T = j) = 0$. The defective distribution $W_j(\cdot)$ is computed as

$$W_j(k) = \begin{cases} W_{j-1}(k-1)p_{k-1,j} + W_{j-1}(k)q_{k,j}, & \text{if } k > \frac{j-m}{2}; \\ 0, & \text{if } k \leq \frac{j-m}{2}. \end{cases} \qquad (23)$$

This recursion allows us to compute the distribution $P(T = j)$, $j = 1, 2, \ldots$, and the defective distributions $W_j(k)$, $k = 1, \ldots, n$, $j = 1, 2, \ldots$, while storing only the values of $W_j(\cdot)$ at stage j. As j increases, $W_j(\cdot)$ loses mass.

This algorithm can be used for any finite number N of individuals in the population. If N approaches infinity and simultaneously λ approaches one, with suitable related rates, the distribution can be found using a diffusion approximation. For this, we define new random variables X_t^N and Y_t^N by

$$\frac{S_t}{N} = 1 - \frac{X_t^N}{N^\alpha},$$
$$I_t = Y_t^N N^\beta,$$

and let $\lambda_N = 1 + a/N^\gamma$. Martin Löf [39] found exponents α, β and γ such that X_t^N and Y_t^N converge weakly to a limiting diffusion, see [39] or [22] for details. Appropriate values for these exponents are $\alpha = \beta = \gamma = 1/3$. After re-scaling time as $s = tN^{-2/3}$ and letting $N \to \infty$, X_t^N and Y_t^N converge weakly to diffusions X_s and Y_s, which satisfy the stochastic differential equations

$$dX_s = (1 + 2\theta)ds,$$
$$dY_s = (a - X_s)ds + \sqrt{2}\,dW_s,$$

where $a = \lim_{N \to \infty} N^{1/3}(\lambda_N - 1)$.

The process X_s is deterministic linear drift, $X_s = (1 + 2\theta)s$, so that Y_s is defined by

$$dY_s = (a - (1 + 2\theta)s)ds + \sqrt{2}\,dW_s.$$

After integration,

$$Y_s = b + as - (1 + 2\theta)s^2/2 + \sqrt{2}\,W_s, \qquad (24)$$

a diffusion with parabolic drift starting at

$$b = \lim_{N,m \to \infty} m/N^{1/3}. \qquad (25)$$

The limiting epidemic stops when the right hand side of (24) is equal to zero, or in other words, when the Brownian motion $\sqrt{2}\,W_s$ hits the parabola $b + as - (1 + 2\theta)s^2/2$ for the first time.

Epidemic size defines a continuous functional with respect to the topology of weak convergence of stochastic processes. Hence the weak convergence of the pre-limit processes to Y implies convergence of the distribution of epidemic size for finite N to a distribution associated with the time Brownian motion hits a parabola.

Pre-limit and limiting distribution curves are shown in Fig. 3. In the figure we can observe the convergence of epidemic size distributions and get an idea of the size of N necessary for the pre-limit to approximate the limit to a certain degree of accuracy. We compare the distributions obtained using the algorithm (22) and (23) for the pre-limit and the limiting diffusion obtained in [39] for different values of parameters a and b, with $\theta = 0$. For the pre-limit, λ and m are chosen according to $\lambda = 1 + a/N^{1/3}$, $b = m/N^{1/3}$. We see that the shape of the distribution is highly sensitive to the values of the parameters a and b when the model is slightly super-critical, that is, when $\lambda > 1$ is very close to 1. The degree of agreement between the limit distribution and the pre-limit for $N = 50,000$ and for $N = 500,000$ is not as precise as one might have expected.

The effect of vaccination in our model can be observed in Fig. 4. Vaccination pushes the mass of the distribution in the direction of smaller epidemic size, but the bimodality of the distribution persists. Increasing θ pushes the distribution towards zero, as one would expect.

A scaling parameter less than 1/3 can also be used and leads to the limit one would obtain from a branching process model. The limiting epidemic size distribution using this scaling is not bimodal, [20].

The embedded chain in the algorithmic scheme for computing the distribution of the final size, as presented in this section, ignores the amount of time between events. This suggests that latency periods in infected individuals might not affect

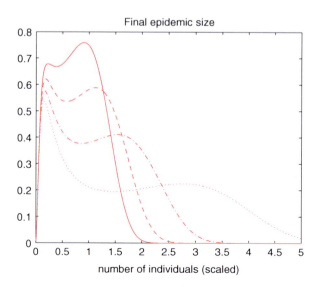

Fig. 4 Distribution of the final epidemic size for $N = 30,000$. The vaccination levels are $\theta = 0$ (*dots*), $\theta = 0.5$ (*dash-dot*), $\theta = 1$ (*dashes*) and $\theta = 1.5$ (*solid*). The other parameters are $a = 1$ and $b = 1$. Vaccination pushes the mass of the distribution to the region of short outbreaks. Similar behavior can be observed for other values of the parameters a and b, [22]

the distribution of the final size. In Section 6 we see that this is true in a very general setting, where homogeneity of the susceptible and infectious classes is abandoned.

5 Stochastic Sustained Oscillations

In this section we will consider the model defined in Section 3, Example 3. As mentioned before, when the basic reproductive number is greater than one, the deterministic system has two equilibrium points, one unstable with no infectives, and a stable endemic point with a positive number of infectives. It can be observed, and shown analytically, that the solutions of the deterministic model oscillate around the endemic point and rapidly damp to the endemic equilibrium as time increases. However time-course data of diseases like measles or chickenpox show periodic oscillations that do not damp as time goes by. It is possible [24, 32] to produce deterministic models which have more slowly damped, or even sustained, oscillations by including, for instance, age structure, quarantine, multiple strains of infectious agents or delays. Of course seasonal periodic forcing produces seasonal oscillations in a deterministic epidemic.

Simulations of a stochastic SIR model follow the damped deterministic trajectory for a certain time after which the stochastic path remains oscillatory, with a varying amplitude, as can be seen in Fig. 5 below.

The oscillations of stochatic SIR paths have a frequency distribution, evidenced by the power spectral density of the process of infectives, and a stochastically varying amplitude. This phenomenon, in which random fluctuations sustain nearly periodic oscillations in a system which has a stable constant equilibrium in the deterministic limit, has been called *coherence resonance* or *autonomous stochastic resonance*. Coherence resonance has been observed in a number of experimental studies of electrical, chemical and physiological phenomena, [43].

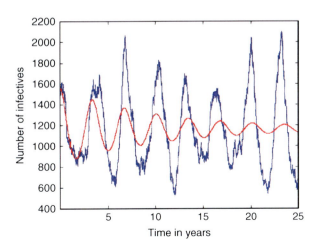

Fig. 5 A sample path of the infective process of stochastic SIR with demography contrasted to the damped oscillations of the corresponding deterministic system with the same initial point. The parameters are $N = 2,000,000$, average life span $1/\mu = 80$ years, $R_0 = 15$, average time of infectiousness $1/\gamma = 15$ days. Notice that the stochastic path initially follows the deterministic trajectory

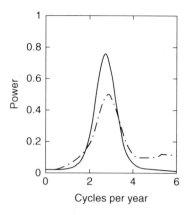

Fig. 6 The power spectral density of the process of infectives in the stochastic SIR model (*dot-dash*) and the multi-scale approximation (*solid*). The values used are $R_0 = 15$, $N = 500,000$, $1/\mu = 55$ years and $1/\gamma = 25$ days

Although coherence resonance has been recognized as a possible occurrence in the presence of noise when a dynamical system has a small or hidden inherent periodicity, the phenomenon is only beginning to be understood quantitatively, from the stochastic process viewpoint. In [4], Aparicio and Solari give a convincing explanation of the non-damping of stochastic SIR in terms of the average change in a Liapunov function as the process moves inside and outside a parabola in phase space. In [31] we use multi-scale analysis to show that a stationary version of the system (16) and (17) can be rather closely approximated, in a neighborhood of the endemic equilibrium, for a suitable range of the parameters β, γ and μ, by a linear combination of sinusoids, where the coefficient processes in this approximation are Ornstein-Uhlenbeck processes running on a slower time scale.

The accuracy of the multiscale approximation to (16), (17) for a particular choice of parameters can be evaluated by comparing the power spectral densities of the two processes as in Fig. 6.

6 Effects of Varying Infectiousness

If an individual becomes infected at time t, he may not become infectious immediately. There may be a latent period during which he is asymptomatic and/or remains uninfectious to others. More generally, infectiousness may vary in a variety of patterns following the event of disease transmission. In [23] we defined for each individual, a function which quantifies how infectious he is at time t following the event of his infection. This function may depend on many factors, including a latent period, the response of the individual's immune system, the effects of medical treatments, etc. In epidemic modeling, it is natural to question how the pattern of infectiousness affects disease dynamics. In particular we are interested to see how the final size of an epidemic may be affected by how infectiousness varies.

In fact, a latency period does not influence the distribution of the final size of the stochastic SIR. This result has been shown in various contexts, see for example

[1, 3, 8]. In [23] we proposed a more general formulation and showed that the final size depends only on the *integrated infectiousness*. Here are the main points of the argument.

The individuals in a population of constant size are labelled with the values $1, \ldots, N$, for identification. We think of individuals as distributed in space and related by a network of social or other connections, or as moving in space and encountering one another with pair independent frequencies. The numbers $c_{ij} \geq 0$ measure the rates of contact from individual i to individual j for all pairs (i, j) with $1 \leq i, j \leq N$. Notice that $c_{ji} \neq c_{ij}$ in general. Our model assumption is that the time T_{ij} of first infectious contact from i to j happens in the time interval $[t, t + \Delta t]$ with probability

$$P(T_{ij} \in [t, t + \Delta t] | T_{ij} > t, \mathcal{F}_i) = c_{ij} X_i(t) \Delta t + o(\Delta t). \tag{26}$$

Time in (26) runs according to a clock which starts at the first infectious contact made to individual i. The *infectiousness* process of individual i, $X_i(t)$, measures, at each time t, the probability that a contact made by i at time t is effective in transmitting the disease. The collection of sets $\mathcal{F}_i$ represents the information generated by the entire history of the random infectiousness process X_i, not including its start time. The infectiousness clock of individual i may start at time 0, but it may be that $X_i(0) = 0$, so that i is not actually infectious at time 0. Nevertheless we refer to such individuals as *initial infectives*. The product in (26) should be read as the probability of contact from i to j in the time increment $[t, t + \Delta t]$, $c_{ij} \Delta t + o(\Delta t)$, times the conditional probability of transmission of disease, given that contact is made, $X_i(t)$. The random function $c_{ij} X_i(t)$ is a random hazard function, which satisfies

$$P(T_{ij} > t | \mathcal{F}_i) = e^{-\int_0^t c_{ij} X_i(s) ds}, \tag{27}$$

for every $t \geq 0$. Notice that conditioning on $\mathcal{F}_i$ allows us to write a specific sample path, $X_i(s)$. If we let

$$D_i = \int_0^\infty X_i(s) ds < \infty, \tag{28}$$

the probability that an individual j has no infectious contact from individual i, given a sample path of the process X_i, is

$$P(\text{no infection from } i \text{ to } j \,|\, \mathcal{F}_i) = e^{-c_{ij} D_i}.$$

We say that an individual i is *nominally contacted* when an infectious contact to i occurs. This may not be the first infectious contact. Let $\mathcal{F} = \bigcup_i \mathcal{F}_i$ be the σ-algebra generated by the infectiousness processes of all individuals in the population. $\mathcal{F}$ contains the information of the patterns of infectiousness of the entire population. Let $\mathcal{P}$ denote the set of all individuals in the population and let $\mathcal{X}_k$ and $\mathcal{Y}_k$, $k = 0, 1, 2, \ldots$ be

$\mathcal{X}_0 = \{\text{initial infectives}\}$,

$\mathcal{Y}_0 = \mathcal{P} - \mathcal{X}_0$,

$\mathcal{X}_1 = \{j : j \in \mathcal{Y}_0, \exists i \in \mathcal{X}_0 \text{ such that } j \text{ is nominally contacted by } i\}$,

$\mathcal{Y}_1 = \mathcal{Y}_0 - \mathcal{X}_1$,

$\cdots$.

We can see that $\mathcal{Y}_0 \supset \mathcal{Y}_1 \supset \ldots$ and that the set of all nominally contacted individuals, $\bigcup_{k=0}^{\infty} \mathcal{X}_k$, where $\mathcal{X}_i \cap \mathcal{X}_j = \emptyset$ if $i \neq j$, is equal to the set of all individuals who become infected. The size of this set is the total epidemic size. Thus, if we let $\mathcal{X} \subset \mathcal{Y}_0$, the probability that the random set $\mathcal{X}_1$ is exactly $\mathcal{X}$, given $\mathcal{F}$, is

$$P(\mathcal{X}_1 = \mathcal{X}|\mathcal{F}) = \prod_{j \in \mathcal{X}} \left(1 - \prod_{i \in \mathcal{X}_0} e^{-D_i c_{ij}} \right) \cdot \prod_{j \in \mathcal{Y}_0 - \mathcal{X}} \prod_{i \in \mathcal{X}_0} e^{-D_i c_{ij}}.$$

The distributions of $\mathcal{X}_k$, given $\mathcal{X}_{k-1}, k = 2, 3, \ldots$ can be computed similarly. Therefore, the probability distribution of the number of individuals that have nominal contacts, given all the patterns of infectiousness, is

$$P\left(|\cup_k \mathcal{X}_k| = n|\mathcal{F}\right) = \sum_{\substack{\mathcal{X} \subset \mathcal{P} \\ |\mathcal{X}| = n}} P\left(\cup_k \mathcal{X}_k = \mathcal{X}|\mathcal{F}\right),$$

which depends only on the random variables $D_i, i = 1, \ldots, N$ and the c_{ij}'s.

7 Stochastic and Deterministic Dynamics are Complementary

In this final section of the chapter we point out some useful general relationships between compartmental stochastic and deterministic epidemic models. The two types of model are alternate viewpoints on the same phenomenon, offering complementary insights.

The class of stochastic epidemic models of this chapter is defined by two properties: first, the dynamics can be described by a compartmental diagram such as Fig. 2, with inputs and outputs, and second, the process is a vector-valued continuous time Markov process. This class of models is extremely large. For instance, to Examples 1, 2, and 3 can be added compartments which correspond to the latent, the asymptomatic, those quarantined, those vaccinated, the presence of multiple diseases, or classes of vectors such as mosquitoes which carry infectious agents.

We have indicated in Section 3, using an SIR example, how each such model corresponds to a deterministic model. One can write the stochastic increment equations as in (16) and (17), and then take the conditional expected value of each increment given the process at the beginning of that increment to obtain deterministic increment equations. Or one can divide each state variable by N to obtain equations for the proportion of individuals in each class at time t, and apply the law of large numbers to these equations [29].

On the other hand, starting with a family of ordinary differential equations, which describes a dynamical system, one can arrive at a variety of corresponding stochastic models by interpreting some or all the deterministic rates as stochastic rates in the sense of (1), (2).

Each of these model formulations, the stochastic and the deterministic dynamical system, augments our understanding of the other. The ODE model can be thought of as a deterministic skeleton of any corresponding stochastic model. An indispensable step in understanding the behavior of a stochastic model is the analysis of the dynamics of the ODE model. A dramatic example is the one described in Section 5. In fact, the analysis of stochastically sustained oscillations involves the details of the damped deterministic oscillations. Here are two additional examples.

In epidemic theory deterministic analysis often starts with the basic reproductive number, R_0. In Example 3, if R_0 is less that one, the unique equilibrium has no infectives. However in certain other models [2, 17], there is a more complex bifurcation structure in which, for a range of R_0 below one, there are two locally stable equilibria, one with no infectives and one with a positive number of infectives, separated by an unstable equilibrium. This structure is sometimes called a *backward bifurcation* because of the shape of the bifurcation diagram, Fig. 7. An example is the model with susceptible, infected, and vaccinated individuals, defined by Brauer [17]. The dynamics tell us that a deterministic path is attracted to the equilibrium which is on the same side of the unstable equilibrium as the initial point of the path. However, a stochastic path started in a neighborhood of the unstable equilibrium will have probability about one half of being attracted to either equilibrium in the stochastic version of Brauer's model [33]. The authors of [33] continue to study the details of

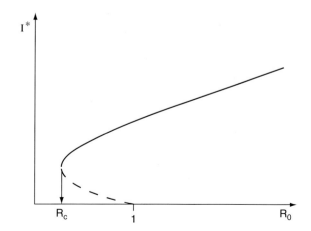

Fig. 7 A typical backward bifurcation diagram. I^* is the value of the infectives at the equilibrium. The *solid lines* stand for stability while *dashed lines* for instability. Taken with permission from [45]

this problem. Of interest, for example, is the function which describes the probability of attraction of the process of infectives to each locally stable equilibrium as the distance of the starting point from the unstable equilibrium increases.

The deterministic susceptible-infected-susceptible (SIS) models are a bit simpler than those of Examples 2 and 3. For $R_0 > 1$, there is a stable equilibrium of the ODE, and the convergence of the path of susceptibles to this equilibrium is monotone rather than by damped oscillations as in Example 3. In fact this is a logistic model, whose susceptible class converges to a saturation point. The paths of the stochastic model lie near the deterministic path and continue to vary randomly around the deterministic equilibrium for a rather long time with high probability. The existence of an absorbing state, $I_t = 0$, in the finite state space means, according to general Markov chain theory, that ultimately the Markov process goes to the absorbing state.

Even in the simple SIS model the deterministic dynamic skeleton shows us a great deal about the behavior of the stochastic paths, and brings to our attention questions which pertain to the stochastic model: What is the nature of the stochastic path of I_t as it varies near the deterministic equilibrium? Starting from the deterministic equilibrium, what is the distribution of the time until the stochastic path hits 0? These questions have been studied by Nåsell [41] for the SIS and other processes.

We should point out, in closing, that the stochastic models we have discussed here are simple ones, involving no more than two linked stochastic equations. The difficulty of a stochastic model grows closely in step with the difficulty of its companion ODE model. Additional stochastic models related to systems of ODE's result from the introduction of stochastic structure to parameters.

References

1. Addy CL, Longini IM, Harber M (1991) A generalized stochastic model for the analysis of infectious disease final size data. Biometrics 47(3):961–974.
2. Allen L, van den Driessche P (2006) Stochastic epidemic models with a backward bifurcation. Mathematical Biosciences 3:445–458.
3. Andersson H, Britton T (2000) *Stochastic epidemic models and their statistical analysis.* Lecture Notes in Statistics, 151. Springer-Verlag, New York.
4. Aparicio JP, Solari HG (2001) Sustained oscillations in stochastic systems. Mathematical Biosciences 169:15–25.
5. Bailey NTJ (1953) The total size of a general stochastic epidemic. Biometrika 40(1/2):177–185.
6. Bailey NTJ (1975) *The mathematical theory of infectious diseases and its applications, Third ed.*, Oxford University Press, Oxford.
7. Ball F (1985) Deterministic and stochastic epidemics with several kinds of susceptibles. Advances in Applied Probability 17:1–22.
8. Ball F (1986) A unified approach to the distribution of total size and total area under the trajectory of infectives in epidemic models. Advances in Applied Probability 18:289–310.
9. Ball F, Clancy D (1993) The final size and severity of a generalized stochastic multitype epidemic model. Advances in Applied Probability 25:721–736.
10. Ball F, Nåsell I (1994) The shape of the size distribution of an epidemic in a finite population. Mathematical Biosciences 123:167–181.

11. Ball F, Mollison D, Scalia-Tomba G (1997) Epidemics with two levels of mixing. Annals of Applied Probability 7:46–89.
12. Barbour AD (1972) The principle of diffusion of arbitrary constants. Journal of Applied Probability 9:519–541.
13. Barbour AD (1974) On a functional central limit theorem for Markov population processes. Advances in Applied Probability 6:21–39.
14. Bartlett MS (1949) Some evolutionary stochastic processes. Journal of the Royal Statistical Sociey Series B 11:211–229.
15. Becker N (1989) *Analysis of infectious disease data.* Chapman and Hall, London.
16. Becker N, Dietz K (1995) The effect of the household distribution on transmission and control of highly infectious diseases. Mathematical Biosciences 127:207–219.
17. Brauer F (2004) Backward bifurcations in simple vaccination models, Journal of Mathematical Analysis and Applications 298:418–431.
18. Daley DJ, Gani J (1999) *Epidemic modeling: an introduction.* Cambridge Studies in Mathematical Biology, 15. Cambridge University Press, Cambridge.
19. Diekmann O, Heesterbeek JAP (2000) *Mathematical epidemiology of infectious diseases. Model building, analysis and interpretation.* Wiley Series in Mathematical and Computational Biology. John Wiley & Sons, Ltd., New York.
20. Dolgoarshinnykh RG, Lalley SP (2006) Critical scaling for the simple SIS stochastic epidemic. Journal of Applied Probability. 43:892–898.
21. Grenfell BT, Dobson AP (1996) *Ecology of infectious diseases in natural populations.* Cambridge University Press, Cambridge.
22. Gordillo LF, Marion SA, Martin Löf A, Greenwood PE (2007) Bimodal epidemic size with vaccination. Bulletin of Mathematical Biology 70:589–602.
23. Gordillo LF, Marion SA, Greenwood PE (2008) The effect of patterns of infectiousness on epidemic size. Mathematical Biosciences and Engineering 5(3):429–435.
24. Hethcote HW, Levin SA (1989) Periodicity in epidemiological models. In: Gross L, Hallam TG, Levin SA (eds) Applied Mathematical Ecology, Springer, Berlin pp. 193–211.
25. Irwin JO (1963) The place of mathematics in medical and biological statistics. Journal of the Royal Statistical Society. Series A (General) 126(1):1–45.
26. Isham V, Medley G (eds.) (1996) *Models for infectious human diseases: their structure and relation to data.* Cambridge University Press, Cambridge.
27. Kendall DG (1956) Deterministic and stochastic epidemics in closed populations. Proceedings of the Third Berkeley Symposium Mathematical Statistics and Probability 4:149–165. University of California Press, Berkeley.
28. Kermack WO, McKendrick AG (1927) A contribution to the mathematical theory of epidemics, Proceedings of the Royal society of London. Series A 115(772):700–721.
29. Kurtz TG (1978) Strong approximation theorems for density dependent Markov chains. Stochastic Processes and their Applications 6:223–240.
30. Kurtz TG (1981) *Approximation of population processes.* CBMS-NSF Regional Conference Series in Applied Mathematics, 36. Society for Industrial and Applied Mathematics (SIAM), Philadelphia, PA.
31. Kuske R, Gordillo LF, Greenwood PE (2007) Sustained oscillations via coherence resonance in SIR, Journal of Theoretical Biology 245:459–469.
32. Levin SA, Dushoff J, Plotkin J (2004) Evolution and persistence of influenza A and other diseases. Mathematical Biosciences 188:17–28.
33. Lopez R, Dembele B (2007) Stochasticity in Vaccination, manuscript.
34. Lefèvre C, Picard P (1990) A non-standard family of polynomials and the final size distribution of reed-frost epidemic processes. Advances in Applied Probability 22(1): 25–48.
35. Lefèvre C, Picard P (1996) Collective epidemic models. Mathematical Biosciences 134: 51–70.
36. Ludwig D (1974) *Stochastic population theories.* Lecture Notes in Biomathematics, 3. Springer-Verlag, New York.

37. Marion S, Greenwood PE (1999) Computation of the size of an epidemic in a finite hetero-geneous population. *Second European Conference on Highly Structured Stochastic Systems* 183–185.
38. McKendrick AG (1926) Applications of mathematics to medical problems. Proceedings of the Edinburgh Mathematical Society 14:98–130.
39. Martin-Löf A (1998) The final size of a nearly critical epidemic and the first passage time of a Wiener process to a parabolic barrier. Journal of the Applied Probability 35(3):671–682.
40. Mollison D (ed) (1995) *Epidemic Models: Their Structure and Relation to Data.* Cambridge University Press, Cambridge.
41. Nåsell I (1996) The quasi-stationary distribution of the closed endemic SIS model. Advances in Applied Probability 28(3):895–932.
42. Nåsell I (2002) Endemicity, persistence, and quasi-stationarity. In: *Mathematical approaches for emerging and reemerging infectious diseases: an introduction (Minneapolis, MN, 1999),* 199–227, IMA Vol. Math. Appl., 125, Springer, New York.
43. Neiman A (2007) Coherence Resonance, Scholarpedia, Art. 1442.
44. Picard P, Lefèvre C (1990) A unified analysis of the final size and severity distribution in collective reed-frost epidemic processes. Advances in Applied Probability 22(2):269–294.
45. Sánchez F, Wang X, Castillo-Chavez C, Gorman D, Gruenewald P (2006) Drinking as an epidemica simple mathematical model with recovery and relapse. In Therapists Guide to Evidence-Based Relapse Prevention: Practical Resources for the Mental Health Professional, Katie A. Witkiwitz G. Alan Marlatt (eds.), Academic Press, Burlington.
46. Scalia-Tomba G (1985) Asymptotic final size distribution for some chain-binomial processes. Advances in Applied Probability 17(3):477–495.
47. Scalia-Tomba G (1986) Asymptotic final size distribution of the multitype Reed-Frost process. Journal of Applied Probability 23(3):563–584.
48. Sellke T (1983) On the asymptotic distribution of the size of the stochastic epidemic. Journal of Applied Probability 20:390–394.
49. Stroud PD, Sydoriak SJ, Riese JM, Smith JP, Mniszewski SM, Romero PR (2006) Semi-empirical power-law scaling of new infection rate to model epidemic dynamics with inhomogeneous mixing. Mathematical Biosciences 203:301–318.

Two Critical Issues in Quantitative Modeling of Communicable Diseases: Inference of Unobservables and Dependent Happening

Hiroshi Nishiura, Masayuki Kakehashi, and Hisashi Inaba

Abstract In this chapter, we discuss two critical issues which must be remembered whenever we examine epidemiologic data of directly transmitted infectious diseases. Firstly, we would like the readers to recognize the difference between *observable* and *unobservable* events in infectious disease epidemiology. Since both infection event and acquisition of infectiousness are generally not directly observable, the total number of infected individuals could not be counted at a point of time, unless very rigorous contact tracing and microbiological examinations were performed. Directly observable intrinsic parameters, such as the incubation period and serial interval, play key roles in translating observable to unobservable information. Secondly, the concept of *dependent happening* must be remembered to identify a *risk* of an infectious disease or to assess vaccine efficacy. Observation of a single infected individual is not independent of observing other individuals. A simple solution for dependent happening is to employ the transmission probability which is conditioned on an exposure to infection.

Keywords Incubation period · Serial interval · Latent period · Generation time · Vaccine efficacy · Vaccine effectiveness · Herd immunity

1 Introduction

What is special about infectious disease epidemiology? Whenever researchers statistically analyze infectious disease data, two important epidemiologic aspects, which differ from the epidemiology of non-communicable diseases, must be remembered.

The first is concerned with observable events. Whereas onset events (e.g. onset of fever and appearance of rash) are directly observable in the field (with or without reporting delay), both infection event and acquirement of infectiousness are unobservable without very rigorous contact tracing and experimental (e.g. microbiological) efforts. Besides, almost all models for the population dynamics

H. Nishiura (✉)
Theoretical Epidemiology, University of Utrecht, Yalelaan 7, 3584 CL, Utrecht, The Netherlands
e-mail: h.nishiura@uu.nl

G. Chowell et al. (eds.), *Mathematical and Statistical Estimation Approaches in Epidemiology*, DOI 10.1007/978-90-481-2313-1_3,
© Springer Science+Business Media B.V. 2009

of infectious diseases have employed a number of assumptions for unobservable events. Observable intrinsic parameters, which characterize the natural history of infection and epidemiologic characteristics of the spread of disease in the absence of public health interventions, must be systematically quantified and employed for infering unobservable events in order to appropriately describe the transmission dynamics.

The second issue is the so-called dependent happening, i.e., observation of a single infected individual is not independent of observing other individuals. Because of the dependence, our population can enjoy herd immunity. Moreover, a necessity arises for theoretical epidemiologists to study infectious disease dynamics using non-linear models. To conduct sound statistical analyses, we should always bear in mind that it is inappropriate to directly apply the concept of relative risk and odds ratio in epidemiology of non-communicable diseases to any assessments of communicable diseases (especially, when the diseases are not endemic). For example, when we evaluate vaccine efficacy, it is far more feasible to employ the ratio of (conditional) probabilities of infection per contact among vaccinated to unvaccinated than directly using the relative risk of infection (which would inform population effectiveness of vaccination).

This chapter is composed as follows. In Section 2, epidemiologic definitions of two observable intervals, i.e., incubation period and serial interval, are discussed. For illustration, we show how the incubation period and serial interval inform infection events in the simplest settings. In Section 3, these two epidemiologic measurements are effectively used to capture the dynamics of infectious diseases. The backcalculation method and the estimation of the generation time are briefly reviewed. In Section 4, the concept and definition of vaccine efficacy and effectiveness of vaccination are considered. Dependent happening is comprehensively reviewed in light of causal inference (i.e. identification and quantification of the average causal parameter of effect in a population). A simple methodological solution for the dependent happening follows in Section 5. In particular, the usefulness of household secondary attack rates for estimating vaccine efficacy is reviewed, and the impact of different types of vaccine efficacy on the reproduction number is discussed using a simple dynamic model.

2 Incubation Period and Serial Interval

The first issue is motivated by a need to improve limited practical utility of the well-known SEIR (susceptible-exposed-infectious-recovered) model with respect to the assumption of intrinsic parameters (e.g. latent and infectious periods) and its use in quantifying the transmission potential. As we mentioned above, the event of acquiring infectiousness is not directly observable (i.e. in reality, individuals in latent and infectious periods are not distinguishable without microbiological and contact-frequency information), whereas symptom onset of an apparent disease is readily observed and reported. In addition, infection events are not directly observable for the majority of directly transmitted diseases (an exception is seen in sexually transmitted infections where the contact is countable by recall effort). Although several theoretical studies have implicitly assumed that the latent period is exactly the same as the incubation period, acquisition of infectiousness and symptom onset differ clearly by definition and are not directly related [5, 73]. These facts considerably affect the applicability of previous SEIR models that did not take into account these differences. Besides, compartments I and/or R of classical SIR and SEIR models have been fitted to the observed (and mostly onset) data to derive some parameter estimates, although the observed data do not necessarily measure either the theoretically defined I or R. Therefore, it should be noted that both SIR and SEIR models do not clearly highlight the observable events in field epidemiology. This complicates the application of theoretical models to observed data.

To resolve this issue, it is essential to understand how the observable intrinsic measures are defined and how we should effectively use these epidemiologic measurements to translate observable to unobservable information. Since onset event is directly observable, two epidemiologic intervals, both of which are concerned with symptom onset of a disease, would be useful. The first is the *incubation period*, defined as the time from infection with a microorganism to symptom development [16, 73]. The second is the *serial interval*, defined as the time since onset of a primary case to onset of the secondary case caused by the primary case [41]. In the following subsections, these two intervals are separately discussed in relation to the identification (i.e. statistical inference) of infection events.

2.1 Incubation Period

The incubation period of infectious diseases ranges from the order of a few hours, which is common for toxic food poisoning, to a decade (or a few decades) as seen in the case of tuberculosis, AIDS and variant Creutzfeldt-Jakob disease (vCJD). Since symptom onset reflects pathogen growth and invasion, and excretion of toxins and initiation of host-defense mechanisms, the length of the incubation period varies largely according to the replication rate of the pathogen, the mechanism of disease development, the route of infection and other underlying factors.

The incubation period of infectious diseases offers various insights into clinical and public health practices, as well as being important for epidemiologic and ecological studies. In clinical practice, the incubation period is useful not only for making rough guesses as to the causes and sources of infection of individual cases, but also for developing treatment strategies to extend the incubation period (e.g. antiretroviral therapy for HIV infection [16]) and for performing early projection of disease prognosis when the incubation period is clearly associated with clinical severity due to dose-response mechanisms (e.g. diseases caused by exotoxin) [74]. Moreover, during an outbreak of a newly emerged directly transmitted disease, the incubation period distribution permits determination of the length of quarantine required for a potentially exposed individual (i.e. by restricting movement of an exposed individual for a duration sufficiently longer than the incubation period) [36]. Further, if the time lag between acquiring infectiousness and symptom onset appears long (i.e., if the incubation period is relatively long compared to the latent period), it implies that isolation measures (e.g. restriction of movement until the infectious individual loses infectiousness) are likely to be ineffective, complicating disease control [42].

Understanding the incubation period distribution also enables statistical estimation of the time of exposure during a point source outbreak [90] as well as a hypothesis-testing to determine whether the outbreak has ended [20]; the former is discussed below. The distribution is also useful in statistical approaches of epidemic curve reconstruction and short-term predictions of slowly progressing diseases; the backcalculation method uses the incubation period to estimate HIV prevalence and project the future incidence of AIDS [19] . During the last decade, this method has also been extended to prion diseases such as Bovine Spongiform Encephalopathy (BSE) [31] and vCJD [24]. The backcalculation method is briefly discussed in the next section. This approach has also recently diverged to quantification of the transmission potential of diseases with an acute course of illness [35] and infectiousness relative to disease-age [78]. Moreover, in cases such as the short and long incubation periods of *Plasmodium vivax* malaria in temperate zones, the incubation period also enhances ecological understanding of adaptation strategies; in temperate zones, clearly separate bimodal peaks with approximate lengths of 2 and 50 weeks are observed [79], helping malaria transmissions continue over the winter season when transmission is usually greatly reduced due to seasonal entomologic characteristics.

The epidemiologist Philip E. Sartwell (1908–1999) contributed most to the foundation of the incubation period distribution modeling [73, 90]. Dr. Sartwell initially found that the incubation period of acute infectious diseases tends to follow a lognormal distribution, and applied such distribution to various diseases. Observing that the distributions often skewed to the right, Dr. Sartwell suggested the use of two parameters (i.e. an estimated *median*, which is also the *geometric mean* due to the characteristics of the lognormal distribution, and a *dispersion factor* as a measure of variability) rather than the sample mean and standard deviation. The lognormal distribution has a probability density function (pdf) of the form:

$$f(x; \mu, \sigma^2) = \frac{1}{x\sigma\sqrt{(2\pi)}} \exp\left(-\frac{(\ln(x) - \mu)^2}{2\sigma^2}\right) \tag{1}$$

for $x > 0$, where μ and σ are the mean and standard deviation of the variable's logarithm. The lognormal assumption for the incubation period was further extended to the estimation of the time of exposure during a point source outbreak. The theoretical basis is illustrated in Fig. 1, the logic of which is explained in the following.

Since all cases in a point source outbreak share the same time of exposure, the epidemic curve, which is drawn according to the time of onset (i.e. incidence), is equivalent to the incubation period distribution (Fig. 1). Suppose that the median point of the case frequency was observed x days after exposure and, further, that there are 100α percentile points on both sides of the observed distribution (upper and lower percentiles 100α where $0 \leq \alpha \leq 1$) with the distances from the median to both percentiles points being a and b days, respectively, the following relationship

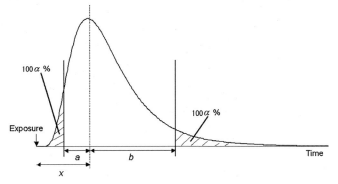

Fig. 1 A method for estimating the time of exposure during a point source outbreak. The *horizontal axis* shows the time since exposure and the distribution the frequency of cases according to the time of onset. The *vertical dashed line* is the median incubation period observed x days after exposure. The remaining two *vertical lines* indicate the times when fractions α and $1 - \alpha$ of cases developed the disease. The intervals between the median and other two *vertical lines* represent a and b, respectively

is given (because the logarithm follows normal distribution)

$$\ln(x) - \ln(x - a) = \ln(x + b) - \ln(x) \tag{2}$$

which is rearranged as

$$\frac{x}{x - a} = \frac{x + b}{x} \tag{3}$$

Consequently, the time of exposure can be inferred using the distance from the time of exposure to the median, x, by taking the distances to any equal percentiles on both sides

$$\hat{x} = \frac{ab}{b - a} \tag{4}$$

Since recall bias (i.e. the extent of imperfection by recalling events in the past) is unavoidable in retrospective epidemiologic studies of food poisoning requiring huge efforts of food traceback, this method appears to be very useful in determining the most plausible time of exposure and narrowing down the amount of information to be traced.

The classic method likely includes sampling errors and does not achieve acceptable precision. More precisely, estimation of the time of exposure is addressed, statistically, by precise solution of the three-parameter lognormal distribution [58, 95]. Let γ be the time of exposure, the pdf of the three-parameter lognormal distribution is given by

$$f(x; \gamma, \mu, \sigma^2) = \frac{1}{(x - \gamma)\sigma \sqrt{(2\pi)}} \exp\left(-\frac{(\ln(x - \gamma) - \mu)^2}{2\sigma^2}\right) \tag{5}$$

for $x > \gamma$. In other words, the statistical issue of the estimation of time of exposure can be replaced by the estimation of the threshold parameter of a standard 3-parameter distribution of the incubation period.

It should be noted that we have limited explicit explanations for the biological validity of assuming lognormal distribution for the incubation period. The fundamental biological reason to assume a lognormal distribution is related to an inoculation study of ectromelia virus (mouse pox) [38], which suggested exponential growth of pathogens within the host during the initial phase. Another similar study suggested that a fixed threshold of pathogen load likely exists when the host response is observed [71]. In other words, what we have learnt to date can be described as follows: *if the growth rate of a microorganism is implicitly assumed to follow normal distribution, and if there is a fixed threshold of pathogen load at which symptoms are revealed due to the host response, exponential growth of microorganisms should result in an incubation period sufficiently approximated by a lognormal distribution* [73]. However, the host-defense mechanism, which is almost entirely responsible for symptom onset, was later shown to be far more complex than previously expected. For example, fever is induced by very complex reactions and by several factors including circulating cytokines such as interluekin-2 [72]. Thus, whereas the lognormal distribution may be applied to the incubation periods of many acute infectious diseases, it is necessary to bear in mind that the assumption is supported only by previous experience. When other distributions (e.g. gamma and Weibull distributions) are alternatively chosen to model the incubation period, at least, the statistical issue of inferring time of exposure (during a point source outbreak) can be addressed by estimating threshold parameter for these distributions (i.e. as it can be done with Equation (5)).

2.2 Serial Interval

The serial intervals are observed when contact tracing is performed as a control measure. The transmission network is then observed, which represents the chain of transmission as a function of calendar time that yields the information of *who acquired infection from whom*. This type of information has been explored to assess the number of secondary transmissions over the course of an epidemic [56] and to evaluate individual variations in transmission [66], but it also enables us to obtain the serial interval [32, 65, 80, 97]. Using this information, here we consider a method to infer the relative infectiousness of infected individuals to certain *disease-age* (i.e. the time elapsed since onset of disease).

Specifically, we consider a situation when researchers would like to gain some information of the relative frequency of infectiousness or of secondary transmissions with respect to the time elapsed since infection or since onset of disease. Here we give an example of the relative infectiousness of smallpox to disease-age.

The infectious period has traditionally been defined as the period in which pathogens are discharged [7]. It presently refers to the period in which infected individuals are capable of generating secondary cases. Knowledge of the infectious period allows us to determine for how long known cases need to be isolated and what should be the latest time point after exposure at which newly infected individuals should be in isolation. However, as we mentioned above, *infectiousness* itself is unobservable, and thus, some inferential techniques to quantify this complicated index are called for.

One approach to addressing this issue is to quantify how the pathogen load changes over time using the most sensitive microbiological techniques (e.g. polymerase chain reaction), but such observations are usually limited to the period after onset of symptoms. Several attempts have been made to measure the distribution of the virus-positive period of smallpox cases [32, 89], but sample sizes were small and only very few samples could be obtained during the early stage of illness. Moreover, linking *virus-positive* results to the probability of causing secondary transmission is difficult without further information, especially about infectious contact (e.g. frequency, mode and degree of contact).

Another way of addressing this complicated issue is to determine the frequency of secondary transmission relative to disease-age [78]. An estimate of the *relative infectiousness* is obtained by analyzing historical data in which it is known who acquired infection from whom. The known transmission network permits serial intervals to be extracted, i.e. the times from symptom onset in a primary case to symptom onset in the secondary case [41, 80]. Given the length of the serial interval s and the corresponding length of the incubation period f, the disease-age l from onset of a symptom in primary case to secondary transmission satisfies

$$s = l + f \tag{6}$$

Considering the statistical distributions for each length results in a convolution equation:

$$s(t) = \int_0^t l(t - \tau) f(\tau) \, d\tau \tag{7}$$

The frequency $l(t - \tau)$ of secondary transmission relative to disease-age can be backcalculated by extracting the serial interval distribution $s(t)$ from a known transmission network, and by using the incubation period distribution $f(\tau)$ which is assumed known. This concept is illustrated in Fig. 2A. If we have information on the length t_i of the serial interval for n cases, the likelihood function is given by

$$L = \prod_{i=1}^n s(t_i) \tag{8}$$

$$= \prod_{i=1}^n \int_0^{t_i} l(t_i - \tau) f(\tau) \, d\tau$$

The parameters that describe the frequency of secondary transmission relative to disease-age can be estimated by maximizing this function.

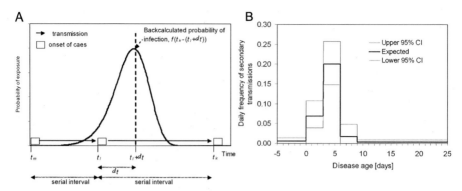

Fig. 2 Relative frequency of secondary transmissions of smallpox by disease-age. A. Backcalculation of the transmission probability: case m infected case l who subsequently infected case k. Their times of onset are t_m, t_l and t_k, respectively. Using the difference of the disease onset (serial interval) $t_k - t_l$ together with the distribution of the incubation period, the disease-age specific probability of transmission from case l to case k is obtained. **B.** Expected daily frequency of secondary transmissions with corresponding 95% confidence intervals. The disease-age $t = 0$ denotes the onset of fever. The illustration was drawn by the author with reference to [76, 78]

Figure 2B shows the back-calculated infectiousness of smallpox relative to disease-age [76, 78]. When the frequency is discussed as a function of disease-age of smallpox, day 0 represents the onset of fever. Before onset of fever (i.e. between day -5 and day -1) altogether only 2.7% of all transmissions occurred. Between day 0 and day 2 (i.e. in the prodromal period before the onset of rash) a total of 21.1% of all transmissions occurred. The daily frequency of passing on the infection was highest between day 3 and day 5, yielding a total of 61.8% of all transmissions. These estimates help determine the latest time by which cases should be in isolation. If each primary case infects on average 6 individuals (i.e. $R_0 = 6$), and if the efficacy of isolation is 100%, the isolation of a primary case before the onset of rash reduces the expected number of victims to $6 \times (0.027 + 0.211) = 1.428$. In other words, Fig. 2B implies that isolation could be extremely effective if performed before onset of rash and that delayed isolation of symptomatic smallpox cases could still be effective if performed within a few days after onset of rash. Consequently, we can expect that optimal isolation could substantially reduce the number of secondary cases, and the outbreak could quickly be brought under control by additional countermeasures (e.g. contact tracing [34]).

Nevertheless, it should be noted that the relative frequency of secondary transmissions tends to be biased by various factors in observation: small sample size of serial intervals may have been influenced by local factors such as differences in contact behavior and mobility of cases. Unless extrinsic factors (e.g. isolation measure and behavioral changes) were explicitly adjusted in the statistical model with more detailed data, the estimated infectiousness several days after appearance of rash would be underestimated. This could partly explain a disagreement of Fig. 2B with a previous epidemiologic study [35] in which the number of secondary cases generated during the prodromal period was estimated as 8.2% of the overall transmission potential.

3 Backcalculation and Estimation of the Generation Time

We then consider how the incubation period and serial interval play their roles in translating observable to unobservable information. Two practical issues are discussed as examples. The first is the so-called *backcalculation* method which has been effectively employed to estimate the total number of HIV-infected individuals in a population using the incubation period of AIDS and AIDS incidence [75]. The second is concerned with the statistical estimation and mathematical definition of the *generation time* which is interpreted as the time interval between infection of a primary case and infection of a secondary case caused by the primary case [94]. As will be shown using *Euler-Lotka equation* in the second subsection, probability density function of the generation time would be a critically important distribution for the estimation of the basic reproduction number, R_0, using the intrinsic growth rate of an epidemic. In line with this, analytical insights into the relationship between the serial interval and generation time are discussed.

3.1 Backcalculation

Whereas the number of AIDS cases is thought to be relatively accurately reported and documented in industrialized countries, asymptomatic HIV infections are seldom noticed unless the infected individual undertakes a voluntary blood test or develops the disease. Backcalculation uses the statistical distribution of the incubation period as key information, and is frequently applied to HIV/AIDS in industrialized countries where the previous AIDS incidence can be assumed to be confidently diagnosed and reported [17, 18, 43]. The epidemic curve for HIV is reconstructed using AIDS incidence and the incubation period, enabling estimation of HIV prevalence and short-term projections of AIDS incidence.

The long incubation period of HIV infection enables assessment of the extent of the epidemic during its course. Backcalculation uses AIDS incidence data at calendar time t, $a(t)$, and the incubation period distribution at time τ after infection, $\omega(\tau)$, to reconstruct the number of HIV infections with calendar time. Assuming that documentation of diagnosed AIDS cases is not significantly delayed, and assuming the impact of antiretroviral therapy on the length of the incubation period is negligible in the simplest setting, the fundamental relationship is given by the following convolution equation

$$a(t) = \int_0^t h(t - u)\omega(u)\,du \qquad (9)$$

where $h(t - u)$ is the number of HIV infections at calendar time $t - u$. The basic idea of backcalculation is to estimate $h(t)$ using known $a(t)$ and $\omega(u)$. It should be noted that the structure of this simple convolution equation is principally the same as what we discussed with Equation (7). Here, to ease understanding of the deconvolution procedure, Equation (9) is considered in discrete time [10, 26]. Since surveillance-based data of AIDS incidence is obtained for a certain interval, t (e.g. every 2 or 3 months), the following equation is obtained

$$a_t = \sum_{u=1}^{t} h_{t-u} \omega_u \tag{10}$$

Assuming that h_t is generated by a nonhomogeneous Poisson process, a_t is an independent Poisson variate. Thus, the likelihood, which is needed to estimate HIV infections (and, sometimes, the parameters of incubation period distribution), is proportional to

$$\prod_{t=1}^{T} \left(\sum_{u=1}^{t} h_{t-u} \omega_u \right)^{r_t} \exp\left(-\sum_{u=1}^{t} h_{t-u} \omega_u \right) \tag{11}$$

where r_t is the observed number of AIDS cases at calendar time t and T is the most recent time of observation. The shape of the curve of HIV infections, h_t, is usually modeled parametrically or non-parametrically [11, 14]. The main sources of uncertainty arise from uncertainties in the incubation period distribution, the shape of the HIV infection curve, and AIDS incidence data [87]. Short-term predictions are obtained based on estimated numbers of HIV infected individuals who have not yet developed AIDS. However, it should be noted that backcalculation such as this provides no information about future infection rates and little information about recent infection rates [39]. Further details of the backcalculation method are described elsewhere [19, 23, 61].

3.2 Generation Time

We consider the generation time using a *renewal equation*:

$$j(t) = \int_0^\infty A(\tau) j(t - \tau) \, d\tau \tag{12}$$

where $j(t)$ is the number of new infections (i.e. incidence) at calendar time t and $A(\tau)$ is the integral kernel informing the rate of secondary transmissions per single primary case at *infection-age* τ (i.e. the time elapsed since infection). When the incidence increases with constant (intrinsic) growth rate r_0 (i.e. when $j(t) = k \exp(r_0 t)$ where k is constant), the Equation (12) is simplified as

$$1 = \int_0^\infty A(\tau) \exp(-r_0 \tau) \, d\tau \tag{13}$$

which is referred to as the Euler-Lotka equation. Since the integral kernel $A(\tau)$ directly informs R_0, defined as the average number of secondary cases generated by a single primary case in a fully susceptible population [28–30], by

$$R_0 = \int_0^\infty A(\tau)\,d\tau \tag{14}$$

and because the density function of the generation time, $g(\tau)$, can be interpreted as the frequency of secondary transmission relative to infection-age τ, i.e.,

$$g(\tau) = \frac{A(\tau)}{\int_0^\infty A(\tau)\,d\tau} \tag{15}$$

the Euler-Lotka equation (13) offers an interpretation,

$$\frac{1}{R_0} = \int_0^\infty \exp(-r_0\tau)g(\tau)\,d\tau \tag{16}$$

representing the relationship between R_0 and the probability density function of the generation time, $g(\tau)$. From the initial growth phase of an epidemic, the intrinsic growth rate, r_0, i.e. the intrinsic rate of (natural) increase for infected individuals [33], is estimated, and R_0 can be subsequently estimated using the Equation (16). Thus, the generation-time distribution has been recognized as playing a key role in estimating the transmission potential of a disease [86, 96]. In many instances, R_0 has been inferred from real-time growth data by using the estimate of r_0 and by assuming that the generation-time distribution is known.

However, it is very difficult to estimate the generation-time distribution in practice, because infection events are seldom directly observable. Indeed, the estimation methods of the generation time and its sampling scheme have yet to be developed. Previously, the distribution of the generation time (or, at least, the mean generation time) was implicitly (and wrongly) assumed to correspond exactly to that of serial interval. However, this is not the case when the incubation period of the primary case depends on the time from onset to secondary transmission [94] and even the means are different when we deal with diseases with asymptomatic secondary transmissions (which will be discussed below).

Figure 3 illustrates an interpretation of the relationship between serial interval S, incubation periods F_1 and F_2, and generation time G in the absence of asymptomatic cases (i.e. where there is no infected individual who does not exhibit any symptoms throughout the course of infection). We denote the time from onset of primary case to secondary transmission by L (note that L can be negative if pre-symptomatic transmission occurs). The serial interval S is given by

$$S = G + F_2 - F_1 \tag{17}$$

which is interpreted as the sum of the generation time and incubation period of the secondary case minus the incubation period of the primary case. Thus, if G, F_1 and F_2 were independent random variables, the serial interval distribution would be

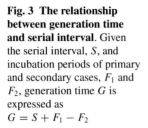

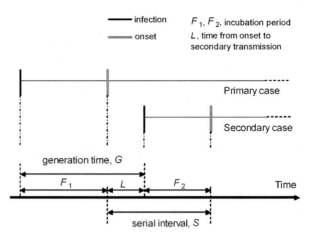

Fig. 3 The relationship between generation time and serial interval. Given the serial interval, S, and incubation periods of primary and secondary cases, F_1 and F_2, generation time G is expressed as

$$G = S + F_1 - F_2$$

the convolution of the generation time and incubation period distributions followed by the cross-correlation of this convolution and the incubation period distribution (However, it should be noted that it is frequently biologically more natural to assume that F_1 and G are dependent). As it is intuitively clear from Equation (17), the mean serial interval would be expected to be identical to the mean generation time, provided that all infected individuals developed symptoms.

In the presence of asymptomatic secondary transmissions, caused by those who were infected and have not developed symptoms yet, and also by those who were infected and will not become symptomatic throughout the course of infection, the interpretation of relationship between S and G is confused [60]. Figure 4 illustrates the most precise, but yet simplistic, model of a directly transmitted disease, accounting for the presence of asymptomatic secondary transmission. Following infection, asymptomatic individuals, $i_1(t, \tau)$, develop disease at the rate $\eta(\tau)$ or recover from infection without developing any symptoms at the rate $\gamma_1(\tau)$, where τ is the infection-age. Symptomatic individuals, $i_2(t, \sigma)$ recover from (or die of) infection at the rate $\gamma_2(\sigma)$ where σ is the disease-age. Assuming further that the rates

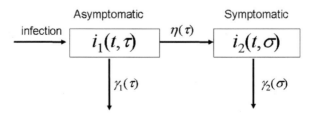

Fig. 4 Compartment model for symptom development of a disease. Following infection, all infected individuals experience asymptomatic state $i_1(t, \tau)$ where τ is infection-age representing the time elapsed since infection. Asymptomatic infected individuals will either develop symptom at the rate $\eta(\tau)$ or recover from infection without developing disease at the rate $\gamma_1(\tau)$. Symptomatic individuals are denoted by $i_2(t, \sigma)$ where σ is the disease-age representing the time elapsed since onset of a disease

of asymptomatic and symptomatic secondary transmissions are, respectively, $\beta_1(\tau)$ and $\beta_2(\sigma)$ and that the initial number of susceptibles is S_0, the linearlized system (for initial growth phase of an epidemic) is governed by the following *McKendrick equations*:

$$\left(\frac{\partial}{\partial t} + \frac{\partial}{\partial \tau}\right) i_1(t, \tau) = -(\eta(\tau) + \gamma_1(\tau))i_1(t, \tau), \tag{18}$$

$$i_1(t, 0) = S_0 \int_0^\infty \beta_1(\tau)i_1(t, \tau)d\tau + S_0 \int_0^\infty \beta_2(\sigma)i_2(t, \sigma)d\sigma, \tag{19}$$

$$\left(\frac{\partial}{\partial t} + \frac{\partial}{\partial \sigma}\right) i_2(t, \sigma) = -\gamma_2(\sigma)i_2(t, \sigma), \tag{20}$$

$$i_2(t, 0) = \int_0^\infty \eta(\tau)i_1(t, \tau)d\tau. \tag{21}$$

Integrating the McKendrick Equations (18), (19), (20), (21) along the characteristic lines, and ignoring contribution from the initial data, we get the following renewal equations:

$$j_1(t) = \int_0^t A_1(\tau)j_1(t - \tau)d\tau + \int_0^t A_2(\sigma)j_2(t - \sigma)d\sigma, \tag{22}$$

$$j_2(t) = \alpha \int_0^t f(\tau)j_1(t - \tau)d\tau, \tag{23}$$

where $j_1(t)$ and $j_2(t)$ are, respectively, the numbers of new infections and new onsets at calendar time t (i.e., $j_1(t) := i_1(t, 0)$ and $j_2(t) := i_2(t, 0)$) and the remaining functions are defined as

$$A_1(\tau) := S_0\beta_1(\tau)\exp\left(-\int_0^\tau (\eta(x) + \gamma_1(x))\,dx\right), \tag{24}$$

$$A_2(\sigma) := S_0\beta_2(\sigma)\exp\left(-\int_0^\sigma \gamma_2(s)ds\right), \tag{25}$$

$$\alpha := \int_0^\infty \eta(x)\exp\left(-\int_0^x (\eta(s) + \gamma_1(s))\,ds\right)dx, \tag{26}$$

$$f(\tau) := \frac{\eta(\tau)\exp\left(-\int_0^\tau (\eta(x) + \gamma_1(x))\,dx\right)}{\alpha}. \tag{27}$$

Thus, $A_1(\tau)$ and $A_2(\sigma)$ are interpreted as the rate of asymptomatic and symptomatic secondary transmissions, respectively, per single primary case at infection-age τ and disease-age σ. α is the probability that an infected individual ever develops symptoms. $f(\tau)$ gives the probability density of the incubation period of length τ.

Replacing $j_2(t)$ in the right-hand side of (22) by that of (23), we get

$$j_1(t) = \int_0^t A_1(\tau)j_1(t-\tau)d\tau + \alpha \int_0^t \left(A_2(\sigma) \int_0^{t-\sigma} j_1(t-\sigma-\tau)f(\tau)d\tau \right) d\sigma,$$

$$= \int_0^t A_-(\tau)j_1(t-\tau)d\tau, \tag{28}$$

where

$$A_-(\tau) = A_1(\tau) + \alpha \int_0^\tau A_2(\tau-\sigma)f(\sigma)d\sigma \tag{29}$$

The Equation (28) describes the renewal process of newly infected individuals, and thus, the basic reproduction number, R_0, is given by

$$R_0 = \int_0^\infty A_-(\tau)d\tau \tag{30}$$

Consequently, the mean generation time, T_g, is calculated as

$$T_g = \frac{1}{R_0} \int_0^\infty \tau A_-(\tau)d\tau \tag{31}$$
$$= \theta L_1 + (1-\theta)(L_2 + F),$$

where θ is the proportion of asymptomatic transmissions ($0 \leq \theta \leq 1$) among the total number of secondary transmissions, i.e.,

$$\theta := \frac{1}{R_0} \int_0^\infty A_1(\tau)\tau \tag{32}$$

and L_1, L_2 and F are

$$L_1 := \frac{\int_0^\infty \tau A_1(\tau)d\tau}{\int_0^\infty A_1(x)dx}, \tag{33}$$

$$L_2 := \frac{\int_0^\infty \sigma A_2(\sigma)d\sigma}{\int_0^\infty A_2(y)dy}, \tag{34}$$

$$F := \int_0^\infty \tau f(\tau)d\tau, \tag{35}$$

which are interpreted as the mean infection-age of asymptomatic transmission, the mean disease-age of symptomatic transmission and the mean incubation period, respectively.

Although we omit further technical details for simplicity (see [60] for original descriptions, in particular, of the analytical expression of the integral kernel $A+(\sigma)$), the mean serial interval, $T_{s,multi}$, can be analytically derived from another renewal equation of symptomatic infected individuals:

$$j_2(t) = \int_0^t A_+(\sigma)j_2(t - \sigma)d\sigma, \tag{36}$$

which leads to

$$T_{s,multi} = \frac{\int_0^\infty \sigma A_+(\sigma)d\sigma}{\int_0^\infty A_+(s)ds}$$

$$= \frac{R_1}{1 - R_1}L_1 + L_2 + F, \tag{37}$$

where R_1, which is assumed to be less than unity, is the average number of asymptomatic transmissions per single asymptomatic infected individual (i.e. the reproduction number for asymptomatic transmission), expressed as

$$R_1 = \int_0^\infty A_1(\tau)d\tau, \tag{38}$$

which can also be written as θR_0, and $Q := \int_0^\infty A_+(\sigma)d\sigma$ is what we call the state reproduction number for the symptomatic class (i.e. the average number of symptomatic secondary transmissions per single primary symptomatic case during its entire course of infectiousness [60]). Here, it must be noted that $T_{s,multi}$ is what we call *multi-step serial interval* defined as the average length from the primary symptomatic cases to the secondary symptomatic cases who are infected either *directly* from the primary case or *indirectly* by way of asymptomatic cases. Rather than this, classic definition of the mean *one-step serial interval*, $T_{s,one}$, is the period from observation of symptom onset in one case to observation of symptom in a second case *directly* infected from the first (i.e. indirect transmission is unobservable, and thus, was not explicitly taken into account in the tranditional definitions given by Pickles [84], Hope Simpson [59] and Bailey [7]). $T_{s,one}$ is much easier than (37), and expressed as

$$T_{s,one} = L_2 + F \tag{39}$$

which is exactly what we discussed in Section 2.2 using Equation (6).

Consequently, we get the following relationship

$$T_g \leq T_{s,one} \leq T_{s,multi} \tag{40}$$

where equality holds if there is no asymptomatic transmission (which leads to $R_1 = 0$ or $\theta = 0$; see [60] for further details). In other words, it is analytically proven that the mean lengths of one-step and multi-step serial intervals are longer than the mean generation time, as long as asymptomatic transmission exists.

In this way, key unobservable information has to be estimated mainly by extracting observable and quantifiable parameters. If one would like to focus on *symptom onset* as observable event, then the incubation period and serial interval, both definitions of which are concerned with onset event, would play the most important roles among all epidemiologic measurements to translate observables to unobservables. To widen the applicability of mathematical models of infectious diseases, it is essential to construct a theory by observable ingredients and derive an estimator to address the issue of unobservability of infection event and acquirement of infectiousness.

4 Dependent Happening

As seen in the origin of field epidemiology (i.e. an identification of the source of environmental contamination with cholera, which is believed to have been initially suggested by John Snow), *causal inference* has played a central role among all epidemiologic disciplines. In particular, epidemiologic studies of chronic illness have been (and will be) focused on the *cause of disease* to find potentially effective preventive measures and therapeutic methods. The challenges posed by chronic illness have pointed out to epidemiologists the multifactorial complex nature of disease causality, which has been referred to as a *web of causality*. Appropriate epidemiologic designs and sound statistical approaches to address the relevant issue have been the main interests among general epidemiologists [44, 57].

Of course, efforts on the similar point have to be made for clarifying useful prevention strategies against infectious diseases, but it must be remembered that the epidemiology of directly transmitted infectious diseases is rather different from other (e.g. chronic) non-communicable diseases in that the disease spreads from person-to-person. That is, observation of a single infected individual is not independent of observing other individuals in a population of interest [63]. If this is the case, the usual formulation of risk assessment parameters, such as odds ratio, relative risk and risk difference, which are so useful in chronic disease epidemiology, do not offer stable assessments of risk for factors that affect contagion [64]. We first illustrate this concept in the next subsection and thereafter discuss the definitions and properties of vaccine efficacy, and direct and indirect effects of vaccination.

4.1 What Would Matter Due to Dependence?

In the epidemiology of non-communicable diseases, causal relationship between disease and a single risk factor is usually measured by examining relative risk (synonymous: risk ratio) or attributable risk (which will be denoted by RR and AR, respectively). For example, supposing that the frequencies of lung cancer among smokers and non-smokers are p_1 and p_0, RR and AR of smoking with respect to the development of lung cancer are calculated as

$$RR = \frac{p_1}{p_0} \qquad (41)$$

$$AR = p_1 - p_0 \qquad (42)$$

Therefore, if the risk ratio is greater than 1, we suspect that *smoking elevated the risk of lung cancer*, which is useful to discuss the causality. Moreover, the attributable risk is useful to quantify the impact (or contribution) of smoking on (to) development of lung cancer.

The similar simple discussion can be applied to the frequencies of Japanese encephalitis cases among vaccinated and unvaccinated individuals, denoted by p_v and p_u, respectively. Since the natural reservoir of Japanese encephalitis is believed to be swine (and other animals including birds), and because human is belived to be dead-end host (i.e. who does not generate secondary infections including infection among mosquitoes), we can ignore the issue of dependence, at least, for now. Then, the relative risk of vaccination with respect to infection with Japanese encephalitis virus is given by RR in Equation (41) and, subsequently, the *vaccine efficacy*, VE, is evaluated as

$$VE = 1 - RR \qquad (43)$$
$$= 1 - \frac{p_v}{p_u}$$

which has been a fundamental idea in field epidemiology [45, 83] . Here's an example:

Vaccination program for prevention against Japanese encephalitis was conducted in a population where the disease is endemic. The cases are constantly observed over time and, thus, we assume the disease is in an endemic equilibrium. Among vaccinated individuals, 20% experienced infection. On the other hand, 80% of unvaccinated individuals experienced infection. The relative risk is

$$RR = \frac{0.2}{0.8} = 0.25 \qquad (44)$$

and thus, we expect that the vaccination was effective because RR < 1. Further, the vaccine efficacy is

$$VE = 1 - RR = 0.75 \qquad (45)$$

From these, we conclude that *the risk of Japanese encephalitis among vaccinated individuals was 0.25 times as large as that among unvaccinated individuals* and moreover, *the vaccine efficacy was estimated at 75%*.

This simple discussion required two of the key assumptions. The first is the endemic equilibrium in which the frequency of infection would not be influenced by time effect. The second is the independence between individuals. In statistical terms, the latter is referred to as *no interference* [25] or *stability assumptions* [88].

Epidemiology should have been much easier, if we could directly attribute the population effectiveness to the average causal effect at an individual level. In addition to the basics, infectious disease epidemiologists have to account for dependent happening, the simplest illustration of which is given in Fig. 5. We consider the generation of cases, where each primary case causes 2 secondary cases in the absence of vaccination (Fig. 5A).

What happens if a portion of this population was vaccinated? In Fig. 5B, two individuals were vaccinated prior to the outbreak and were uninfected. Not only these two vaccinated individuals, but also unvaccinated two individuals (who had been expected to be cases in the absence of vaccination) were uninfected, due to the protection of a vaccinated individual. Protection among the two unvaccinated individuals can be deemed *indirect effect* of vaccination, which was caused by dependence between individuals [54].

We consider this issue using response variables X_0 and X_1 for unvaccinated and vaccinated populations, following a series of studies by Halloran [53–55]. Since the response of interest is infection, which is dichotomous, we write $X_i = 1$ if infected under treatment i and $X_i = 0$ if uninfected under treatment i where $i = 1$ or 0. The causal effect of vaccination, T, is usually measured by attributable risk (see Equation (42)) as the average of the individual effects, and more strictly speaking, is expressed as the difference between the expected value of the potential outcomes

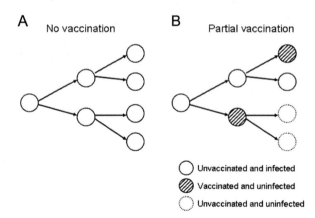

Fig. 5 Theoretical initial courses of a communicable disease outbreak following a geometric growth. A. The infection tree (i.e. transmission network) is shown by generation. Each primary case generates 2 secondary cases. **B**. Infection tree under partial vaccination. Vaccination was conducted prior to the outbreak among 2 individuals (i.e. two *striped circles*) who resulted in non-infection. Due to the prevention of a vaccinated individual, two other unvaccinated individuals (i.e. two *dashed circles*), who had been expected to be cases without vaccination, did not experience infection, which is deemed indirect effect of vaccination

if everyone received one treatment and the expected value of the potential outcomes if everyone received the other treatment. That is,

$$T = E(X_0) - E(X_1) = E(X_0 - X_1) \tag{46}$$

Since we cannot observe the potential outcomes of each individual under each intervention, we have to rewrite Equation (46) to reflect each individual's potential outcome under the intervention that she/he used. Let Y be the particular intervention that an individual used (i.e. $Y = 1$ and 0 for vaccinated and unvaccinated), the actual observable difference, A, is

$$A = E(X_0 \mid Y = 0) - E(X_1 \mid Y = 1) \tag{47}$$

where $E(X_i \mid Y = i)$ is the average of the potential outcomes among individuals who received intervention i. Under two assumptions, i.e., non-interference and independence, T and A are assumed equal [50].

Nevertheless, if the population expected value depends on fraction of vaccinated (due to indirect effect), the relation does not hold, i.e.,

$$T = E(X_0 - X_1) \neq E(X_0 \mid Y = 0) - E(X_1 \mid Y = 1) = A \tag{48}$$

Therefore, directly applying risk assessment parameters, such as relative risk and attributable risk, to the assessment of a specific risk (or evaluation of vaccine efficacy) of communicable diseases would be unfortunately flawed [53, 64].

4.2 Herd Immunity and the Concept of Effectiveness

Let us compare two different small populations, each with 25 individuals (Fig. 6). The vaccination coverage of population A is 20%, whereas that of population B

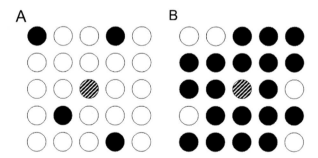

Fig. 6 Small populations with different vaccination coverage. Each circle represents an individual. Black (and the striped individual in the center) denotes vaccinated, whereas white is unvaccinated. The vaccination coverages of populations **A** and **B** are, respectively, 20 and 80%. Assuming that the contact patterns are homogeneous and not different between A and B, the risk of infection for a striped individual in population B is smaller than that in population A

is 80%. Suppose that the contact pattern is homogeneous in both populations, and assuming that the frequencies of contact are not different between A and B, how different are the risks of infection of a vaccinated individual in the center of these populations? Obviously, the risk in population A is higher than that in B, because individuals surrounding striped (vaccinated) individual in population A are mainly unvaccinated. In other words, even if the vaccination does not offer perfect protection, individuals in population B can enjoy better community benefit compared to that in population A.

The community benefit extends to those who would have been infected by the vaccinee, had he developed the disease. Consequently, vaccinees are not only protected to their own benefit, but to the benefit of the community, and moreover, unvaccinated individuals are susceptible not only to their own adversity, but to the adversity of the community. The degree of community protection is referred to as *herd immunity* [40, 62, 77]. When it comes to the assessment of vaccination, this is also referred to as *indirect effect of vaccination*. Because of the presence of herd immunity, disease eradication (e.g. of smallpox) was (and can be for other diseases) achieved without vaccinating all susceptible individuals. And, this concept indeed results in a well known *control relation* to achieve a vaccination coverage, c, which is sufficient to eradicate a disease in a randomly mixing population, i.e.,

$$c > \kappa = \frac{1}{\epsilon}\left(1 - \frac{1}{R_0}\right) \tag{49}$$

where κ is referred to as *critical coverage* of vaccination for eradication, ϵ is vaccine efficacy and R_0 is the basic reproduction number of a disease [2, 93].

It should be noted that the threshold principle itself may better account for individual heterogeneity (i.e. variance of contact frequency) to precisely reflect realistic contact patterns. Let the mean and variance of contact rate be m and σ^2, respectively, and let us assume that the transmission mechanism is described by the so-called *frequency dependence* [15, 27, 70]. If the distribution of contact rate is explicitly taken into account, R_0 in the heterogeneouxly mixing population is expressed as

$$R_0 = R_{0,random}\left(1 + \left(\frac{\sigma}{m}\right)^2\right) \tag{50}$$

where $R_{0,random}$ denotes the basic reproduction number without individual heterogeneity (where $\sigma^2 = 0$) [1, 6]. Assuming that the vaccination takes place independently (i.e. independent of contact) and that the vaccine effect is irrelevant to secondary transmission (i.e. not reducing infectiousness of vaccinated individuals), R_0 in Equation (50) directly applies to the right-hand side of Equation (49) [37]. If the distribution is extremely right-skewed (e.g. $\sigma \to \infty$), this leads $R_0 \to \infty$, making it impossible to control the disease by means of mass vaccination only [22, 69].

Rather than discussing the herd immunity threshold of a disease using mathematical models (which can be found elsewhere [3, 4, 40, 81]), here we emphasize the issue of dependent happening which complicates statistical estimation of vaccine efficacy using epidemiologic observations. Although the *effectiveness* of vaccination reflects the result of protection of a vaccinated population and can be measured using observed data, this would not be connected to average causal effect at an *individual level* (i.e. vaccine efficacy) which would have been identical to the effectiveness under the stability assumption.

The definitions of direct and indirect effectiveness of vaccination (i.e. protection at a population level) were formulated using final sizes of an epidemic (i.e. fraction of those who experienced infection during an epidemic among a total of susceptible individuals) among vaccinated and unvaccinated groups, z_v and z_u [47] and the relevant discussions on epidemiologic study design have been made using these definitions (which can be found elsewhere [51, 55]). The definition also uses another final size which would have been observed in the absence of vaccination, z_c. The direct effectiveness, DE, indirect effectiveness, IE, and the total effetiveness, TE, of vaccination are respectively defined as

$$\text{DE} = 1 - \frac{z_v}{z_u} \tag{51}$$

$$\text{IE} = 1 - \frac{z_u}{z_c} \tag{52}$$

$$\text{TE} = 1 - \frac{z_v}{z_c} \tag{53}$$

which measures the benefit to an vaccinated individual, the overall benefit of the vaccination program to unvaccinated people and vaccinated people, respectively. Moreover, if we define the average risk of infection in the study population, z_0, as

$$z_0 = (1 - p)z_u + pz_v \tag{54}$$

where p is the vaccination coverage, the average effectiveness is defined as

$$\text{AE} = 1 - \frac{z_0}{z_c} \tag{55}$$

which measures the overall benefit of the vaccination program to the entire population. Since DE does not directly inform vaccine efficacy, VE, because of dependent happening, another definition of *field efficacy*, FE, has to be defined as

$$\text{FE} = 1 - \frac{\beta_v}{\beta_u} \tag{56}$$

as a solution, where β_v and β_u are the transmission rates among vaccinated and unvaccinated, respectively (please continue reading for the details of their roles in a population).

In a randomly mixing population, the relationship between FE and DE is analytically interpretable [47]. Here we consider this relationship as well as an analytical interpretation of IE. Specifically, we theoretically consider two different types of vaccines. The first is the so-called *leaky* vaccine which would not offer perfect protection from disease but would reduce the susceptibility among vaccinated. The second is *all-or-nothing* type which offer perfect protection among a portion of vaccinated individuals.

Let the numbers of vaccinated susceptible, infectious and recovered individuals be S_v, I_v and R_v, respectively. Similarly, the numbers of unvaccinated susceptible, infectious and recovered individuals are, respectively, denoted by S_u, I_u and R_u. When a leaky vaccine is considered, we assume $S_v(0) = N_v$ and $S_u(0) = N_u$ where N_v and N_u are the total number of vaccinated and unvaccinated individuals, respectively. Assuming that the recovery rate γ is independent of vaccination, the dynamics of vaccinated individuals are described by

$$\frac{dS_v}{dt} = -\beta_v S_v (I_v + I_u) \tag{57}$$

$$\frac{dI_v}{dt} = \beta_v S_v (I_v + I_u) - \gamma I_v \tag{58}$$

$$\frac{dR_v}{dt} = \gamma I_v \tag{59}$$

Similarly, the dynamics of unvaccinated individuals are described by

$$\frac{dS_u}{dt} = -\beta_u S_u (I_v + I_u) \tag{60}$$

$$\frac{dI_u}{dt} = \beta_u S_u (I_v + I_u) - \gamma I_u \tag{61}$$

$$\frac{dR_u}{dt} = \gamma I_u \tag{62}$$

As written above, because we assume that there was no immune individuals (due to infection) prior to an epidemic, $R_v(0) = R_u(0) = 0$. The final size equations are subsequently derived as

$$\ln(1 - z_v) = -\frac{\beta_v}{\gamma} (R_v(\infty) + R_u(\infty)) \tag{63}$$

$$= -\frac{\beta_v N}{\gamma} (p z_v + (1 - p) z_u)$$

$$\ln(1 - z_u) = -\frac{\beta_u}{\gamma} (R_v(\infty) + R_u(\infty)) \tag{64}$$

$$= -\frac{\beta_u N}{\gamma} (p z_v + (1 - p) z_u)$$

where $p(:= N_v/(N_u + N_v))$ is vaccination coverage (as utilized in (54)). Taking the ratio of (63) to (64), we get

$$\text{FE} = 1 - \frac{\beta_v}{\beta_u} = 1 - \frac{\ln(1 - z_v)}{\ln(1 - z_u)} \tag{65}$$

From (65), we observe that DE approximates FE of leaky vaccine in a randomly mixing population, but it is also clear that DE is always smaller than FE and that FE is more appropriate estimator to attribute observation at a population level to the average individual effect (i.e. efficacy) of vaccination. Therefore, we'd better use the ratio of transmission rates (and, more precisely, the ratio of transmission probabilities per contact; see next section) among vaccinated to unvaccinated, rather than using the ratio of the numbers of infected individuals, to appropriately interpret the causal effect of vaccination.

When an all-or-nothing vaccine is considered, we assume $S_v(0) = (1 - \alpha)N_v$, $R_v(0) = \alpha N_v$ and $S_u(0) = N_u$ where α is regarded as field efficacy under the all-or-nothing assumption ($0 \leq \alpha \leq 1$). Since vaccines of this type (theoretically) do not reduce susceptibility, we assume that the transmission rates are identical, i.e., $\beta := \beta_v = \beta_u$. Assuming again that the recovery rate γ is independent of vaccination, the final sizes satisfy

$$\ln\left(1 - \frac{z_v}{1 - \alpha}\right) = -\frac{\beta}{\gamma}(R_v(\infty) - R_v(0) + R_u(\infty)) \tag{66}$$

$$\ln(1 - z_u) = -\frac{\beta}{\gamma}(R_v(\infty) - R_v(0) + R_u(\infty)) \tag{67}$$

It should be noted that $z_v = (R_v(\infty) - R_v(0))/N_v$. The Equations (66) and (67) result in

$$\alpha = 1 - \frac{z_v}{z_u} \tag{68}$$

which conincides with DE.

In reality, the leaky assumption may reflect the so-called *imperfect vaccines* (e.g. vaccines against influenza, malaria and various bacterial diseases), whereas the all-or-nothing assumption may be the case for vaccines against viral diseases with narrow antigenic diversity (e.g. measles and smallpox).

Estimation of indirect effect, IE, has to consider another theoretical epidemic in the absence of vaccination. The final size, z_c, in the absence of vaccination satisfies

$$\ln(1 - z_c) = -z_c \frac{\beta_u N}{\gamma} \tag{69}$$

where β_u is assumed to be smaller than β_v for the leaky assumption, and is assumed identical to that among vaccinated ($= \beta$ in (66) and (67)) for the all-or-nothing assumption. No explicit analytical solution can be obtained from (69), but this can be iteratively solved (and it should be noted that $\beta_u N / \gamma$ in the right hand side is defined as the basic reproduction number, R_0). Subsequently, IE is estimated from (52). It should be noted that even when the transmission rate among vaccinated is identical to that among unvaccinated (i.e. all-or-nothing vaccine), IE is always positive due to dependent happening (as long as we ignore demographic stochasticity which could yield negative IE by chance). Conditional assessment for causal inference (which is aimed at an appropriate estimation of vaccine efficacy) will be further elaborated in the next section. Further technical details on the relevant modeling exercises can be found elsewhere [47].

To be strict, it should be noted that the above mentioned definitions of (mainly direct) effectiveness are flawed. Especially, DE is not precise as it contains indirect effect in its definition (because the above mentioned arguments consider only indirect effects on unvaccinated individuals). More appropriate definitions should take into account the indirect effects on both vaccinated and unvaccinated individuals, which yields three different definitions of IE, i.e., among vaccinated, unvaccinated and the entire population, and two different definitions of DE, i.e., among vaccinated and the entire population. Theoretical foundations on this matter have been developed by Haber [46] and Becker [13].

5 Addressing Dependent Happening

Because of the dependent happenings, quantitative modeling of infectious diseases has an important role in appropriately predicting the likely population effectiveness of a single intervention, yet mathematically separating the population effectiveness from the individual effect (i.e. efficacy). In other words, we should always remember that the need to assess causal effect or to simulate population effectiveness arises from this complicated principle of infectious diseases. When it comes to the causal inference, it is frequently the case that researchers have to clarify the average causal effect using observed data and clearly (and possibly analytically) bridge between an estimate at a population level and that at an individual level. This point is relevant to the estimation of vaccine efficacy from observed data in field epidemiology [50].

In this section, we discuss a method to address dependent happening using a conditional epidemiologic measurement. The method utilizes the *household secondary attack rate* (SAR) [49], which has been traditionally regarded as a measure of infectiousness [21]. We first show that the use of SAR can separately estimate the reductions in susceptibility and infectiousness among vaccinated individuals compared to unvaccinated individuals, and then prove that the combined effect directly and equally contribute to the reduction in the reproduction number.

5.1 Household Secondary Attack Rate

To address the dependence, recall causal effects under stability assumption T and A in subsection 4.1. Since T $\neq$ A in (48), we have to consider alternative strategies for inference. One of the simplest methods to resolve dependent happening is to employ *conditional direct causal effect* for examining the effect of a preventive measure (e.g. vaccination) on susceptibility which is conditioned on a specified exposure to infection [54]. That is, let K denote the exposure to infection where $K = +$ represents positive exposure to infection and $K = -$ represents no exposure to infection. We condition the expected values of potential outcomes among vaccinated and unvaccinated on K; i.e., let $E(X_1 \mid K = +)$ and $E(X_0 \mid K = +)$ be the expected outcomes in the population, respectively, if everyone were vaccinated and exposed to infection, and if everyone were unvaccinated and exposed to infection, the average conditional causal effect of the vaccine in the population compared to that without vaccination, $T_{conditioned}$, is

$$T_{conditioned} = E(X_0 \mid K = +) - E(X_1 \mid K = +) \tag{70}$$

As we discussed with Equation (47), we have to rewrite (70) to reflect observation (in real world scenarios) where only a portion of the population is vaccinated. In the presence of an intervention, exposure to infection is influenced by the treatment assignment (e.g. due to epidemiologic study design or irregular distribution of vaccination in the population), and thus, to be more precise, we write the exposure K as a function of assignments Y, i.e., $K(Y)$. Using this Y denoting the particular intervention that an individual used, Equation (70) can be rewritten as

$$E(X_0 \mid K = +) - E(X_1 \mid K = +) = E(X_0 \mid Y = 0, K(Y) = +) - E(X_1 \mid Y$$
$$= 1, K(Y) = +) \tag{71}$$

That is, causal effect of the vaccination (i.e. which leads to an estimator of vaccine efficacy) can be defined by conditioning the outcome on exposure to infection [54], which would be extremely useful to fill in the gap between individual and population effects.

Furthermore, the average conditional indirect effect, $IE_{conditioned}$, can also be defined in a similar way:

$$IE_{conditioned} = E(X_0 \mid K(Y = 0 \mid +)) - E(X_0 \mid K(Y = 1 \mid +)) \tag{72}$$

where $K(Y = 0 \mid +)$ and $K(Y = 1 \mid +)$ are, respectively, the exposure to an unvaccinated infectious individual and to a vaccinated infectious individual. In other words, the Equation (72) measures the reduction in infectiousness among vaccinated cases compared to unvaccinated cases.

In observation, this conditional measurement can be achieved, in the simplest manner, using the household secondary attack rate. The secondary attack rate, SAR, is the probability that infection occurs among susceptible individuals following a known contact with an infected person (or another infectious source) [49]. In other words, the SAR is conditional on the contact between an infectious source and a susceptible host (it should be noted that the term with *rate* is a misnomer, because this is actually a proportion). Thus, we write

$$SAR = \frac{\text{number of individuals exposed who developed disease}}{\text{total number of susceptible exposed individuals}} \quad (73)$$

When estimating SAR from epidemiologically observed data, we have to account for the correlation of susceptibles exposed to the same infectious source in order to appropriately quantify SAR.

The ratio of two SARs would be extremely useful to estimate the relative infectiousness and susceptibility of two types of populations [48]. Suppose that SAR_{ij} denotes the household secondary attack rate where i and j, respectively, give the previous vaccination histories of the secondary and primary case (i.e. i or $j = 1$ represents previously vaccinated, whereas i or $j = 0$ represents unvaccinated individuals). Vaccine efficacy for susceptibility, VE_S, and infectiousness, VE_I, can be estimated using the following ratios:

$$VE_S = 1 - \frac{SAR_{10}}{SAR_{00}} \quad (74)$$

$$VE_I = 1 - \frac{SAR_{01}}{SAR_{00}} \quad (75)$$

Moreover, we also get

$$VE_T = 1 - \frac{SAR_{11}}{SAR_{00}} \quad (76)$$

$$= 1 - (1 - VE_S)(1 - VE_I)$$

which is interpreted as a combined effect of susceptibility and infectiousness and can be thought of as the *naive susceptible equivalent* of a vaccinated compared to an unvaccinated individual [49]. We consider the following household transmission data of smallpox, which were observed in India [76, 85]:

The household SARs caused by unvaccinated primary cases among unvaccinated and vaccinated contacts were estimated to be $SAR_{00} = 40/650 = 0.0615$ and $SAR_{10} = 11/583 = 0.0189$, respectively. Those caused by vaccinated primary cases among unvaccinated and vaccinated household contacts were $SAR_{01} = 10/499 = 0.0200$ and $SAR_{11} = 2/421 = 0.0048$, respectively. The crude efficacy of vaccine in reducing susceptibility VE_S, infectiousness VE_I, and a combined effect of both VE_T is then estimated by

$$VE_S = 1 - \frac{SAR_{10}}{SAR_{00}} = 0.693 \quad (77)$$

$$VE_I = 1 - \frac{SAR_{01}}{SAR_{00}} = 0.674 \quad (78)$$

$$VE_T = 1 - \frac{SAR_{11}}{SAR_{00}} = 0.923 \qquad (79)$$

If we make the simplifying assumption that the biological effect of vaccination was identical for all vaccinated individuals, vaccination reduced susceptibility by 69.3%, infectiousness by 67.4%, and the combined effect was 92.3%.

Limiting our interest to the household transmission data (or conditioning observation on those with household contact which would not be too different by individual), and stratifying the vaccination histories of both primary and secondary cases, we can appropriately estimate not only the reduction in susceptibility but also that in infectiousness among vaccinated individuals [55]. This method is useful not only for assessing vaccine efficacy but also for estimating other treatment effect at an individual level such as epidemiologic effects of antiviral agents against influenza transmission [52].

In this way, although comparison of two groups (i.e. with and without intervention) have been simply assessed by popualtion data for non-communicable diseases (as long as their frequencies of exposures are identical), dependent happening in communicable diseases confuses the interpretation of the population effectiveness. The confusion is caused by indirect effect. To address this issue in infectious disease epidemiology and attribute observation at a population level to an average causal effect at an individual level, conditional measurement can be deemed extremely useful to appropriately analyze epidemiologic datasets.

5.2 The Impact of Reductions in Susceptibility and Infectiousness on the Transmission Dynamics

In relation to the conditional measurement in households, we lastly consider the impact of different effects of vaccination (e.g. reductions in susceptibility and infectiousness) on the transmission dynamics using SIR model. Specifically, we consider a vaccine which elicits both all-or-nothing and leaky effects. The following model simplifies the previously published exercise by Simon and Koopman [92]. As we have done with Equations (57), (58), (59), (60), (61), (62), let S_v, I_v, S_u and I_u be the numbers of vaccinated susceptible and infectious individuals and of unvaccinated susceptible and infectious individuals, respectively. Rather than investigating an epidemic which ignores background demographic dynamics, here we consider the system with constant per capita birth rate, μ, which is assumed equivalent to the natural mortality rate. Vaccination is assumed to take place at birth with the coverage p. Because of all-or-nothing effect, the fraction $p\alpha$ of newborns becomes permanently immune, and the remaining fraction $p(1 - \alpha)$ is susceptible. Since we assume that the population sizes of both vaccinated and unvaccinated individuals are constant over time, we ignore the recovered individuals, R_v and R_u, for simplicity. We also assume that the recovery rate γ is independent of vaccination, because duration effect is seldom reported [76, 91] and moreover, such observations tend to be limited to the symptomatic period (not infectious period). Then, the four equations of the system, representing the transmission dynamics in a randomly mixing population, are

$$\frac{dS_v}{dt} = \mu p(1 - \alpha)N - \beta \lambda_S S_v (\lambda_I I_v + I_u) - \mu S_v \tag{80}$$

$$\frac{dI_v}{dt} = \beta \lambda_S S_v (\lambda_I I_v + I_u) - (\gamma + \mu)I_v \tag{81}$$

$$\frac{dS_u}{dt} = \mu(1 - p)N - \beta S_u (\lambda_I I_v + I_u) - \mu S_u \tag{82}$$

$$\frac{dI_u}{dt} = \beta S_u (\lambda_I I_v + I_u) - (\gamma + \mu)I_u \tag{83}$$

where β is the transmission rate which is assumed identical among vaccinated and unvaccinated individuals. However, due to leaky effect, susceptibility of vaccinated individuals is reduced by a factor λ_S and infectiousness of vaccinated cases is reduced by λ_I, both of which are assumed to lie in the range of $0 \leq \lambda_S, \lambda_I \leq 1$. If $\alpha = 0$, it should be noted that λ_S and λ_I, respectively, correspond to $1 - \text{VE}_S$ and $1 - \text{VE}_I$ in the last subsection, both of which are also referred to as *transmission probability ratio* [48].

We combine Equations (81) and (83) to explore $\lambda_I I_v + I_u$, i.e.,

$$\lambda_I \frac{dI_v}{dt} + \frac{dI_u}{dt} = \beta(\lambda_S \lambda_I S_v + S_u)(\lambda_I I_v + I_u) - (\gamma + \mu)(\lambda_I I_v + I_u) \tag{84}$$

Replacing $\lambda_I I_v + I_u$ by I_c (where the subscript c is intended to represent *combined*), Equation (84) is simplified as

$$\frac{dI_c}{dt} = I_c \left(\beta(\lambda_S \lambda_I S_v + S_u) - (\gamma + \mu) \right)$$

$$= \beta I_c \left(\lambda_S \lambda_I S_v + S_u - \frac{N}{R_0} \right) \tag{85}$$

where $R_0 = \beta N / (\gamma + \mu)$ and N is the total population size (here, $N = N_v + N_u$ under vaccination). Since we know that

$$\lambda_S \lambda_I S_v + S_u \leq \lambda_S \lambda_I (1 - \alpha)pN + (1 - p)N, \tag{86}$$

if

$$(1 - p) + \lambda_S \lambda_I (1 - \alpha)p < \frac{1}{R_0} \tag{87}$$

or

$$R_0 \left(1 - (1 - \lambda_S \lambda_I (1 - \alpha))p \right) < 1 \tag{88}$$

the parenthesized term in the right hand side of Equation (85) will always be negative. Then, $I_c(t) \to 0$ as $t \to \infty$, and every solution of system (80), (81), (82), (83) coverges to the disease-free equilibrium

$$(S_u, S_v, I_u, I_v, R_u, R_v) = ((1 - p)N, p(1 - \alpha)N, 0, 0, 0, p\alpha N) \qquad (89)$$

when the condition (88) holds. In other words, to achieve eradication of a disease in question, the vaccination coverage p should satisfy

$$p > \frac{1}{1 - \lambda_S \lambda_I (1 - \alpha)} \left(1 - \frac{1}{R_0}\right) \qquad (90)$$

Nevertheless, if

$$(1 - p) + \lambda_S \lambda_I (1 - \alpha) p > \frac{1}{R_0} \qquad (91)$$

the solutions of the system (80), (81), (82), (83) move away from (89), indicating that the disease-free equilibrium is unstable.

If everyone is vaccinated so that $p = 1$, the threshold condition (90) to eradicate the disease is

$$\lambda_S \lambda_I (1 - \alpha) R_0 \leq 1 \qquad (92)$$

From Equations (90) and (92), we clearly see that the different vaccine effects (i.e. all-or-nothing effect and leaky effects in reducing susceptibility and infectiousness) act mathematically in the same way to reduce the critical vaccination fraction. Moreover, if $\alpha = 0$, it should be noted that $\lambda_S \lambda_I$ in (90) is equivalent to $1 - \text{VE}_T$ in (76), which makes (90) idential to (49). From (90), we observe that the more potent the vaccine (i.e., the smaller is $\lambda_S \lambda_I (1 - \alpha)$), the smaller the vaccination coverage p needs to be to achieve the herd immunity threshold. The use of I_c is what we call the Lyapounov function approach, more detailed exercise on this matter (with other types of biological effects of vaccination) can be found elsewhere [92].

This kind of expectation (of different types of vaccine efficacy) arose from field trials of vaccination against HIV/AIDS and malaria [67, 68], both of which have yet to be developed. As we have seen, it has been very striking that the different biological effects would work as the product to contribute to lower R_0. Nevertheless, it has to be remembered that this *equality* of vaccine effects does not hold for non-randomly mixing population. In heterogeneously mixing populations, no single vaccination fraction can define the threshold level of vaccination. Therefore, the challenging issue is that the eradition threshold in such a population will be achieved by vaccinating different subgroups at different levels. In any case, to quantitatively address the issue of estimating different types of vaccine efficacy, the use of household data would be recommended, because household outbreaks contain some information about the possible source of infection and the data reasonably permit assuming homogeneous mixing within the household [12].

6 Conclusion

In this chapter, we discussed two critical issues which have to be remembered whenever researchers analyze observed data of infectious diseases. First, since many unobservable events would always be the source of uncertainty in all mathematical models of the transmission dynamics, observable statistical distributions must be effectively employed to translate observables to unobservables. For this reason, the incubation period and serial interval are deemed critically important epidemiologic measurements, if symptom onset is observable for a disease in question. Therefore, it is essential to make sure that systematically collected data are aggregated and stored for posterity in order to appropriately discuss the dynamics of infectious diseases using observed data. Second, transmission probabilities (or other conditional epidemiologic measurements) per exposure to infection should be effectively employed to address the dependence between individuals, as long as we deal with directly transmitted infectious diseases (i.e. communicable diseases). Although our example of dependent happening was focused on an assessment of vaccine efficacy, the readers are advised to remember (to gain some sense of quantitative modeling) that the need for mathematical modeling in all practical settings arises due to this complicated issue. Rather than numerical computations of complicated models with lots of unsupported assumptions, it is often the case that an analytical approach to conveniently address this issue or useful dataset which is conditioned on infection event may work better to answer to key questions in the field of medical epidemiology and public health.

One important future work still remains with respect to the issue of observability. Although our framework permits estimating various unobservable epidemiologic variables (e.g. the generation time), statistical and biological validity to assume a specific distribution has yet to be clarified. For this reason, it is necessary to understand the detailed natural history of an infection, especially, as to *what is happening within infected host*. Symptom onset is not only determined by pathogen dynamics within host but also regulated by complex immune responses [82]. For example, an explicit reason why lognormal distribution fits well with the incubation period of diseases with acute course of illness, and the similar reason for assuming Weibull distribution for the incubation period of AIDS, have yet to be offered.

Since this chapter was intended to summarize the issue of dependent happening in a rudimentary fashion, and because of the space limitation, we did not discuss the details of heterogeneously mixing populations on this matter. Whereas various types of effectiveness of vaccination during an epidemic were defined using final size equations, final size would be greatly confused by heterogeneous contact patterns. For example, even when we consider household transmission, dependence between households must be addressed using an appropriate mathematical approach [9]. Although a mathematical foundation of household transmission has been developed and well-formulated [8], a quantitative method to effectively utilize the model (e.g. to derive an estimator) has yet to be offered. Given that the final size is always confused by contact heterogeneity, observational approaches to conditionalize key epidemiologic measurements on exposure to infection would play a crucial role in many epidemiological and statistical studies.

Much work remains to be carried out for powerful general analyses to give insights into the transmission dynamics of communicable diseases using observed data.

Acknowledgments The work of HN was supported by The Netherlands Organisation for Scientific Research (NWO).

References

1. Anderson, R.M. (1991) Populations and infectious diseases: Ecology or epidemiology? *J. Anim. Ecol.* 60:1–50
2. Anderson, R.M., May, R.M. (1982) Directly transmitted infectious diseases: Control by vaccination. *Science* 215:1053–1060
3. Anderson, R.M., May, R.M. (1985) Vaccination and herd immunity to infectious diseases. *Nature* 318:323–329
4. Anderson, R.M., May, R.M. (1990) Immunisation and herd immunity. *Lancet* 335: 641–645
5. Anderson, R.M., May, R.M. (1991) *Infectious Diseases of Humans: Dynamics and Control.* Oxford University Press, Oxford
6. Anderson, R.M., Medley, G.F., May, R.M., Johnson, A.M. (1986) A preliminary study of the transmission dynamics of the human immunodeficiency virus (HIV), the causative agent of AIDS. *IMA J. Math. Appl. Med. Biol.* 3:229–263
7. Bailey, N.T.J. (1975) *The Mathematical Theory of Infectious Diseases and Its Applications* (2nd Ed). Charles Griffin, London
8. Ball, F., Lyne, O. (2006) Optimal vaccination schemes for epidemics among a population of households, with application to variola minor in Brazil, *Stat. Methods. Med. Res.* 15: 481–497
9. Ball, F., Mollison, D., Scalia-Tomba, G. (1997) Epidemics with two levels of mixing, *Ann. Appl. Prob.* 7:46–89
10. Becker, N. (1995) Part 5: Data analysis: Estimation and prediction. Statistical challenges of epidemic data. In: Mollison, D. (ed.) *Epidemic Models: Their Structure and Relation to Data,* pp. 339–349. Cambridge University Press, Cambridge
11. Becker, N.G. (1997) Uses of the EM algorithm in the analysis of data on HIV/AIDS and other infectious diseases. *Stat. Methods. Med. Res.* 6:24–37
12. Becker, N.G., Britton, T., O'Neill, P.D. (2003) Estimating vaccine effects on transmission of infection from household outbreak data. *Biometrics.* 59:467–475
13. Becker, N.G., Britton, T., O'Neill, P.D. (2006) Estimating vaccine effects from studies of outbreaks in household pairs. *Stat. Med.* 25:1079–1093
14. Becker, N.G., Watson, L.F., Carlin, J.B. (1991) A method of non-parametric back-projection and its application to AIDS data. *Stat. Med.* 10:1527–1542
15. Begon, M., Bennett, M., Bowers, R.G., French, N.P., Hazel, S.M., Turner, J. (2002) A clarification of transmission terms in host-microparasite models: Numbers, densities and areas. *Epidemiol. Infect.* 129:147–153
16. Brookmeyer, R. (1998) Incubation period of infectious diseases. In: Armitage, P., Colton, T. (eds.) *Encyclopedia of Biostatistics*, pp. 2011–2016. Wiley, New York

17. Brookmeyer, R., Gail, M.H. (1986) Minimum size of the acquired immunodeficiency syndrome (AIDS) epidemic in the United States. *Lancet* 2:1320–1322
18. Brookmeyer, R., Gail, M.H. (1988) A method for obtaining short-term projections and lower bounds on the size of the AIDS epidemic. *J. Am. Stat. Assoc.* 83:301–308
19. Brookmeyer, R., Gail, M.H. (1994) *AIDS Epidemiology: A Quantitative Approach* (Monographs in Epidemiology and Biostatistics). Oxford University Press, New York
20. Brookmeyer, R., You, X. (2006) A hypothesis test for the end of a common source outbreak. *Biometrics* 62:61–65
21. Chapin, C.V. (1912) *The Sources and Modes of Infection* (2nd Edition). John Wiley and Sons, New York
22. Colgate, S.A., Stanley, E.A., Hyman, J.M., Layne, S.P., Qualls, C. (1989) Risk behavior-based model of the cubic growth of acquired immunodeficiency syndrome in the United States. *Proc. Natl. Acad. Sci. USA* 86:4793–4797
23. Colton, T., Johnson, T., Machin, D. (Eds) (1994) Proceedings of the Conference on Quantitative Methods for Studying AIDS, held in Blaubeuren, Germany, June 14–18, 1993. In: *Stat. Med.* 13:1899–2188
24. Cousens, S.N., Vynnycky, E., Zeidler, M., Will, R.G., Smith, P.G. (1997) Predicting the CJD epidemic in humans. *Nature* 385:197–198
25. Cox, D.R. (1958) *Planning of Experiments*. John Wiley and Sons, New York
26. Day, N.E., Gore, S.M., McGee, M.A., South, M. (1989) Predictions of the AIDS epidemic in the U.K.: The use of the back projection method. *Philos. Trans. R. Soc. Lond. Ser. B.* 325: 123–134
27. de Jong, M.C.M., Diekmann, O., Heesterbeek, J.A.P. (1995) How does transmission of infection depend on population size? In: Mollison, D. (ed.) *Epidemic Models: Their Structure and Relation to Data*, pp. 84–94. Cambridge University Press, Cambridge
28. Diekmann, O., Heesterbeek, J.A.P.: (2000) *Mathematical Epidemiology of Infectious Diseases: Model Building, Analysis and Interpretation*. Wiley, New York
29. Diekmann, O., Heesterbeek, J.A., Metz, J.A. (1990) On the definition and the computation of the basic reproduction ratio R_0 in models for infectious diseases in heterogeneous populations. *J. Math. Biol.* 28:365–382
30. Dietz, K. (1993) The estimation of the basic reproduction number for infectious diseases. *Stat. Methods. Med. Res.* 2:23–41
31. Donnelly, C.A., Ferguson, N.M., Ghani, A.C., Anderson, R.M. (2003) Extending backcalculation to analyse BSE data. *Stat. Methods. Med. Res.* 12:177–190
32. Downie, A.W., St Vincent, L., Meiklejohn, G., Ratnakannan, N.R., Rao, A.R., Krishnan, G.N., Kempe, C.H. (1961) Studies on the virus content of mouth washings in the acute phase of smallpox. *Bull. World Health Organ.* 25:49–53
33. Dublin, L.I., Lotka, A.J. (1925) On the true rate of natural increase. *J. Am. Stat. Assoc.* 151:305–339
34. Eichner, M. (2003) Case isolation and contact tracing can prevent the spread of smallpox. *Am. J. Epidemiol.* 158:118–128
35. Eichner, M., Dietz, K. (2003) Transmission potential of smallpox: Estimates based on detailed data from an outbreak. *Am. J. Epidemiol.* 158:110–117
36. Farewell, V.T., Herzberg, A.M., James, K.W., Ho, L.M., Leung, G.M. (2005) SARS incubation and quarantine times: When is an exposed individual known to be disease free? *Stat. Med.* 24:3431–3445
37. Farrington, C.P. (2003) On vaccine efficacy and reproduction numbers. *Math. Biosci.* 185: 89–109
38. Fenner, F. (1948) The pathogenesis of the acute exanthems. An interpretation based upon experimental investigation with mouse-pox (infectious ectromelia of mice). *Lancet* ii:915–920
39. Ferguson, N.M., Donnelly, C.A., Woolhouse, M.E., Anderson, R.M. (1997) The epidemiology of BSE in cattle herds in Great Britain. II. Model construction and analysis of transmission dynamics. *Phil. Trans. R. Soc. Lond. Ser. B.* 352:803–838

40. Fine, P.E. (1993) Herd immunity: history, theory, practice. *Epidemiol. Rev.* 15:265–302
41. Fine, P.E. (2003) The interval between successive cases of an infectious disease. *Am. J. Epidemiol.* 158:1039–1047
42. Fraser, C., Riley, S., Anderson, R.M., Ferguson, N.M. (2004) Factors that make an infectious disease outbreak controllable. *Proc. Natl. Acad. Sci. USA* 101:6146–6151
43. Gail, M.H., Brookmeyer, R. (1988) Methods for projecting course of acquired immunodeficiency syndrome epidemic. *J. Natl. Cancer. Inst.* 80:900–911
44. Greenland, S., Brumback, B. (2002) An overview of relations among causal modelling methods. *Int. J. Epidemiol.* 31:1030–1037
45. Greenwood, M., Yule, G.U. (1915) The statistics of anti-typhoid and anti-cholera inoculations, and the interpretation of such statistics in general. *Proc. R. Soc. Med.* 8:113–190
46. Haber, M. (1999) Estimation of the direct and indirect effects of vaccination. *Stat. Med.* 18:2101–2109
47. Haber, M., Longini, I.M., Halloran, M.E. (1991) Measures of the effects of vaccination in a randomly mixing population. *Int. J. Epidemiol.* 20:300–310
48. Halloran, M.E. (1988) Concepts of infectious disease epidemiology. In: Rothman, K.J., Greenland, S. (eds.) *Modern Epidemiology*, 2nd Edition, pp. 529–554. Lippincott Williams and Wilkins, New York
49. Halloran, M.E. (1988) Secondary attack rate. In: Armitage, P., Colton, T. (eds.) *Encyclopedia of Biostatistics*, pp. 4025–4029. Wiley, New York
50. Halloran, M.E. (2001) Overview of study design. In: Thomas, J.C., Weber, D.J. (eds.) *Epidemiologic Methods for the Study of Infectious Diseases*, pp. 86–115. Oxford University Press, New York
51. Halloran, M.E., Haber, M.J., Longini, I.M., Struchiner, C.J. (1991) Direct and indirect effects in vaccine field efficacy and effectiveness. *Am. J. Epidemiol.* 133:323–331
52. Halloran, M.E., Hayden, F.G., Yang, Y., Longini, I.M., Monto, A.S. (2007) Antiviral effects on influenza viral transmission and pathogenicity: Observations from household-based trials. *Am. J. Epidemiol.* 165:212–221
53. Halloran, M.E., Struchiner, C.J. (1991) Study designs for dependent happenings. *Epidemiology* 2:331–338
54. Halloran, M.E., Struchiner, C.J. (1995) Causal inference in infectious diseases. *Epidemiology* 6:142–151
55. Halloran, M.E., Struchiner, C.J., Longini, I.M. (1997) Study designs for evaluating different efficacy and effectiveness aspects of vaccines. *Am. J. Epidemiol.* 146: 789–803
56. Haydon, D.T., Chase-Topping, M., Shaw, D.J., Matthews, L., Friar, J.K., Wilesmith, J., Woolhouse, M.E. (2003) The construction and analysis of epidemic trees with reference to the 2001 UK foot-and-mouth outbreak. *Proc. R. Soc. Lond. Ser. B.* 270:121–127
57. Hernan, M.A., Robins, J.M. (2006) Instruments for causal inference: An epidemiologist's dream? *Epidemiology* 17:360–372
58. Hill, B.M. (1963) The three-parameter lognormal distribution and Bayesian analysis of a point-source epidemic. *J. Am. Stat. Assoc.* 58:72–84
59. Hope Simpson, R.E. (1948) The period of transmission in certain epidemic diseases: An observational method for its discovery. *Lancet.* 2:755–760
60. Inaba, H., Nishiura, H. (2008) The state-reproduction number for a multistate class age structured epidemic system and its application to the asymptomatic transmission model. *Math. Biosci.* 216:77–89
61. Jewell, N.P., Dietz, K., Farewell, V.T. (1992) *AIDS Epidemiology: Methodological Issues.* Birkhauser, Berlin
62. John, T.J., Samuel, R. (2000) Herd immunity and herd effect: New insights and definitions. *Eur. J. Epidemiol.* 16:601–606
63. Koopman, J.S., Longini, I.M. (1994) The ecological effects of individual exposures and nonlinear disease dynamics in populations. *Am. J. Public. Health.* 84: 836–842

64. Koopman, J.S., Longini, I.M., Jacquez, J.A., Simon, C.P., Ostrow, D.G., Martin, W.R., Wood-cock, D.M. (1991) Assessing risk factors for transmission of infection. *Am. J. Epidemiol.* 133:1199–1209

65. Lipsitch, M., Cohen, T., Cooper, B., Robins, J.M., Ma, S., James, L., Gopalakrishna, G., Chew, S.K., Tan, C.C., Samore, M.H., Fisman, D., Murray, M. (2003) Transmission dynamics and control of severe acute respiratory syndrome. *Science.* 300:1966–1970

66. Lloyd-Smith, J.O., Schreiber, S.J., Kopp, P.E., Getz, W.M. (2005) Superspreading and the effect of individual variation on disease emergence. *Nature* 438:355–359

67. Longini, I.M., Datta, S., Halloran, M.E. (1996) Measuring vaccine efficacy for both suscepti-bility to infection and reduction in infectiousness for prophylactic HIV-1 vaccines. *J. Acquir. Immune. Defic. Syndr. Hum. Retrovirol.* 13:440–407

68. Longini, I.M., Sagatelian, K., Rida, W.N., Halloran, M.E. (1998) Optimal vaccine trial design when estimating vaccine efficacy for susceptibility and infectiousness from multiple populations. *Stat. Med.* 17:1121–1136

69. May, R.M., Lloyd, A.L. (2001) Infection dynamics on scale-free networks. *Phys. Rev. E. Stat. Nonlin. Soft. Matter. Phys.* 64:066112

70. McCallum, H., Barlow, N., Hone, J. (2001) How should pathogen transmission be modelled? *Trends. Ecol. Evol.* 16:295–300

71. Meynell, G.G., Meynell, E.W. (1958) The growth of micro-organisms in vivo with par-ticular reference to the relation between dose and latent period. *J. Hyg. (Lond)* 56: 323–346

72. Netea, M.G., Kullberg, B.J., Van der Meer, J.W. (2000) Circulating cytokines as mediators of fever. *Clin. Infect. Dis.* 31:S178–S184

73. Nishiura, H. (2007) Early efforts in modeling the incubation period of infectious diseases with an acute course of illness. *Emerg. Themes. Epidemiol.* 4:2

74. Nishiura, H. (2006) Incubation period as a clinical predictor of botulism: analysis of previ-ous izushi-borne outbreaks in Hokkaido, Japan, from 1951 to 1965. *Epidemiol. Infect.* 135: 126–130

75. Nishiura, H. (2007) Lessons from previous predictions of HIV/AIDS in the United States and Japan: epidemiologic models and policy formulation. *Epidemiol. Perspect. Innov.*4:3

76. Nishiura, H., Brockmann, S.O., Eichner, M. (2008) Extracting key information from his-torical data to quantify the transmission dynamics of smallpox. *Theor. Biol. Med. Model.* 5:20

77. Nishiura, H., Dietz, K., Eichner, M. (2006) The earliest notes on the reproduction number in relation to herd immunity: Theophil Lotz and smallpox vaccination. *J. Theor. Biol.* 241: 964–967

78. Nishiura, H., Eichner, M. (2007) Infectiousness of smallpox relative to disease age: estimates based on transmission network and incubation period. *Epidemiol. Infect.* 135: 1145–1150

79. Nishiura, H., Lee, H.W., Cho, S.H., Lee, W.G., In, T.S., Moon, S.U., Chung, G.T., Kim, T.S. (2007) Estimates of short and long incubation periods of Plasmodium vivax malaria in the Republic of Korea. *Trans. R. Soc. Trop. Med. Hyg.* 101:338–343

80. Nishiura, H., Schwehm, M., Kakehashi, M., Eichner, M. (2006) Transmission potential of primary pneumonic plague: time inhomogeneous evaluation based on historical documents of the transmission network. *J. Epidemiol. Community. Health.* 60:640–645

81. Nokes, D.J., Anderson, R.M. (1988) The use of mathematical models in the epidemiological study of infectious diseases and in the design of mass immunization programmes. *Epidemiol. Infect.* 101:1–20

82. Nowak, M., May, R.M. (2000) *Virus Dynamics: Mathematical Principles of Immunology and Virology.* Oxford University Press, Oxford

83. Orenstein, W.A., Bernier, R.H., Hinman, A.R. (1988) Assessing vaccine efficacy in the field. Further observations. *Epidemiol. Rev.* 10:212–241

84. Pickles, W. (1939) *Epidemiology in Country Practice.* John Wright & Sons, Bristol

85. Rao, A.R., Jacob, E.S., Kamalakshi, S., Appaswamy, S., Bradbury (1968) Epidemiological studies in smallpox. A study of intrafamilial transmission in a series of 254 infected families. *Indian. J. Med. Res.* 56:1826–1854

86. Roberts, M.G., Heesterbeek, J.A. (2007) Model-consistent estimation of the basic reproduction number from the incidence of an emerging infection. *J. Math. Biol.* 55:803–816

87. Rosenberg, P.S., Gail, M.H. (1990) Uncertainty in estimates of HIV prevalence derived by backcalculation. *Ann. Epidemiol.* 1:105–115

88. Rubin, D.B. (1990) Comment: Neyman (1923) and causal inference in experiments and observational studies. *Stat. Sci.* 5:472–480

89. Sakar, J.K., Mitra, A.C., Mukherjee, M.K., De, S.K., Mazumdar, D.G. (1973) Virus excretion in smallpox. 1. Excretion in the throat, urine, and conjunctiva of patients. *Bull. World Health Organ.* 48:517–522

90. Sartwell, P.E. (1950) The distribution of incubation periods of infectious diseases. *Am. J. Hyg.* 51:310–318

91. Satou, K., Nishiura, H. (2007) Evidence of the partial effects of inactivated Japanese encephalitis vaccination: analysis of previous outbreaks in Japan from 1953 to 1960. *Ann. Epidemiol.* 17:271–277

92. Simon, C.P., Koopman, J.S. (2001) Infection transmission dynamics and vaccination program effectiveness as a function of vaccine effects in individuals. In: Blower, S., Castillo-Chavez, C., van den Driessche, P., Yakubu, A.A. (eds.) *Mathematical Approaches for Emerging and Reemerging Infectious Diseases : Models, Methods and Theory*, pp. 143–155. Springer-Verlag, New York

93. Smith, C.E. (1964) Factors in the transmission of virus infections from animal to man. *Sci. Basis. Med. Annu. Rev.* i:125–150

94. Svensson, A. (2007) A note on generation time in epidemic models. *Math. Biosci.* 208: 300–311

95. Tango, T. (1998) Maximum likelihood estimation of date of infection in an outbreak of diarrhea due to contaminated foods assuming lognormal distribution for the incubation period. *Jpn. J. Public. Health.* 45:129–141

96. Wallinga, J., Lipsitch, M. (2007) How generation intervals shape the relationship between growth rates and reproductive numbers. *Proc. R. Soc. Lond. Ser. B.* 274:599–604

97. Wallinga, J., Teunis, P. (2004) Different epidemic curves for severe acute respiratory syndrome reveal similar impacts of control measures. *Am. J. Epidemiol.* 160:509–516

The Chain of Infection, Contacts, and Model Parametrization

Stephen Tennenbaum

Abstract Contact rates and transmission probabilities are based on complicated environmental conditions, and biological and social dynamics. There are many types of models that capture different aspects of these dynamics. Estimating contact related parameter values and transmission probabilities requires a good understanding of the details of the transmission process and the class of model being used to describe it. In this paper we review the basic classes of models, the connection between the chain of infection and the descriptions of the infection process including the meaning of "contacts" in the various modeling approaches. Some suggestions as to ways to better tie together the biological and mechanistic aspects of the infection process and the more phenomenological descriptions of model parameters are discussed.

Keywords Chain of infection · Contact rates · Mixing · Model parametrization · Modes of transmission · Portal of entry · Portal of exit · Proportionate mixing

1 Modeling Infection

Infectious diseases, are primarily social phenomena. As such there are necessarily interactions between individuals that take place enabling the transmission of the pathogenic organism from one person to another. The many forms of this process can be modeled in multiple ways. G.P. Garnett [16] for instance, provides the following characterization of the modeling process. There are compartmental models where the population is broken down into specific disease stages such as "susceptible", "latent", "symptomatic", etc. versus distributional models where the disease would be described by some gradation of severity or immune response. There are discrete time models versus continuous time models, the former can be described by difference equations or a Markov process (for example) and the state

S. Tennenbaum (✉)
Mathematical, Computational and Modeling Sciences Center, Arizona State University, Tempe, AZ 85287-1904, USA
e-mail: set1@asu.edu

G. Chowell et al. (eds.), *Mathematical and Statistical Estimation Approaches in Epidemiology*, DOI 10.1007/978-90-481-2313-1_4,
© Springer Science+Business Media B.V. 2009

of the population is updated in steps, while the latter can described by differential equations and the state of the population is "updated" continuously. There are deterministic models where parameter values are fixed; relationships are defined by specific functions and the result (if simulated) is the same each time for the same starting values. In contrast stochastic models encompass both models where the occurrence of events are simulated as the result of some random process and models where parameters are expressed in terms of probability distributions (rather than point estimates) in a system of differential equations resulting in stochastic differential equations. Populations can be represented by averages (mean field models) where we look at the numbers of persons in a particular state, or as probability distributions of particular states at a particular time, or dispersion of numbers across states, or represented as individuals (agent based models) where we keep track of each person's state over time. We can have models that are linear where the states of the system are simple (linear) functions (deterministic – Markov process, or stochastic – Kolmogorov equations), or models that have more complex (and harder to analyze) non-linear terms. Results can be analytical or numerical and/or the result of simulations. Models can have varying levels of structure from the simple SIS (susceptible-infected-susceptible) model to those where we break down the population by age, geographic location, activity, or other classification scheme in addition to the state of infection. And by detailing the population even further structures can be layered over each other or expressed in a hierarchy. For example we can create a metapopulation model where cities are connected by transportation networks that operate on different time scales than the disease dynamics of the populations within those cities. Given all these complications, we can briefly describe a few examples of the ways disease transmission can be handled.

One simple description of contagion employs the mass action assumption (see for example Anderson and May [3]). This assumes that the population is well-mixed and any two individuals are equally likely to encounter each other.

$$\frac{dS}{dt} = -\beta SI, \text{ and } \frac{dI}{dt} = \beta SI.$$

Here, S is the number of susceptible individuals; I is the number of infected individuals and β is known as the transmission rate. If this model is reformulated in terms of the proportion of the contacts that a susceptible person has with infected people [22] then we have

$$\frac{dS}{dt} = -(\beta N) S \frac{I}{N}, \text{ and } \frac{dI}{dt} = (\beta N) S \frac{I}{N}.$$

where N is the total size of the population. It is apparent here that the per capita rate of infection (βN) increases in direct proportion to the population size. This may at first sight seem plausible however the exact relationship is dependent on how people are infected through their daily encounters. For a variety of childhood infectious diseases where direct contact is important the per capita rate of infection is, for the most part, independent of community size [22]. Using a per capita rate of infection of the form βN^v Anderson and May [3] found that data for communities with population sizes from 1,000 to 400,000 gave values of v between 0.03 and 0.07. This strongly suggests that for these situations, the standard per capita rate of infection corresponding to $v = 0$ where people have a fixed number of contacts per day is more realistic approximation than per capita rate of infection corresponding to $v = 1$. Thus we have the more often seen result

$$\frac{dS}{dt} = -\beta S \frac{I}{N}, \text{ and } \frac{dI}{dt} = \beta S \frac{I}{N}.$$

There are many modifications of this basic infection mechanism. For example vertical infection wherein newborns are infected by their mothers, models with population and subpopulation size – dependent contact functions have also been considered [6]. Contact rates are most tractable when based on proportionate mixing, that is the probability of a person contacting another from a given group is proportional to that group's weighted fractional representation in the population [8]. Various other forms of nonlinear incidences have been considered. Some lead to periodicity in the disease prevalence; these necessarily involve loss of immunity or some other form of renewal of susceptibles by birth or immigration. Models with age structure of the population also lead to non-linearities in the infection rates when there are differences in infectivity or shifts in infectious periods associated with that structure [27]. The latter can occur due to non-exponentially distributed waiting times in the compartments. These distributed delays lead to epidemiology models with integral or integrodifferential or functional differential equations or delay-differential Equations [22]. Detailed models of AIDs transmission or TB can include some or all these aspects since the diseases are so long lasting and change their character so significantly over the course of the infection [4].

Another effect is seasonal variations in transmission. These are modeled by allowing the transmission parameter β, to be a function of time (usually measured in years). For example many authors use a sinusoidal forcing function for the seasonality $\beta(t) = \beta_0 (1 + \beta_1 \cos 2\pi t)$ where β_0 is the baseline level of transmission and β_1 determines the amplitude of the seasonal variation (the "strength" of seasonality). This forcing can result in quite complicated patterns of outbreaks over longer periods of time as the amplitude of the forcing function increases, eventually leading to chaotic dynamics under the right conditions [30].

In most of these mean field modeling approaches the transmission rates are given a specific form based broadly on a hypothesized mathematical relationship. The conceptual basis of that form is usually, loosely based around some mechanistic analogy to a physical process, e.g. mass action, or sinusoidal forcing function, etc. The unknown parameters are almost always determined by inverse methods that find the values that best fit the model to data.

Another, probabilistic, approach for very small populations (households or small communities) is the use of "chain binomial models". These models look at the probability that, for a fixed household size n, the infection will be transmitted from the first person to a number of susceptibles based on the given probability of transmission to a single person at that time. In the Reed-Frost approach [11, 35] the probability of infection of a single person is equal to $q^{I(t)}$ where q is the probability of a single infected person infecting another person. In the Greenwood approach [11, 18] the probability of infection of a single person is equal to q, that is, it is fixed and not dependent on the number of people already infected (a single infected can saturate the environment with contagion) [15]. A more sophisticated extension of this approach was used by Longini et al. in their agent based models of pandemic influenza [28].

Other complicating factors are involved in the study of vector transmitted diseases. The transmission process is thus multi-population, multi-stage, and quite often seasonal. Macroparasite diseases (where "infectious load" – the number of infectious organisms per host – becomes an important aspect of the transmission process) are metapopulation models in a very literal sense. Sexually transmitted diseases are akin to vector transmitted diseases in that they are multi-population and multi-stage, in addition most theoreticians have added serial monogamy between sexes which requires a conservation of contacts constraint that is often built into the transmission terms. Models that also include sexual preferences (based on age, race or other social distinctions) can become quite complicated [7].

The result of Anderson and May [3] that showed independence of infectivity from population size may be derived from the fact that the populations and population sizes considered are above certain size or density thresholds. That is, they are at levels where people in those populations are already making contacts at near the maximum possible per-capita average number. Contact rates and by extension transmission rates are in fact saturating functions of population density. Defining density as $\delta(N) \equiv N/\text{area}$ and setting

$$\beta(N) = \beta \frac{\delta(N)}{\kappa + \delta(N)}$$
$$= \beta \frac{N}{\kappa \cdot \text{area} + N},$$

leads to a typical model of a saturating function. The above observation begs the question – what do we mean by "area" or even "population" (N) for that matter? For individuals that are limited to the range of movement in a given period (time scales on the order of the generation time of the disease or less) and that encounter one another in a random manner (within the period have the same probability of meeting anyone), the "area" is the space in which this mixing takes place and "population" refers to the groups of individuals within that space, susceptibles are the members of the population at risk, and so on. Of course once heterogeneities are introduced such as long distance travel, individual preferences, or other assorting or associating pressures, then the meanings of area or population are not so clear. In addition the model itself may change as infectives change behavior or susceptibles act to minimize risk. Direct measurements of these parameters become even more difficult, and with increasing heterogeneity they become little more than fitted phenomenological constants that have little connection to basic principles. In order to maintain a firm grounding another approach is needed. To this end there have been a large number of models that use a *network* approach by which individuals or subpopulations are modeled as nodes of a directed graph and the edges are the social or transportation connections [29, 31]. Most recently much of this work has focused on "small world" networks deriving from observations on social and communication networks [1, 2, 34]. A useful practical group of studies (although strictly heuristic as far as disease is concerned) is the spread of computer viruses over the World Wide Web [1, 10, 26]. Rather than attempting to here explain the construction, measures, and properties of the various network models of disease, we will simply describe the main categories and types of these models and leave the more detailed explanations for future work. These models are of three general sorts, as enumerated by Keeling and Eames, 2005 [25].

First there are what Keeling and Eames call *real networks* (ostensibly a description of an actual community or population from a network perspective). A complete description of a real network is almost impossible even for the smallest populations; however, the sampling of these networks may provide an accurate picture of the structure and function of disease spread among real people. Data for these studies come from infection tracing, where the source of infection for each case in an epidemic is determined [21]; contact tracing, where all the contacts of a source individual, the index case, are identified in order to head off progression of the disease and further potential transmission [17]; and diary-based studies, where subjects keep a record of contacts they make throughout the day. This allows for a larger number of individuals to be sampled in detail [14].

Second we have *simulation models* incorporating networks. These simulations are relatively straightforward and there have been a number of very good studies incorporating networks [13, 20]. These model are typically agent based models that keep track of each individual in the population and simulate their contacts (and disease transmission) over time.

Third there are a plethora of studies involving *idealized networks*. These look at some of the topological characteristics of networks constructed under given constraints and examine the effect that those characteristics have on the spread of a disease. They include random networks where individuals represent nodes with connections that are assigned at random according to some algorithm, for example a fixed number of unique contacts for each node. The dynamics of diseases on random networks can be studied as a simple branching process [12]. In lattice networks, individuals are the nodes in a regular grid, and a fixed number of the adjacent individuals are connected. Lattices are spatially localized and homogeneous and thus highly clustered [19]. Small-world networks are midway between lattices and random networks. Some algorithm is used to take a regular lattice and "rewire" a certain number of connections randomly. At a certain level of rewiring, these networks exhibit both the local dynamics of the regular lattice and the global dynamics of random networks [34]. Spatial networks position individuals within a given space and connected with a probability that depends on their distance according to some rule. In scale-free networks, new individuals are added to a network one by one with each new individual connecting preferentially to individuals that are already highly connected. The result is a power-law distribution of contacts per individual [25]. And in exponential random graphs the probability of a connection between any two nodes is fixed and independent of the probability of a connection between of any other pair of nodes [5].

The essence of all these network approaches is that the edges of the network represent connections or contacts in the context of disease transmission. The different approaches try to preserve some essential feature of the transactions and contacts of the population being described while being as parsimonious as possible about possible architectures. Since the nodes (usually) represent individuals, the whole issue of defining the population and area of interest is implicit in these models. As in the chain binomial models and the agent based models discussed above transmission probabilities are estimated from data that are matched as closely as possible to the particular class of connection being modeled [13].

2 The Chain of Infection

No matter what modeling approach is used, it is the elements of the chain of infection that must be understood if the spread of a particular disease is to be controlled or prevented. The chain of infection consists of six components: (1) pathogens, (2) reservoirs or carriers, (3) portals of exit, (4) modes of transmission, (5) portals of entry, and (6) hosts (susceptibles).

The transmission process begins at the "portal of exit". Table 1 lists the portals of exit [1] and the common means by which the pathogen exits (Fig. 1).

The next link in the chain is the transmission of the pathogen by direct or indirect means to a new host. Table 2 shows the portals of exit and the associated modes of transmission. Transmission by coughing or sneezing, etc. is considered direct if source and recipient are less than a meter apart, other then that *direct* transmission is by physical contact. *Air droplets* are airborne fluids containing an infectious agent,

Table 1 Portals of exit and the activities or processes that enable exit

Portal of exit	Some activities that enable exit
Respiration	Coughing, sneezing and talking
Oral	Saliva – spitting, talking, kissing
Genital	Sexual activity
Intravenous	Bites, needles, and wounds
Urinary	Sexual activity, urination, poor hygiene, poor sanitation
Skin	Lesions, wounds
Gastrointestinal	Feces, vomitus, saliva – poor hygiene, poor sanitation
Cardiovascular (rare)	Possible blood transfusion
Conjunctival	Rubbing eyes, contact with objects
Transplacental	Mother to fetus

[1] Portals of entry and exit are listed in order of the frequency of pathogen *entry* [33].

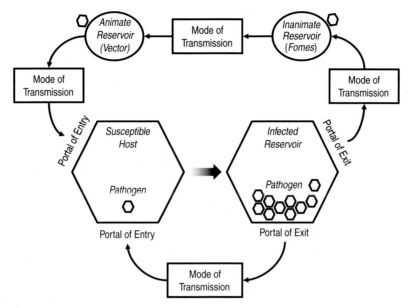

Fig. 1 The "chain of infection". Reservoirs can be any source of infection living or inanimate. In the *bottom loop* the host becomes the next reservoir in the chain; in the *top loop* there are multiple intermediate reservoirs

usually from coughing or sneezing, that has traveled over one meter away from the reservoir. Air transport of the pathogen in dust or by itself is what is meant by *"air dust"*. *Water* and *food* are similarly self explanatory. *Fomites* (fomes sing.) are any inanimate objects or surfaces that can serve as reservoirs, they can be stationary or move. A *vector* is any living organism that serves as a reservoir – *biological* means that the pathogen lives in and possibly causes disease (but not necessarily) in the carrier, *mechanical* means that the pathogen resides on the surface or tissues of the carrier without using the carrier's tissues for nutrition or reproduction.

Table 2 Portals of exit and the modes of transmission. (x's are the most common modes)

Portal of exit	Mode of transmission							
	Direct	Air droplet	Air dust	Water	Fomites	Food	Vector mechanical	Vector biological
Respiratory	< 1*m*	x	x		x	x		
Oral	x			x	x	x		
Genital	x			x	x			
Intravenous					x			x
Urinary	x			x	x			
Skin	x			x	x	x	x	x
Gastrointestinal	x		x	x	x	x	x	x
Cardiovascular		x	x					
Conjunctival	x							
Transplacental	x							

Table 3 Portals of entry and the modes of transmission (x's are the most common modes)

Portal of entry	Direct	Air droplet	Air dust	Water	Fomites	Food	Vector mechanical	Vector biological
Respiratory	$< 1m$	x	x					
Oral	x			x	x	x	x	x
Genital	x			x	x			
Intravenous					x			x
Urinary	x							
Skin	x		x	x	x		x	x
Gastrointestinal	x			x	x	x		
Cardiovascular		x	x					
Conjunctival	x	x	x	x	x			
Transplacental	x							

Finally only certain modes of transmission are usually effective at delivering the pathogen to an appropriate portal of entry – the means by which a new host can become infected (Table 3) [33].

Entry by skin or mucosa is usually via a cut or lesion although some organisms (insects, worms, molds, fungi, etc.) can penetrate through unbroken epithelium. Respiratory entry is in the bronchial passages and lungs themselves, whereas cardiovascular entry is into the bloodstream via the lungs.

Actual transmission from one diseased organism (infected) to new host (susceptible) can occur via multiple steps in the chain of transmission. For example, a dog roles on a dead squirrel picking up a pathogen, then a person pats the dog transferring the pathogen to hands, then the person prepares or handles food, which is eaten by another unwary (and unfortunate) susceptible person. There are at least 4 reservoirs in this chain before reaching the final host.

3 Contact and Transmission Rates

Portals of exit and entry, mode of transmission, social mixing, and social structure, effect the communicability of a disease. The environmental conditions (temperature, humidity, light and other factors) affect the resilience and durability of the pathogen. The ability of the pathogen to penetrate barriers and protections at the portals of entry determine the invasiveness of the disease. And the virulence is the strength of pathogenicity[33], the ability of an inoculate to cause, and the severity of the subsequent disease measured relative to the response of the affected population.

For a typical structured compartmental model the "transmission rate" (β) absorbs much of this information in a single parameter that phenomenologically describes the rate at which new cases are formed from already existing ones. The other part of the communicability is the number of susceptible people that can potentially pick up the disease. This is a function of some sort of communication (direct or indirect) of the pathogen between an infected carrier and the potential host.

Starting with the rate at which one individual comes in contact with another,[2] we begin with a basic conservation principle that contacts are reciprocal [7]. The total number of contacts of group i with group j must be the same as the total number of contacts of group j with group i. In symbols,

n is the number of groups.

c_{ij} is the contact rate of "i" with "j" (units: contacts per person per unit time).

c_i is the total contact rate of "i"; $c_i = \sum_j c_{ij}$ (units: contacts per person per unit time).

p_{ij} is the fraction of "i's" contacts with "j" (or in other words "i's" probability of contacting someone who is a member of "j" given that a contact has taken place); since $p_{ij} = c_{ij}/c_i$ (unitless) then $\sum_j p_{ij} = 1$.

N_i is the number of individuals in group "i" (units: number of people).

The total number of contacts per unit time between "i" and "j" is the same as the total number between "j" and "i", which is

$$c_{ij} N_i = c_{ji} N_j$$
$$p_{ij} c_i N_i = p_{ji} c_j N_j. \qquad (1)$$

Summing over all j

$$\sum_j p_{ji} c_j N_j = \sum_j p_{ij} c_i N_i$$
$$= c_i N_i \sum_j p_{ij}$$
$$= c_i N_i$$

Dividing both sides of the conservation of contacts Equation (1) by $c_i N_i$

$$\frac{p_{ij} c_i N_i}{c_i N_i} = \frac{p_{ji} c_j N_j}{c_i N_i}$$
$$p_{i,j} = \frac{p_{ji} c_j N_j}{\sum_k p_{ki} c_k N_k}. \qquad (2)$$

If we assume that the probability of the member of any group i contacting a member of any other group j (including their own) $p_{i,j}$ is *separable*, that means it is the product of a function of i times a function of j (i.e. $p_{ij} = u_i v_j$) then

$$1 = \sum_j p_{ij} = \sum_j u_i v_j = u_i \sum_j v_j,$$

---

[2] For now we'll use a intuitive sense of what "contact" means and leave more detailed analysis for later.

or

$$u_i = \frac{1}{\sum_j v_j} \text{ for each } i.$$

This implies that u_i is constant for all i, that is $u_i = u$, and that $p_{i,j}$ is a function of just j,

$$p_{ij} = u_i v_j = u v_j = \frac{v_j}{\sum_k v_k}.$$

Using the relationship from Equation (2) we find that

$$p_{ij} = \frac{p_{ji} c_j N_j}{\sum_k p_{ki} c_k N_k} = \frac{u v_i c_j N_j}{\sum_k u v_i c_k N_k} = \frac{c_j N_j}{\sum_k c_k N_k}.$$

Define *proportionate mixing* by

$$\rho_j \equiv \frac{c_j N_j}{\sum_k c_k N_k}, \quad j = 1, 2, \ldots, n,$$

that is, the probability (conditioned on a meeting occurring) that someone from group i meets someone from group j is the same as someone from group h contacting someone from group j. It is equal to the fraction of j's contacts out of all contacts by everyone in the population. The total number of contacts per unit time between i and j in the proportionate mixing case is

$$p_{ij} c_i N_i = \frac{c_i c_j N_i N_j}{\sum_k c_k N_k}$$

$$c_{ij} N_i = \frac{c_i c_j N_i N_j}{\sum_k c_k N_k}.$$

As a brief aside, this last relationship lets us test if the contact probabilities are separable, that is, if the mixing is proportionate. This is important because separability often allows for much simpler analysis of the models. In general the total contacts per unit time of everyone in group i with group j is $c_{ij} N_i = C_{ij} = c_{ji} N_j = C_{ji}$. The contact matrix $\mathbf{C} = [C_{ij}]$ is symmetric, and the column sums and the row sums are the same ($\sum_j C_{ij} = \sum_j C_{ji} = C_i$). The total of all contacts per unit time is $\sum_k c_k N_k = \sum_i \sum_j C_{ij} = C_T$. Thus if the contact probabilities are separable then we should have

$$C_{ij} \approx \frac{C_i C_j}{C_T}.$$

The deviations of the observed elements of the contact matrix (C_{ij}) from the expected elements $C_i C_j C_T^{-1}$ are

$$\delta_{ij} = C_{ij} - \frac{C_i C_j}{C_T}.$$

Note that the sum of the deviations always adds to zero,

$$\sum_j \delta_{ij} = \sum_j \left(C_{ij} - \frac{C_i C_j}{C_T} \right)$$

$$= C_i - \frac{C_i}{C_T} \sum_j C_j$$

$$= C_i - \frac{C_i}{C_T} C_T = 0$$

We can use Pearson's chi-square goodness of fit test, where the test statistic is

$$\chi^2 = C_T \sum_j \sum_i \frac{\delta_{ij}^2}{C_i C_j}$$

to find the probability that the observed contact matrix is consistent with the null hypothesis of proportionate mixing.

In order to calculate the rate of new infections in the general case, let π_j be the probability of an infected person in group "j" transmitting the pathogen given a contact (probability of an effective contact)$(\pi_j c_{is,jI})$. And let ξ_i be the probability of a susceptible person in group "i" getting infected given an *effective* contact . The total number of new infections of susceptibles "i" from all infectives "j" is $\xi_i \pi_j c_{is,jI} S_i$ or equivalently $\xi_i \pi_j p_{is,jI} c_{is} S_i$.[3] The total rate of new infections of susceptibles "i" from all infectives is

$$\text{new cases per unit time in group } i \text{ is} \qquad \xi_i c_{is} S_i \sum_j \pi_j p_{is,jI}$$

Letting $\xi_i c_{S_i} = \beta_i$ so that the transmission rate scales with c_{S_i}, leads to the following expression for the new cases per unit time in group i

$$\beta_i S_i \sum_j \pi_j p_{is,jI}$$

In the separable case with "M" denoting a generic non-susceptible, non-infected class we have

$$p_{is,jI} = \frac{c_{jI} I_j}{\sum_k c_{ks} S_k + c_{kI} I_k + c_{kM} M_k},$$

---

[3] The sub-subscripts are just indicators that the contacts (and contact rates) are between susceptibles and infectives and do not affect the cardinality of the group indices. For example, in an age classified model susceptibles age i_S and infecteds age i_I are both the same age $– i$.

so we can write

$$\text{new cases per unit time in group } i \text{ is } \quad \frac{\beta_i S_i \sum_j \pi_j c_{j_l} I_j}{\sum_k c_{k_S} S_k + c_{k_I} I_k + c_{k_M} M_k}.$$

Now how does all this relate back to the chain of transmission? π – the probability of an infected person transmitting the pathogen given a contact is a function of the portal(s) of exit for the disease, and the mode of transmission. For a given population or group this function would be a weighted average based on the actual frequency of all the possible portals and modes. What is defined as a "contact" and thus contact rate (c_{ij}) is also dependent on the disease's mode of transmission, portals of exit and entry, and the social and technological morphology of the population in question. And ξ – the probability of a susceptible person getting infected is a function of the condition of the susceptible person or group, the virulence of the pathogen, the portal of entry, and mode of transmission. It would be no small achievement to catalogue all of the possible values for these parameters for the most common infectious diseases. Another approach might be to further break down these parameters into factors determined by (i) the pathogen, (ii) the host (iii) local and current environmental conditions and (iv) portals, and modes of transmission alone (independent of the other 3 factors). The components of each can be set up as products of conditional probabilities. For example a possible model for the transmission might look like

$$\pi = \pi_{\text{pathogen}} \cdot \pi_{\text{reservoir}} \cdot \pi_{\text{portal}} \cdot \pi_{\text{transmission}} \cdot \pi_{\text{env}} + error.$$

Each of these components could be analyzed in a generalized linear model from data taken from as many different events as possible. The catalogue of different values for each of the components could then be recombined to match the circumstances of any new outbreak or pending epidemic in order to provide reasonable model results without having to wait for data to come back from the current event.

4 Conclusions

By understanding the process of transmission and particular expression of the components that come together to make up the transmission rate researchers and public health officials have been able to make insightful recommendations about controlling or preventing the spread of a disease. Currently there exists a variety of resources to obtain information about plant, animal and human pathogens (see for example [9, 23, 32]). These include such information as taxonomy, lifecycle, genetic information, epidemiology, hosts, vectors, disease progression, treatments, diagnostic tests, etc. Much information for the modeling of a disease outbreak or epidemic can be gleaned from these sources such as latency and incubation periods, stage progression, recovery periods, infective dose via common portal of entry. However, there is no central database or publication organizing information for the modeling of the infectivity itself for broad range of diseases. By breaking down the infectivity into separate components that can be related back to the chain of infection it may be possible to assemble those parts that are disease independent and those that are disease specific to allow modeling efforts to be possible even if there is very limited information, or different options to be explored under a variety of scenarios. In the mean time, the modeling of contacts between individuals via a matrix **C**, potentially tied to clear social and biological mechanisms, must be seen, in the context of models being fit to data, that is, as a matrix of simply fitted parameters. The potential for incorporating relevant biological and environmental meaning within these parameters exists but so far no clear data-driven methods have been developed to do this.

Acknowledgments I wish to thank Carlos Castillo-Chavez, and Carlos Castillo-Garsow at ASU for their useful and insightful comments. This work was in part supported by funding from The National Science Foundation (DMS-0502349).

References

1. H. Albert, R. Jeong, & A.L. Barabási (1999). Diameter of the world-wide web. Nature 401:130–131.
2. L.A. Amaral, A. Scala, M. Barthelemy, & H.E. Stanley (2000). Classes of small-world networks. Proc. Natl. Acad. Sci. 97(21):11149–11152.
3. R.M. Anderson & R.M. May (1991). Infectious Diseases of Humans: Dynamics and Control. Oxford University Press, Oxford, UK.
4. M. Artzrouni (1990). On transient effects in the HIV/AIDS epidemic. J. Math. Biol. 28: 271–291.
5. B. Bollobás (1985). Random Graphs. Academic Press 516 pgs. London.
6. F. Brauer (1990). Models for the spread of universally fatal diseases. J. Math. Biol. 28: 451–462.
7. C. Castillo-Chavez, S. Busenberg, & K. Gerow (1991). Pair formation in structured populations. In: Differential Equations with Applications in Biology, Physics and Engineering., J. Goldstein, F. Kappel, & W. Schappacher, eds. Marced Dekker, New York pp. 47–65.
8. C. Castillo-Chavez , H.W. Hethcote, V. Andreasen, S.A. Levin, & W.M. Liu (1989). Epidemiological models with age structure, proportionate mixing, and cross-immunity. J. Math. Biol. 27:233–258.
9. Center for Disease Control & Prevention CDC website CDC Atlanta, GA. http://www.cdc.gov/ Cited 12 Dec. 2008
10. F.B. Cohen (1994). A Short Course on Computer Viruses. Wiley 250 pgs. New York.
11. D.J. Daley & J. Gani (1999). Epidemic Modeling: An Introduction Cambridge University Press, N.Y, New York. 228 pgs.
12. O. Diekmann, J.A.P. Heesterbeek, & J.A.J. Metz (1998). A deterministic epidemic model taking account of repeated contacts between the same individuals. J. Appl. Prob. 35:462–468.
13. K.T.D. Eames, & M.J. Keeling (2002). Modeling dynamic and network heterogeneities in the spread of sexually transmitted diseases. Proc. Natl Acad. Sci. 99:13330–13335.
14. W.J. Edmunds, C.J. O'Callaghan, & D.J. Nokes (1997). Who mixes with whom? A method to determine the contact patterns of adults that may lead to the spread of airborne infections. Proc. R. Soc. B 264:949–957.
15. J. Gani, & D. Jerwood (1971). Markov Chain Methods in Chain Binomial Epidemic Models. Biometrics, 27(3):591–603.

16. G.P. Garnett (2002). An introduction to mathematical models in sexually transmitted disease epidemiology. Sex. Transm. Inf. 78:7–12.
17. A.C. Ghani & G.P. Garnett (1998). Measuring sexual partner networks for transmission of sexually transmitted diseases. J. R. Stat. Soc. A 161, 227–238.
18. M. Greenwood (1931). The statistical measure of infectiveness. J. Hygiene, 31: 336–351.
19. B.T. Grenfell, O.N. Bjornstad, & J. Kappey (2001). Travelling waves and spatial hierarchies in measles epidemics. Nature 414:716–723.
20. M.E. Halloran, I.M. Longini, Jr., A. Nizam, & Y. Yang (2002). Containing bioterrorist smallpox. Science 298:1428–1432.
21. D.T. Haydon, M. Chase-Topping, D.J. Shaw, L. Matthews, J.K. Friar, J. Wilesmith, & M.E.J. Woolhouse (2003). The construction and analysis of epidemic trees with reference to the 2001 UK foot-and-mouth outbreak. Proc. R. Soc. B 270:121–127.
22. H.W. Hethcote (2000). The mathematics of infectious diseases. Siam Rev., 42(4):599–653.
23. D. L. Heymann, ed. (2004). Control of Communicable Diseases Manual. American Public Health Association. 700 pgs. Wasington D.C.
24. M.J. Keeling (2005). Implications of network structure for epidemic dynamics. Theor. Popul. Biol. 67:1–8.
25. M.J. Keeling & K.T.D. Eames (2005). Networks and epidemic models. J. R. Soc. Interface 2:295–307.
26. J.O. Kephart, G.B. Sorkin, D.M. Chess, & S.R. White (1997). Fighting computer viruses. Sci. Am. 277(5):88–93.
27. W.O. Kermack & A.G. McKendrick (1927). Contributions to the mathematical theory of epidemics, part 1. Proc. Roy. Soc. London Ser. A, 115:700–721.
28. I.M. Longini, Jr., A. Nizam, S. Xu, K. Ungchusak, J. Hanshaoworakul, D.A.T. Cummings, & M.E. Halloran (2005). Containing Pandemic Influenza at the Source. Science, 309:1083–1087. and online supporting material at www.sciencemag.org/cgi/content/full/309/5737/1078/DC1.
29. R.M. May & A.L. Lloyd (2001). Infection dynamics on scale-free networks. Physical Review E 64:066112.
30. L.F. Olsen & W.M. Schaffer (1990). Chaos Versus Noisy Periodicity:Alternative Hypotheses for Childhood Epidemics. Science 249(4968):499–504.
31. R. Pastor-Satorras & A. Vespignani (2001). Epidemic spreading in scale-free networks. Phys. Rev. E 63:066117.
32. Pathport: The pathogen portal project (2002). Virginia Bioinformatics Institute. Blacksburg, VA. http://pathport.vbi.vt.edu/pathinfo/index.php Cited 12 Dec. 2008
33. T.C. Timmreck (1994). An Introduction to Epidemiology. Jones & Bartlett 484 pgs. Boston.
34. D.J. Watts & S.H. Strogatz (1998). Collective dynamics of 'small-world' networks. Nature 393: 440–442.
35. E.B. Wilson & M.H. Burke (1942). The epidemic curve. Proc. Nat. Acad. Sci. 28(9): 361–367.

The Effective Reproduction Number as a Prelude to Statistical Estimation of Time-Dependent Epidemic Trends

Hiroshi Nishiura and Gerardo Chowell

Abstract Although the basic reproduction number, R_0, is useful for understanding the transmissibility of a disease and designing various intervention strategies, the classic threshold quantity theoretically assumes that the epidemic first occurs in a fully susceptible population, and hence, R_0 is essentially a mathematically defined quantity. In many instances, it is of practical importance to evaluate time-dependent variations in the transmission potential of infectious diseases. Explanation of the time course of an epidemic can be partly achieved by estimating the effective reproduction number, $R(t)$, defined as the actual average number of secondary cases per primary case at calendar time t (for $t > 0$). $R(t)$ shows time-dependent variation due to the decline in susceptible individuals (intrinsic factors) and the implementation of control measures (extrinsic factors). If $R(t) < 1$, it suggests that the epidemic is in decline and may be regarded as being *under control* at time t (vice versa, if $R(t) > 1$). This chapter describes the primer of mathematics and statistics of $R(t)$ and discusses other similar markers of transmissibility as a function of time.

1 Introduction

The basic reproduction number, R_0 (pronounced as *R nought*), is a key quantity used to estimate transmissibility of infectious diseases. Theoretically, R_0 is defined as the average number of secondary cases generated by a single primary case during its entire period of infectiousness in a fully susceptible population [14]. The reproduction number, R, is directly related to the type and intensity of interventions necessary to control an epidemic since the objective of public health efforts is to achieve $R < 1$ as soon as possible. One of the best known utilities of R_0 is in determining the critical coverage of immunization required to eradicate a disease in a randomly mixing population. When an effective vaccine is available against the disease in question, it is of interest to estimate the critical proportion of the

H. Nishiura (✉)
Theoretical Epidemiology, University of Utrecht, Yalelaan 7, 3584 CL, Utrecht, The Netherlands
e-mail: h.nishiura@uu.nl

G. Chowell et al. (eds.), *Mathematical and Statistical Estimation Approaches in Epidemiology*, DOI 10.1007/978-90-481-2313-1_5,
© Springer Science+Business Media B.V. 2009

population that needs to be vaccinated (*i.e.* vaccination coverage) in order to attain $R < 1$ [3, 4, 33]. Considering the so-called *control relation*, $1 - \frac{1}{R_0}$, the protection conferred to the population by achieving a critical vaccination coverage, *herd immunity*, yields the threshold condition for the eradication of a disease [18, 28]. As it is extensively discussed elsewhere [13, 14], the mathematical definition of R_0 is given by using the next generation matrix where R_0 is in the simplest case calculated as the dominant eigenvalue (see Chapter 1). In addition to the threshold phenomena, R_0 has been classically used to suggest the *severity* of an epidemic, because the proportion of those experiencing infection at the end of an epidemic (i.e. *final size*) depends only on R_0 [23]. The basic statistical methods to estimate R_0 from observed epidemiological datasets have been reviewed by Klaus Dietz elsewhere [15].

Although R_0 may be useful for understanding the transmissibility of a disease and designing various intervention strategies, the classic threshold quantity theoretically assumes that the epidemic first occurs in a *fully* susceptible population, and hence, R_0 is essentially a *mathematically defined* quantity. In addition to R_0, it is of practical importance to evaluate time-dependent variations in the transmission potential. Explanation of the time course of an epidemic can be partly achieved by estimating the effective reproduction number, $R(t)$, defined as the actual average number of secondary cases per primary case at calendar time t (for $t > 0$) [6–10, 22, 29, 30, 35]. $R(t)$ shows time-dependent variation due to the decline in susceptible individuals (intrinsic factors) and the implementation of control measures (extrinsic factors). If $R(t) < 1$, it suggests that the epidemic is in decline and may be regarded as being *under control* at time t (vice versa, if $R(t) > 1$). Even when effective interventions against a specific disease are limited, it is plausible that the contact frequency leading to infection varies as a function of time owing to the recognition of epidemics and/or dissemination of the relevant information through mass media. In this chapter, we show how $R(t)$ is mathematically defined and how it can be estimated from the observed epidemiological datasets. In addition, other similar time-dependent threshold quantities, which have been proposed in a few practical settings, are discussed.

2 Renewal Equation Offers the Conceptual Understanding of $R(t)$

2.1 Infection-Age Structured Model

To understand the theoretical concept of $R(t)$, we first consider an *infection-age* structured epidemic model. Hereafter, *infection-age* stands for the time elapsed since infection. Whereas the simple modified version (or widely known form) of the Kermack-McKendrick model is governed by ODEs (e.g. SIR and SEIR models), the very initial model employed the infection-age structured assumption from in 1927 [24]. Nevertheless, the mathematical importance of the original model was recognized only after the 1970s [12, 27]. We denote the numbers of susceptible and recovered individuals by $S(t)$ and $U(t)$ (Note: to avoid any confusions between the effective reproduction number and the recovered individuals, we denote the recovered individuals by $U(t)$ hereafter). Further, let $i(t, \tau)$ be the density of infectious individuals at calendar time t and infection-age τ. The infection-age structured SIR model is given by

$$\frac{dS(t)}{dt} = -\lambda(t)S(t)$$

$$\left(\frac{\partial}{\partial t} + \frac{\partial}{\partial \tau} \right) i(t, \tau) = -\gamma(\tau)i(t, \tau) \tag{1}$$

$$i(t, 0) = \lambda(t)S(t)$$

$$\frac{dU(t)}{dt} = \int_0^\infty \gamma(\tau)i(t, \tau)\, d\tau$$

where $\lambda(t)$ is referred to as the *force of infection* (foi) at calendar time t (i.e. foi is defined as the rate at which susceptible individuals get infected) which is given by:

$$\lambda(t) = \int_0^\infty \beta(\tau)i(t, \tau)\, d\tau \tag{2}$$

and $\beta(\tau)$ and $\gamma(\tau)$ are the rates of secondary transmissions per single infectious case and recovery at infection-age τ, respectively. It should be noted that the above model has not taken into account the background host demography (i.e. birth and death). In a closed population, the total population size N is thus given by

$$N = S(t) + \int_0^\infty i(t, \tau)\, d\tau + U(t) \tag{3}$$

which is independent of calendar time t. The system (1) can be reasonably integrated along the characteristic line

$$i(t, \tau) = \Gamma(\tau)j(t - \tau) \tag{4}$$

for $t - \tau > 0$ (and $\frac{\Gamma(\tau)}{\Gamma(\tau - t)} j_0(\tau - t)$ for $\tau - t > 0$) where

$$j(t) = i(t, 0) \tag{5}$$

and

$$\Gamma(\tau) = \exp\left(-\int_0^\tau \gamma(\sigma)\, d\sigma \right) \tag{6}$$

and $j_0(\tau)$ informs the infection-age distribution of initially infected individuals at the beginning of an epidemic. Accordingly, the number of new infections at calendar time t, $j(t)$, is referred to as the *incidence of infection*. It is not difficult to derive

$$S(t) = S(0) - \int_0^t j(\sigma)\,d\sigma \tag{7}$$

from (1). Thus, the subequation of $i(t, 0)$ in system (1) is rewritten as

$$j(t) = \lambda(t)\left[S(0) - \int_0^t j(\sigma)\,d\sigma\right] \tag{8}$$

Taking into account the initial condition in (4), Equation (8) is rewritten as

$$j(t) = \left[S(0) - \int_0^t j(\sigma)\,d\sigma\right]\left[G(t) + \int_0^t \psi(\tau)j(t - \tau)\,d\tau\right] \tag{9}$$

where

$$\psi(\tau) = \beta(\tau)\Gamma(\tau) \tag{10}$$

$$G(t) = \int_0^\infty \beta(\sigma + t)\frac{\Gamma(\sigma + t)}{\Gamma(\sigma)}j_0(\sigma)\,d\sigma \tag{11}$$

Considering the initial invasion phase (i.e. exponential growth phase of an epidemic), we get a linearized equation

$$j(t) = S(0)G(t) + S(0)\int_0^t \psi(\tau)j(t - \tau)\,d\tau \tag{12}$$

The Equation (12) represents Lotka's integral equation, where the basic reproduction number, R_0, is given by

$$R_0 = S(0)\int_0^\infty \psi(\tau)\,d\tau \tag{13}$$

Thus, the epidemic will grow if $R_0 > 1$ and decline to extinction if $R_0 < 1$. Assuming that the infection-age distribution is stable, we get a simplified renewal equation

$$j(t) = \int_0^\infty A(\tau)j(t - \tau)\,d\tau \tag{14}$$

where $A(\tau)$ is the product of $\psi(\tau)$ and $S(0)$, indicating the rate of secondary transmissions caused by a single primary case at calendar time 0 and infection-age τ. Assuming that we observe an exponential growth of incidence during the initial phase (i.e. $j(t) = k \exp(rt)$ where k and r are, respectively, a constant ($k > 0$) and the intrinsic growth rate), the following relationship is obtained:

$$j(t) = j(t - \tau) \exp(r\tau) \tag{15}$$

Replacing $j(t - \tau)$ in the right hand side of (14) by (15), we get

$$j(t) = \int_0^\infty A(\tau) j(t) \exp(-r\tau) \, d\tau \tag{16}$$

Removing $j(t)$ from both sides of (16), we get the Euler-Lotka characteristic equation:

$$1 = \int_0^\infty e^{-r\tau} A(\tau), d\tau \tag{17}$$

Further, we consider a probability density of the *generation time* (i.e. the time from infection of a primary case to the infection of a secondary case by the primary case [34]), denoted by $w(\tau)$:

$$w(\tau) := \frac{A(\tau)}{\int_0^\infty A(x) dx} = \frac{A(\tau)}{R_0}. \tag{18}$$

Using (18), the Equation (17) is replaced by

$$\frac{1}{R_0} = \int_0^\infty \exp(-r\tau) w(\tau), d\tau \tag{19}$$

The Equations (15), (16), (17), (18), (19) are what Wallinga and Lipsitch have discussed, revisiting the classical theory of Lotka [16, 36], which reasonably suggests the relationship between the generation-time distribution and R_0. Accordingly, the estimator of R_0 using the intrinsic growth rate is given by:

$$\hat{R}_0 = \frac{1}{M(-r)}, \tag{20}$$

where $M(-r)$ is the moment generating function of the generation-time distribution $w(\tau)$, given the intrinsic growth rate r [36]. Equation (20) significantly improved the issue of estimating R_0 using the intrinsic growth rate alone, because (20) permits validating estimates of R_0 by various different distributional assumptions for $w(\tau)$. The importance of realistic assumptions for the distributions of latent and infectious periods has been emphasized in recent studies [25, 26, 32, 37, 39] and indeed, this point is addressed by (20) to gain robust estimate of R_0. It should be noted that the convolution of latent and infectious periods yields $w(\tau)$. Since the assumed lengths of generation time most likely yielded different estimates of R_0, for example, for

Spanish influenza by different studies [30], Equation (20) highlights a critical need to clarify the generation time distribution using observed data.

2.2 Deriving the Estimator of the Effective Reproduction Number

To further derive an estimator of $R(t)$, we consider the non-linear phase of an epidemic. Derivation of R_0 given by (20) assumes an exponential growth which is applicable only during the very initial phase of an epidemic (or, when the transmission is stationary over time), and thus, it is of practical importance to widen the applicability of the above-described renewal equations in order to appropriately interpret the time-course of an epidemic. We explicitly account for the depletion of susceptible individuals, as we deal with an estimation issue with time-inhomogeneous assumptions. Adopting the *mass action* principle of Kermack and McKendrick, we get:

$$j(t) = S(t) \int_0^\infty \psi(\tau) j(t - \tau) \, d\tau$$
$$= \int_0^\infty A(t, \tau) j(t - \tau) \, d\tau \tag{21}$$

where $A(t, \tau)$ is interpreted as the reproductive power at calendar time t and infection-age τ at which an infected individual generates secondary cases. We refer to the Equation (21) as a non-autonomous renewal equation, where the number of new infections at calendar time t is proportional to the number of infectious individuals (as assumed in the renewal equation in the initial phase).

Using Equation (21), the effective reproduction number, $R(t)$ (i.e. the *instantaneous* reproduction number at calendar time t) is defined as:

$$R(t) = \int_0^\infty A(t, \tau) \, d\tau \tag{22}$$

where $A(t, \tau)$ is, in practical terms, decomposed as

$$A(t, \tau) = S(t)\beta(\tau)\Gamma(\tau) \tag{23}$$

Following (23), we can immediately see that $R(t)$ with an autonomous assumption (i.e. where contact and recovery rates do not vary with time) is given by:

$$R(t) = \frac{S(t)}{S(0)} R_0 \tag{24}$$

which is shown in [14]. In practical terms, Equation (24) reflects the temporal decline in the epidemic due to depletion of susceptible individuals. This corresponds to the classic assumption of the Kermack and McKendrick model.

However, as we discussed in the beginning of this chapter, we postulate that human contact behaviors (and other extrinsic factors) modifies the dynamics as a function of epidemic time, assuming that the decline in incidence does reflect not only depletion of susceptibles but also various extrinsic dynamics (e.g. isolation and contact tracing). Thus, instead of the assumption in (21), we assume time-inhomogeneous $\psi(t, \tau)$; *i.e.*

$$
\begin{aligned}
j(t) &= S(t) \int_0^\infty \psi(t, \tau) j(t - \tau) \, d\tau \\
&= \int_0^\infty A(t, \tau) j(t - \tau) \, d\tau
\end{aligned}
\tag{25}
$$

to describe $A(t, \tau)$.

Even so, it is convenient to assume separation of variables for $A(t, \tau)$ to derive simple estimator of $R(t)$ (implicitly assuming that the relative infectiousness to infection-age is independent of calendar time) [20]. Under this assumption, $A(t, \tau)$ is rewritten as the product of two functions $\phi_1(t)$ and $\phi_2(\tau)$:

$$
A(t, \tau) = \phi_1(t)\phi_2(\tau)
\tag{26}
$$

Arbitrarily assuming a normalized density for $\phi_2(\tau)$, *i.e.*,

$$
\int_0^\infty \phi_2(\tau) \, d\tau \equiv 1
\tag{27}
$$

then, it is easy to find that

$$
R(t) = \int_0^\infty A(t, \tau) \, d\tau = \phi_1(t)
\tag{28}
$$

suggesting that the function $\phi_1(t)$ is equivalent to the (instantaneous) effective reproduction number $R(t)$. Another function $\phi_2(\tau)$ represents the density of infection events as a function of infection-age τ. Accordingly, we can immediately see that $\phi_2(\tau)$ is exactly the same as $w(\tau)$, the generation-time distribution. That is, the above arguments suggest that $A(t, \tau)$ (i.e. the rate at which an infectious individual at calendar time t and infection-age τ produces secondary cases) is decomposed as:

$$
A(t, \tau) = R(t)w(\tau)
\tag{29}
$$

Inserting (29) into (25) yields an estimator of $R(t)$ [20]:

$$
\hat{R}(t) = \frac{j(t)}{\int_0^\infty j(t - \tau)w(\tau) \, d\tau}
\tag{30}
$$

Another type of the effective reproduction number as a function of time considers the number of secondary cases per single primary case as a function of calendar time when the primary case experienced infection. Due to this reason, the reproduction number is referred to as the *cohort* reproduction number, $R_c(t)$, defined as

$$R_c(t) = \int_0^\infty A(t + \tau, \tau)\, d\tau \tag{31}$$

If the separable assumption (28) is the case, Equation (31) is rewritten as

$$R_c(t) = \int_0^\infty R(t + \tau)w(\tau)\, d\tau \tag{32}$$

which is interpreted as a smoothed function of the instantaneous reproduction number [20, 21]. The above Equation (32) is exactly what was proposed in applications to SARS [35] and foot and mouth disease [17]. Preceding these definitions in infectious disease epidemiology [20], both $R(t)$ and $R_c(t)$ have been explicitly defined as the period and cohort total fertility rates, respectively, in mathematical demography [1]. The difference between $R(t)$ and $R_c(t)$ is highlighted when a specific event at calendar time t occurs (e.g. a public health intervention starts at calendar time t). Then, $R(t)$ abruptly varies (e.g. declines) with calendar time t, but $R_c(t)$ smoothly varies, because $R_c(t)$ smooth out the timing (i.e. infection-age) of secondary transmissions among a cohort who experienced infection at calendar time t.

Discretizing (30) and (32) to apply them to the daily incidence data (i.e. using j_i incident cases infected between time t_i and time t_{i+1} and descretized generation time distribution w_i),

$$\hat{R}(t_i) = \frac{j_i}{\sum_{j=0}^n j_{i-j} w_j} \tag{33}$$

can be used as the estimator of $R(t)$, and

$$\hat{R}_c(t_i) = \sum_{m=0}^n \frac{j_{i+m} w_j}{\sum_{k=0}^n j_{i+m-k} w_k} \tag{34}$$

as the estimator of $R_c(t)$. However, it should be noted that the study in SARS implicitly assumed that onset data $c(t)$ at calendar time t reflects the above discussed infection event $j(t)$ [35]. That is, supposing that we observed c_i onset cases reported between t_i and t_{i+1}, $R_c(t)$ was calculated as

$$\hat{R}_c(t_i) = \frac{c_i}{\sum_{j=0}^n c_{i-j} s_j} \tag{35}$$

where s_j is the discretized *serial interval* which is defined as the time from onset of a primary case to onset of the secondary cases [19]. The method permits reasonable transformation of an epidemic curve (i.e. temporal distribution of case onset) to the estimates of time-inhomogeneous cohort reproduction number $R_c(t)$. Employing the relative likelihood of case k infected by case l using the density function of serial interval $s(t)$; *i.e.*,

$$p_{(k,l)} = \frac{s(t_k - t_l|\theta)}{\sum_{m \neq k} s(t_k - t_m|\theta)} \tag{36}$$

the expected value and variance of $R_c(t_i)$ are given by the following

$$E(R_c(t_i)) = \frac{1}{n_t^2} \sum_{l:t_l=t} \sum_{k=1}^{n-q} p_{(k,l)} \tag{37}$$

$$\text{Var}(R_c(t_i)) = \frac{1}{n_t^2} \sum_{k=1}^{n-q} \left(\sum_{l:t_l=t} p_{(k,l)}(1 - p_{(k,l)}) - \sum_{l,m:t_l=t_m=t} p_{(k,l)}p_{(k,m)} \right)$$

where n_t is the total number of reported case onsets at calendar time t [11].

Using the above described methods (or similar concepts with similar assumptions), we can transform epidemic curves into the effective reproduction number and assess the impact of control measures on an epidemic. However, whereas the Equations (33) and (35) are similar in theory, we need to explicitly account for the difference between onset and infection event. In fact, when there are many asymptomatic infections and asymptomatic secondary transmissions, serial interval is not equivalent to the generation time, and thus, directly adopting the above methods would be inappropriate.

3 Applying Theory to the Data

3.1 A Simple Example

Here we consider a simplified example of pandemic influenza from 1918 to 1919 in Prussia, Germany [30]. Medical officers in Prussia recorded the daily number of influenza deaths from 29 September 1918 to 1 February 1919 (Fig. 1) [31]; a total of 8911 deaths were reported. Throughout the pandemic period in Germany, the largest number of deaths was seen in this fall wave. Prussia represents the northern part of present Germany and at the time of the pandemic it was part of the Weimer Republic as a free state following World War I. The death data were collected from 28 different local districts surrounding the town of Arnsberg, which, at the time of the epidemic, had a population of approximately 2.5 million individuals (the mortality rate in this period being 0.36%). Although case fatality for the entire observation

Fig. 1 Epidemic curve of pandemic influenza in Prussia, Germany, from 1918 to 1919. Reported daily number of influenza deaths (*solid line*) and the back-calculated temporal distribution of onset cases (*dashed line*). Daily counts of onset cases were obtained using the time delay distribution from onset to death (Fig. 2). Data source: Ref [31]

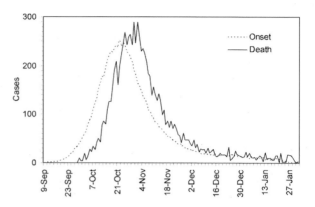

area was not documented, the numbers of cases and deaths during part of the fall wave were recorded for 25 districts. Among a total of 61,824 cases, 1609 deaths were observed, yielding a case fatality estimate of 2.60% (95% CI: 2.48, 2.73). For simplicity, the inflow and outflow of individuals migrating between Prussia and other areas were ignored in the following analysis.

The daily incidence (i.e. daily case onset) was back-calculated using the daily number of influenza deaths (Fig. 1) and the time delay distribution from onset to death (Fig. 2). Given $f(\tau)$, the frequency of death τ days after onset, the relationship between the reported daily number of deaths, $D(t)$, and daily incidence, $C(t)$, at calendar time t is given by:

$$D(t) = p \int_0^t C(t - \tau) f(\tau) \, d\tau \tag{38}$$

where p is the case fatality ratio, which is independent of time. Although the case fatality, p, was not taken into account in Fig. 1, the following model reasonably cancels out the effect of p assuming that the conditional probability of death given infection is independent of time.

Fig. 2 Distribution of the time delay from onset to death during the influenza epidemic in Prussia, Germany, from 1918 to 1919. Time from disease onset (i.e. fever) to death is given for 6233 influenza deaths. A simple 5-day moving average was applied to the original data. Data source: Ref [31]

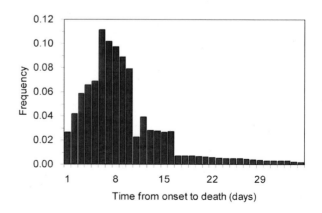

The effective reproduction number can be estimated using estimators (33) and (34), but, unfortunately, detailed information on the distribution of the generation time, $w(\tau)$, has yet to be clarified for pandemic influenza, and historical records often offer only the approximate mean length. Thus, the analyses conducted here simplify the model using various mean lengths of the generation time assumed in previous studies. Supposing that we observed C_i cases in generation i, the expected number of cases in generation $i + 1$, $E(C_{i+1})$ occurring a mean generation time after onset of C_i is given by:

$$E(C_{i+1}) = C_i R_i \tag{39}$$

where R_i is the effective (cohort) reproduction number in generation i. That is, cases in each generation, C_1, C_2, C_3, ..., C_n are given by $C_0 R_0$, $C_1 R_1$, $C_2 R_2$, ..., $C_{n-1} R_{n-1}$ and also by $C_0 R_0$, $C_0 R_0 R_1$, $C_0 R_0 R_1 R_2$, ..., $C_0 \prod_{k=0}^{n-1} R_k$, respectively. By incorporating variations in the number of secondary transmissions generated by each case into the same generation (referred to as the offspring distribution), the model can be formalized using a discrete-time branching process [5]. The Poisson process is conventionally assumed to model the offspring distribution, representing stochasticity (i.e. randomness) in the transmission process. This assumption indicates that the conditional distribution of the number of cases in generation $i + 1$ given C_i is given by:

$$C_{i+1} \mid C_i \sim \text{Poisson}[C_i R_i] \tag{40}$$

For observation of cases from generation 0 to N, the likelihood of estimating R_i is given by:

$$L = \text{constant} \times \prod_{j=0}^{N-1} (C_j R_j)^{C_{j+1}} \exp(-C_j R_j) \tag{41}$$

Since the Poisson distribution represents a one parameter power series distribution, the expected values and uncertainty bounds of R_i can be obtained for each generation. The 95% CI were derived from the profile likelihood. Since the length of the generation time in previous studies ranged from 0.9 to 6 days, three different fixed-length generation times (i.e. 1, 3 and 5 days) are assumed for Equation (41) with respect to the observed data. Although application of the delta function for the generation time suffers some overlapping of cases in successive generations, this exercise ignored this and, rather, focused on the time variation in transmissibility using this simple assumption. That is, assuming that the generation-time distribution of length τ, $w(\tau)$, is given by the following delta function with the mean length 1, 3 or 5 days,

$$w(\tau) = \infty, \quad \text{for } \tau = 1, \ 3 \ or \ 5 \tag{42}$$

and $w(\tau) = 0$ otherwise, and for each assumption of the mean length, the daily number of cases was grouped by the determined generation time length. Whereas the choice of generation time therefore affects estimates of R_i, it does not affect the ability to predict the temporal distribution of cases. It should be noted that this simple model assumes a homogeneous pattern of spread.

Figure 3 shows time variations in the estimated effective reproduction numbers obtained assuming three different generation times (i.e. 1, 3 and 5 days) compared with the corresponding epidemic curve. Epidemic date 0 represents 9 September 1918 when the back-calculated onset of cases initially yielded a value the nearest integer of which was 1. Since the precision of the estimate is influenced by the observed number of cases, wide 95% confidence intervals were observed for estimates using a short generation time. However, these time variations in $R(t)$

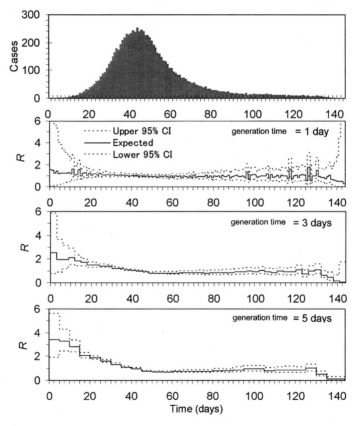

Fig. 3 Epidemic curve and the corresponding effective reproduction numbers (R) with variable generation times. Time variation in the effective reproduction number (the number of secondary infections generated per case by generation) assuming three different generation times is shown. The generation time was assumed to be 1 (second from the top), 3 (*lower middle*) and 5 days (*bottom*). Days are counted from September 9, 1918, onwards

exhibited similar qualitative patterns: (i) although the $R(t)$ was highest at the beginning of the epidemic, the estimates fell below 1 when the epidemic curve came close to the peak (i.e. Days 45–50). For example, the estimated $R(t)$ at Day 50 was 0.92 (95% CI: 0.79, 1.06), 0.82 (0.75, 0.89) and 0.72 (0.67, 0.78), respectively, for a generation time of 1, 3 and 5 days. This period corresponds to the time when public health measures were instituted, e.g. obligatory case reporting, encouragement of mask wearing, and closing of public buildings such as churches and theaters [31]. (ii) Thereafter, $R(t)$ stayed slightly below unity, reflecting a slow decline in the number of onset cases. (iii) Shortly before the end of the epidemic (i.e. Days 90–120), $R(t)$ increased again above 1. (iv) Finally, the expected values of $R(t)$ fell below 1 very close to the end of the epidemic. In this stage, estimates assuming a short generation time exhibited wide uncertainty bounds, reflecting stochasticity due to the small number of cases.

Figure 4 compares the expected values of $R(t)$ assuming each of the generation times employed. Although the possibility of individual heterogeneity (e.g. potential superspreaders in the early stage) cannot be excluded, $R(t)$ at calendar time $t = 0$ is theoretically equivalent to R_0. Assuming generation times of 1, 3 and 5 days, R_0 was estimated to be 1.58 (95% CI: 0.03, 10.32), 2.52 (0.75, 5.85) and 3.41 (1.91, 5.57), respectively. It is remarkable, therefore, to see that $R(t)$ largely depends on the assumed length of the generation time. That is, the longer the generation time, the higher the $R(t)$. It should also be noted that the relationship between $R(t)$ and the generation time is reversed when the epidemic is under control (i.e. when $R(t) < 1$ in the later stage of the epidemic). The finding is analytically interpretable from Equation (20) which suggests that the absolute number of the reproduction number

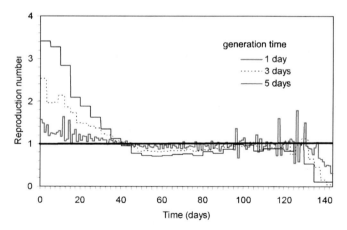

Fig. 4 Comparison of the effective reproduction number assuming different generation times. Expected values of the effective reproduction number with a generation time of 1 (*grey*), 3 (*dashed black*) and 5 days (*solid black*). The *horizontal solid line* represents the threshold value, $R = 1$, below which the epidemic will decline to extinction. Days are counted from September 9, 1918, onwards

is informed by the growth rate of an epidemic as well as the shape and scale of the generation time distribution [32, 36].

3.2 What to do with the Coarsely Reported Data?

Although we usually seek for precisely reported data (e.g. daily counts of cases) to estimate the reproduction number as a function of time, it is impractical in many instances to report observations every day (or to be more precise). If the datasets are reported in a very coarse interval, we have to consider alternative simple algorithms to deal with interval censoring. There are two approaches.

The first is the geometric approximation. As above, we consider that the expected number of cases in generations $0, 1, 2, \ldots, i$ follows a simple geometric series, but with a constant reproduction number, R_k, in a single reporting interval k:

$$a, \ a R_k, \ a R_k^2, \ldots, \ a R_k^i \tag{43}$$

where a denotes the number of index cases in the first generation of reporting interval k. As a special case, suppose that the reporting interval, Δt, is exactly a multiple of the mean generation time (i.e. $\Delta t = ng$ where g and n are the mean generation time and an integer, respectively). In that case, the numbers of cases in k-th and $(k + 1)$-th reports, J_k and J_{k+1}, are

$$J_k = a + a R_k + a R_k^2 + \ldots + a R_k^{n-1} \tag{44}$$

$$= a \sum_{i=0}^{n-1} R_k^i \tag{45}$$

and

$$J_{k+1} = a R_k^n + a R_k^n R_{k+1} + a R_k^n R_{k+1}^2 + \ldots + a R_k^n R_{k+1}^{n-1} \tag{46}$$

$$= a R_k^n \sum_{i=0}^{n-1} R_{k+1}^i \tag{47}$$

where R_k and R_{k+1} are the effective reproduction numbers in reporting intervals k and $k + 1$, respectively. Thus, given an observation of J_k cases in interval k, the expected number of cases in the next interval $k + 1$, $\mathrm{E}(J_{k+1} \mid J_k)$, is given by

$$\mathrm{E}(J_{k+1} \mid J_k) = \frac{(1 - R_k)(1 - R_{k+1}^n) R_k^n J_k}{(1 - R_{k+1})(1 - R_k^n)} \tag{48}$$

It should be noted that n is the number of generations included in each reporting interval.

When the geometric approximation is not feasible (e.g. when the reporting interval is not exactly the multiple of the mean generation time), the exponential approximation should replace the geometric approach. Let r_k and r_{k+1} be the constant growth rates of cases in reporting intervals k and $k + 1$, the conditional expectation (48) is replaced by

$$E(J_{k+1} \mid J_k) = \frac{J_k r_k \exp(r_k \triangle t)}{r_{k+1}} \frac{\exp(r_{k+1} \triangle t) - 1}{\exp(r_k \triangle t) - 1} \qquad (49)$$

where $\triangle t$ is the length of reporting interval. Using the maximum likelihood method, the growth rates r_k are estimated for each reporting interval k. Subsequently, R_k in each reporting interval k is estimated as

$$R_k = \frac{1}{M(-r_k)} \qquad (50)$$

which is analogous to Equation (20).

In this way, even when the reporting interval is coarse (e.g. exceeding the mean generation time), we can still get approximate estimates of R_k which is assumed constant during the single reporting interval. Nevertheless, the linear approximation diminishes precision, and thus, it should be remembered that the observation in more precise reporting interval always gives better insights into the time-course of an epidemic.

4 Incidence-to-Prevalence Ratio and the Actual Reproduction Number

As discussed in the last section, it is frequently the case that the generation time for a specific disease has yet to be estimated, and we do not have the relevant data. Previously, another simple method was proposed; namely, the *incidence-to-prevalence ratio* has been employed in interpreting the time course of an epidemic [2, 38]. In particular, the method has been employed to understand the time course of the HIV epidemic. Although it is true that the problem of long generation times for HIV would complicate the interpretation of the simple method (and thus, the instantaneous and cohort reproduction numbers may always provide better information), here we explicitly consider theoretical backgrounds of this simple method.

As we did in the previous sections, we consider the renewal equation:

$$j(t) = S(t) \int_0^\infty \beta(\tau) i(t, \tau) \, d\tau$$
$$= S(t) \int_0^\infty \beta(\tau) \Gamma(\tau) j(t - \tau) \, d\tau \qquad (51)$$

which employs Kermack and McKendrick type assumption. Following Amundsen et al. [2], here we mathematically define the actual reproduction number, $R_a(t)$. Since the prevalence at calendar time t, $I(t)$, is given by

$$I(t) = \int_0^\infty i(t, \tau) \, d\tau \tag{52}$$

the incidence-to-prevalence ratio, $IPR(t)$, of White et al. [38] at calendar time t is

$$\begin{aligned} IPR(t) &= \frac{j(t)}{I(t)} \\ &= \frac{S(t) \int_0^\infty \beta(\tau) i(t, \tau) \, d\tau}{\int_0^\infty i(t, \tau) \, d\tau} \\ &= S(t) \int_0^\infty \beta(\tau) c(t, \tau) \, d\tau \end{aligned} \tag{53}$$

where

$$c(t, \tau) = \frac{i(t, \tau)}{\int_0^\infty i(t, \tau) \, d\tau} \tag{54}$$

which informs the infection-age distribution (or what we call *age-profile*) of infectious individuals. The actual reproduction number, $R_a(t)$, is defined as

$$R_a(t) = IPR(t)D \tag{55}$$

where

$$D = \int_0^\infty \Gamma(\tau) \, d\tau \tag{56}$$

which informs the average infectious period.

Of course, Equation (55) poses a problem for applying this simple method to HIV epidemiology. If the transmission rate $\beta(\tau)$ was independent of infection-age (and was constant b), $IPR(t)$ would be merely $bS(t)$ and thus

$$R(t) = bS(t)D = R_a(t) \tag{57}$$

Nevertheless, diseases with long generation time usually exhibits strong dependency of infectiousness on infection-age, indicating that the method might not be as useful as the cohort and instantaneous reproduction numbers. Instead, if it is the case that we have both prevalence and incidence in hand for a disease with acute course of illness, $R_a(t)$ still stands as a useful measure of transmissibility as a function of time.

5 Conclusion

In this chapter, we discussed the mathematical and statistical properties of the effective reproduction number as a function of time. We have shown that the renewal theory gives us rich analytical insights into the definition and computation of various time-dependent threshold quantities. The instantaneous and cohort reproduction numbers are explicit measures of the transmissibility, where the former informs the actual number of secondary transmissions at calendar time t, while the latter gives the average number of secondary transmissions among cohort (i.e. infecteds) who were born at calendar time t. These exactly correspond to the period and cohort total fertility rates, respectively, in mathematical demography. The difference between the two is highlighted when a specific event at calendar time t occurs (e.g. a public health intervention starts at calendar time t). Then, $R(t)$ abruptly varies with calendar time t, while $R_c(t)$ smoothly varies. For a disease with long generation time, analysis of both quantities might be called for. We have also provided analytically explicit interpretations of the incidence-to-prevalence ratio and the actual reproduction number. Although it appears that the ratio and the actual reproduction number may not be useful for a disease with long generation time (e.g. HIV/AIDS), these might be extremely useful for a disease with acute course of illness, especially when we have both prevalence and incidence in hand. Applications of the above discussed concepts are seen in other chapters in this volume, and we hope you'll enjoy our statistical approaches to various infectious diseases.

Acknowledgments The work of HN was supported by The Netherlands Organisation for Scientific Research (NWO).

References

1. Alho JM, Spencer BD (2005) Statistical Demography and Forecasting. Springer, New York.
2. Amundsen EJ, Stigum H, Rottingen JA, Aalen OO (2004) Definition and estimation of an actual reproduction number describing past infectious disease transmission: application to HIV epidemics among homosexual men in Denmark, Norway and Sweden. *Epidemiology and Infection* **132**:1139–1149.
3. Anderson RM, May RM (1982) Directly transmitted infectious diseases: control by vaccination. *Science* **215**:1053–1060.
4. Anderson RM, May RM (1991) Infectious Diseases of Humans: Dynamics and Control. Oxford University Press, Oxford.
5. Becker N (1977) Estimation for discrete time branching processes with application to epidemics. *Biometrics* **33**:515–522.
6. Bettencourt LM, Ribeiro RM (2008) Real time bayesian estimation of the epidemic potential of emerging infectious diseases. *PLoS ONE* **3**:e2185.
7. Bettencourt LMA, Ribeiro RM, Chowell G, Lant T, Castillo-Chavez C (2007) Towards real time epidemiology: data assimilation, modeling and anomaly detection of health surveillance data streams. in: Intelligence and security informatics: Biosurveillance. Proceedings of the 2nd NSF Workshop, Biosurveillance, 2007. Lecture Notes in Computer Science. eds F. Zeng et al. Springer-Verlag, Berlin pp. 79–90.

8. Cauchemez S, Boelle PY, Thomas G, Valleron AJ (2006) Estimating in real time the efficacy of measures to control emerging communicable diseases. *American Journal of Epidemiology* **164**:591–597.

9. Cauchemez S, Boelle PY, Donnelly CA, Ferguson NM, Thomas G, Leung GM, Hedley AJ, Anderson RM, Valleron AJ (2006) Real-time estimates in early detection of SARS. *Emerging Infectious Diseases* **12**:110–113.

10. Chowell G, Nishiura H, Bettencourt LM (2007) Comparative estimation of the reproduction number for pandemic influenza from daily case notification data. *Journal of the Royal Society Interface* **4**:155–166.

11. Cowling BJ, Ho LM, Leung GM (2007) Effectiveness of control measures during the SARS epidemic in Beijing: a comparison of the Rt curve and the epidemic curve. *Epidemiology and Infection* **136**:562–566.

12. Diekmann O (1977) Limiting behaviour in an epidemic model. *Nonlinear Analysis, Theory, Methods and Applications* **1**:459–470.

13. Diekmann O, Heesterbeek JAP, Metz JAJ (1990) On the definition and the computation of the basic reproductive ratio R_0 in models for infectious diseases. *Journal of Mathematical Biology* **35**:503–522.

14. Diekmann O, Heesterbeek JAP (2000) Mathematical Epidemiology of Infectious Diseases. Model Building, Analysis and Interpretation. John Wiley and Sons, New York.

15. Dietz K (1993) The estimation of the basic reproduction number for infectious diseases. *Statistical Methods in Medical Research* **2**:23–41.

16. Dublin LI, Lotka AJ (1920) On the true rate of natural increase, as exemplified by the population of the United States, 1920. *Journal of American Statistical Association* **150**: 305–339.

17. Ferguson NM, Donnelly CA, Anderson RM (2001) Transmission intensity and impact of control policies on the foot and mouth epidemc in Great Britain. *Nature* **413**:542–548.

18. Fine PE (1993) Herd immunity: history, theory, practice. *Epidemiologic Reviews* **15**:265–302.

19. Fine PE (2003) The interval between successive cases of an infectious disease. *American Journal of Epidemiology* **158**:1039–1047.

20. Fraser C (2007) Estimating individual and household reproduction numbers in an emerging epidemic. *PLoS ONE* **2**:e758.

21. Grassly NC, Fraser C (2008) Mathematical models of infectious disease transmission. *Nature Review of Microbiology* **6**:477–487.

22. Haydon DT, Chase-Topping M, Shaw DJ, Matthews L, Friar JK, Wilesmith J, Woolhouse ME (2003) The construction and analysis of epidemic trees with reference to the 2001 UK foot-and-mouth outbreak. *Proceedings of the Royal Society of London Series B* **270**: 121–127.

23. Kendall DG (1956) Deterministic and stochastic epidemics in closed populations. In: Newman P (ed) Third Berkeley Symposium on Mathematical Statistics and Probability 4. University of California Press, New York, 1956, pp.149–165.

24. Kermack WO, McKendrick AG (1927) Contributions to the mathematical theory of epidemics – I. *Proceedings of the Royal Society Series A* **115**:700–721 (reprinted in *Bulletin of Mathematical Biology* **53** (1991) 33–55).

25. Lloyd AL (2001a) Destabilization of epidemic models with the inclusion of realistic distributions of infectious periods. *Proceedings of the Royal Society of London Series B* **268**:985–993.

26. Lloyd AL (2001b) Realistic distributions of infectious periods in epidemic models: Changing patterns of persistence and dynamics. *Theoretical Population Biology* **60**:59–71.

27. Metz JAJ (1978) The epidemic in a closed population with all susceptibles equally vulnerable; some results for large susceptible populations and small initial infections. *Acta Biotheoretica* **27**:75–123.

28. Nishiura H, Dietz K, Eichner M (2006) The earliest notes on the reproduction number in relation to herd immunity: theophil Lotz and smallpox vaccination. *Journal of Theoretical Biology* **241**:964–967.

29. Nishiura H, Schwehm M, Kakehashi M, Eichner M (2006) Transmission potential of primary pneumonic plague: time inhomogeneous evaluation based on historical documents of the transmission network. *Journal of Epidemiology and Community Health* **60** (2006) 640–645.

30. Nishiura H (2007) Time variations in the transmissibility of pandemic influenza in Prussia, Germany, from 1918 to 1919. *Theoretical Biology and Medical Modelling* **4**:20.

31. Peiper O (1920) Die Grippe-Epidemie in Preussen im Jahre 1918/19. *Veroeffentlichungen aus dem Gebiete der Medizinalverwaltung* **10**:417–479 (in German).

32. Roberts MG, Heesterbeek JA (2007) Model-consistent estimation of the basic reproduction number from the incidence of an emerging infection. *Journal of Mathematical Biology* **55**:803–816.

33. Smith CE(1964) Factors in the transmission of virus infections from animal to man. *The Scientific Basis of Medicine Annual Reviews* 125–150.

34. Svensson A (2007) A note on generation times in epidemic models. *Mathematical Biosciences* **208**:300–311.

35. Wallinga J, Teunis P (2004) Different epidemic curves for severe acute respiratory syndrome reveal similar impacts of control measures. *American Journal of Epidemiology* **160**:509–516.

36. Wallinga J, Lipsitch M (2007) How generation intervals shape the relationship between growth rates and reproductive numbers. *Proceedings B* **274**:599–604.

37. Wearing HJ, Rohani P, Keeling MJ (2005) Appropriate models for the management of infectious diseases. *PLoS Medicine* **2**:e174.

38. White PJ, Ward H, Garnett GP (2006) Is HIV out of control in the UK? An example of analysing patterns of HIV spreading using incidence-to-prevalence ratios. *AIDS* **20**:1898–1901.

39. Yan P (2008) Separate roles of the latent and infectious periods in shaping the relation between the basic reproduction number and the intrinsic growth rate of infectious disease outbreaks. *Journal of Theoretical Biology* **251**:238–252.

Sensitivity of Model-Based Epidemiological Parameter Estimation to Model Assumptions

A.L. Lloyd

Abstract Estimation of epidemiological parameters from disease outbreak data often proceeds by fitting a mathematical model to the data set. The resulting parameter estimates are subject to uncertainty that arises from errors (noise) in the data; standard statistical techniques can be used to estimate the magnitude of this uncertainty. The estimates are also dependent on the structure of the model used in the fitting process and so any uncertainty regarding this structure leads to additional uncertainty in the parameter estimates. We argue that if we lack detailed knowledge of the biology of the transmission process, parameter estimation should be accompanied by a structural sensitivity analysis, in addition to the standard statistical uncertainty analysis. Here we focus on the estimation of the basic reproductive number from the initial growth rate of an outbreak as this is a setting in which parameter estimation can be surprisingly sensitive to details of the time course of infection.

1 Introduction

Estimation of epidemiological parameters, such as the average duration of infectiousness or the basic reproductive number of an infection, is often an important task when examining disease outbreak data [see, for example, 12, 19, 26]. In many instances, one or more parameters of interest cannot be estimated directly from the available data, so an indirect approach is adopted in which a mathematical model of the transmission process is formulated and is fitted to the data. The resulting parameter estimates will have uncertainty due to noise in the data but they will also depend on the form chosen for the model. Any uncertainties in our knowledge of the biology underlying the transmission process lead to uncertainties in the parameter estimates over and above those that arise from noise in the data.

Standard statistical approaches (see Chapters 1, 5, 7, 10 and 11 of this book) can be used to quantify the uncertainty in parameter estimates that arises from noise in

A.L. Lloyd (✉)
Biomathematics Graduate Program and Department of Mathematics, North Carolina State University, Raleigh, NC 27695, USA
e-mail: alun_lloyd@ncsu.edu

G. Chowell et al. (eds.), *Mathematical and Statistical Estimation Approaches in Epidemiology*, DOI 10.1007/978-90-481-2313-1_6,

the data, but these are not designed to provide insight into the sensitivity of the estimates to the *structure* of the model. In this chapter, we demonstrate that uncertainty due to model structure can, in some instances, dwarf noise-related uncertainty by discussing an estimation problem in which details of the description of the biology of the transmission process can have an important impact. This argues that when there is incomplete knowledge of the biology of the infection, structural sensitivity analysis should accompany statistical uncertainty analysis when model-based approaches are used to interpret epidemiological data.

In this chapter, we illustrate the potential importance of model assumptions by examining the model-based estimation of the basic reproductive number using data obtained from the initial stages of a disease outbreak. We review studies [21, 25, 27, 31, 33, 34] that illustrate that such estimates can be highly sensitive to the assumptions made concerning the natural history of the infection, particularly regarding the timing of secondary transmission events. These results are of major significance in the setting of emerging infectious disease outbreaks, when a rapid quantification of the basic reproductive number is highly desirable to guide control efforts, but when information on the transmission cycle may be scarce. Importantly, the work shows that the use of simple models can greatly underestimate the value of the basic reproductive number, providing overly optimistic predictions for how effective control measures have to be in order to curtail the spread of the disease.

2 The Basic Reproductive Number and Its Estimation Using the Simple SIR Model

The basic reproductive number, R_0, is defined as the average number of secondary infections caused by a typical infective individual in an otherwise entirely susceptible population [see, for example, 11]. In the simplest settings, its value can be calculated as the product of the rate at which such an individual gives rise to infections and the duration of their infectious period. In turn, the infection rate is a product of the rate at which an infective meets susceptible individuals, *i.e.* the contact rate, and the per-contact probability of transmission.

Direct estimation of the basic reproductive number could be undertaken if secondary infections of individual infectives could be quantified. Unfortunately, the most commonly available type of data—aggregated incidence data—does not reveal transmission chains in sufficient detail to identify the source of secondary cases. More detailed data, such as contact tracing data, can elucidate chains of transmission, but is rarely complete enough to allow direct calculation of R_0. In the absence of complete contact tracing data, statistical techniques have been suggested for the estimation of R_0 via reconstruction of transmission chains [13, 32].

The basic reproductive number could also be directly estimated if both the contact rate and transmission probability were known. Again, direct estimation of these quantities is typically difficult. Transmission probabilities can be estimated using certain types of epidemiological data, obtained, for instance, from observation of transmission within families, or other transmission experiments. Such data, however, are often unavailable during the early stages of a disease outbreak.

An alternative approach involves fitting a mathematical model to outbreak data, obtaining estimates for the parameters of the model, allowing R_0 to be calculated. The simplest model that can be used for this purpose is the standard deterministic compartmental SIR model [see, for example, 11]. Individuals are assumed to either be susceptible, infectious or removed, with the numbers of each being written as S, I, and R, respectively. Susceptible individuals acquire infection through contacts with infectious individuals, and the simplest form of the model assumes that new infections arise at rate $\beta SI/N$. Here N is the population size and β is the transmission parameter, which is given by the product of the contact rate and the transmission probability. Recovery of infectives is assumed to occur at a constant rate γ, corresponding to an average duration of infection of $1/\gamma$, and leads to permanent immunity. Throughout this chapter we shall denote the average duration of infectiousness by D_I and assume permanent immunity following infection. We shall also ignore demographic processes (births and deaths), which is a good approximation if the disease outbreak is short-lived and the infection is non-fatal. Ignoring demography leads to the population size N being constant. The model can be written as the following set of differential equations

$$dS/dt = -\beta SI/N \tag{1}$$

$$dI/dt = \beta SI/N - \gamma I \tag{2}$$

$$dR/dt = \gamma I. \tag{3}$$

During the early stages of an outbreak with a novel pathogen, almost the entire population will be susceptible, and, since $S \approx N$, the transmission rate equals βI. The transmission parameter β is the rate at which each infective gives rise to secondary infections and so the basic reproductive number can be written as $R_0 = \beta D_I = \beta/\gamma$. During this initial period, the changing prevalence of infection can, to a very good approximation, be described by the single linear equation $dI/dt = \gamma(R_0 - 1)I$. (We remark that the $S = N$ assumption corresponds to linearizing the model about its infection free equilibrium.) In other words, provided that R_0 is greater than one, which we shall assume to be the case throughout this chapter, prevalence initially increases exponentially with growth rate

$$r = \gamma(R_0 - 1). \tag{4}$$

The incidence of infection is given by $\beta SI/N$ and so, during the early stages of an outbreak, prevalence and incidence are proportional in the SIR setting, so this equation also describes the rate at which incidence grows.

Equation (4) provides a relationship, $R_0 = 1 + rD_I$, between R_0 and quantities that can typically be measured (the initial growth rate of the epidemic and the average duration of infection), and as a result has provided one of the most straightforward ways to estimate R_0.

3 More Complex Compartmental Models

The SIR model of Section 2 employs a very simple, but quite unrealistic, description of the time course of infection. The infectious period is assumed to start immediately upon infection, and the constant recovery rate corresponds to infectious periods being exponentially distributed across the population. In reality, there is a delay—the latent period—between acquisition of infection and the start of infectiousness: an individual typically receives a small dose of an infectious agent and several rounds of replication have to occur within the infected person before they become infectious. The exponential distribution has a much larger variance than infectious period distributions observed in the real world: it predicts that a large number of individuals recover very soon after infection and that a sizeable number of individuals have infectious periods that are much longer than the average. In reality, infectious periods are much more closely centered about their mean [2, 4].

3.1 Inclusion of Latency

A latent period can easily be incorporated within the compartmental framework with the addition of an exposed class (E) of infected but not yet infectious individuals. Assuming that movement between the E and I classes occurs at a constant per-capita rate of σ, we get the standard SEIR model

$$dS/dt = -\beta SI/N \tag{5}$$

$$dE/dt = \beta SI/N - \sigma E \tag{6}$$

$$dI/dt = \sigma E - \gamma I. \tag{7}$$

The latent period here is exponentially distributed with average duration $1/\sigma$. Throughout this chapter, we shall refer to the average duration of latency as D_E. The inclusion of the exposed class does not affect the algebraic expression for the basic reproductive number: we again have $R_0 = \beta D_I = \beta/\gamma$.

The initial behavior of an outbreak can be well described by a linear model, consisting of Equations (6) and (7) with the transmission term being replaced by βI. Provided that R_0 is greater than one, and following an initial transient, prevalence increases exponentially at rate r given by the dominant eigenvalue, the value of which is the larger of the roots of the quadratic

$$r^2 + (\sigma + \gamma)r - \sigma\gamma(R_0 - 1) = 0. \tag{8}$$

Provided that both the average durations of latency and infectiousness are known, Equation (8) can be rearranged to give R_0 in terms of the initial growth rate, giving $R_0 = (1 + rD_E)(1 + rD_I)$ [19, 25]. As for the SIR model, the incidence of infection will also grow at this rate.

Intuitively, it is clear that latency will decrease the initial growth rate of an outbreak: latency delays the start of an individual's infectious period, making their secondary infections occur later than they would if infectiousness were to begin immediately. This can be confirmed mathematically by comparing the roots of Equations (4) and (8). The constant coefficient of the quadratic in Equation (8) is equal to the product of its roots, and, because R_0 is greater than one, its value is negative. The quadratic therefore has one negative and one positive root. The value of the quadratic is negative when $r = 0$ and positive when $r = \gamma(R_0 - 1)$ and so its positive root lies in the interval $(0, \gamma(R_0 - 1))$. The growth rate for the SEIR model is lower than it was for the SIR model.

This effect is illustrated in Fig. 1, where the prevalence of infection seen in an SIR model outbreak (solid curve) is compared to that seen in the corresponding SEIR model (dotted curve). In both cases, the average infectious period is 5 days and R_0 is 5, and for the SEIR model there is a two day average duration of latency. At the initial time the entire population of one million people is taken to be susceptible except for a single infective individual. The latent period has a dramatic effect on the initial growth, and indeed on the entire timecourse, of the outbreak. (We remark that the non-exponential change in prevalence seen at the start of the outbreak in the SEIR model is the transient behavior mentioned above and arises from the second, negative, value for r in Equation 8).

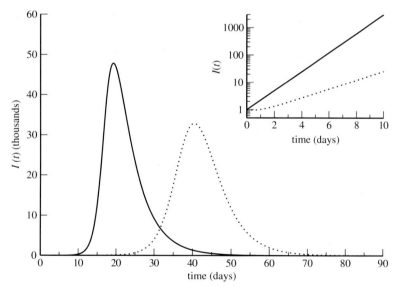

Fig. 1 Impact of latency on a disease outbreak, comparing SIR and SEIR models. *Solid curve*: no latent period (SIR model). *Dotted curve*: exponentially-distributed latent period (SEIR model). The inset (plotted on log-linear axes) focuses on the initial behavior of the two outbreaks, when the epidemics are well-described by linear models, and shows the slower initial growth rate of the SEIR outbreak. The average infectious period is taken to be $D_I = 5$ days, R_0 is 5, and, for the SEIR model, the latent period has an average duration of $D_E = 2$ days. At the initial time, the entire population of $N = 10^6$ is susceptible to the infection, except for one individual who is taken to have just become infectious

3.2 More General Compartmental Models: Gamma Distributed Latent and Infectious Periods

An individual's chance of recovery is not constant over time: typically, the recovery rate increases over time. In terms of a mathematical model, this leads to the complication that the times at which different individuals became infected must be tracked. In contrast, the constant rate assumptions of the SIR and SEIR models are mathematically convenient as their rates of recovery and loss of latency can be written just in terms of the current numbers of infectives and exposeds.

A mathematical trick [1, 10, 17] allows the inclusion of non-exponential distributions within the compartmental framework. The infective class can be subdivided into n stages, arranged in series. Newly infected individuals enter the first infective stage, pass through each in turn, and recover upon leaving the nth stage. It is assumed that progression between stages occurs at constant per-capita rate, leading to an exponential waiting time in each stage and allowing movement between stages to be described by a linear system of differential equations. The stage approach allows the modeler to retain the convenience of the differential equation approach, albeit at the cost of an increased number of state variables and hence dimensionality of the model.

In the simplest setting, the average waiting time (or equivalently the departure rate) in each stage is assumed to be equal: the overall infectious period is then described by the sum of n independent exponential distributions, *i.e.* infectious periods are gamma distributed [10, 17] with shape parameter n, as illustrated in Fig. 2. To allow comparison between models with different numbers of stages, the average duration of infectiousness is often held fixed, meaning that the departure rate is equal to $n\gamma$ for each stage. In a similar way, a non-exponential latent period can be described by the use of m exposed stages. A general form of the SEIR model, which we dub the $SE_m I_n R$ model, is then given by

$$dS/dt = -\beta SI/N \tag{9}$$
$$dE_1/dt = \beta SI/N - m\sigma E_1 \tag{10}$$
$$dE_2/dt = m\sigma E_1 - m\sigma E_2 \tag{11}$$
$$\vdots$$
$$dE_m/dt = m\sigma E_{m-1} - m\sigma E_m \tag{12}$$
$$dI_1/dt = m\sigma E_m - n\gamma I_1 \tag{13}$$
$$dI_2/dt = n\gamma I_1 - n\gamma I_2 \tag{14}$$
$$\vdots$$
$$dI_n/dt = n\gamma I_{n-1} - n\gamma I_n. \tag{15}$$

Here $I = I_1 + I_2 + \cdots + I_n$ is the total number of infectives. We remark that the $SE_m I_n R$ model has just two extra parameters compared to the SEIR model, and

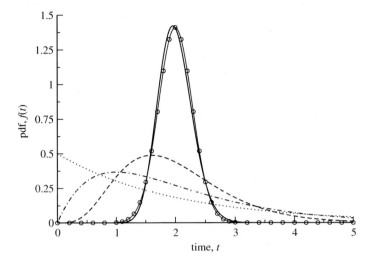

Fig. 2 Gamma distributed infectious periods. The graph illustrates the probability density function (pdf) of gamma distributions with $n = 1$ (*dotted curve*), $n = 2$ (*dot-dashed curve*), $n = 5$ (*dashed curve*) or $n = 50$ (*solid curve*) stages. In each case, the average duration of infection D_I is two days. The variances of the gamma distributions are given by D_I^2/n. As discussed in the text, for large n, the gamma distribution approaches a normal distribution: for comparison, the curve with circles depicts a normal distribution with mean and variance equal to those of the $n = 50$ gamma distribution

that if $n = m = 1$, the model reduces to the standard SEIR model. If either m or n is large, then, by the Central Limit Theorem, the relevant gamma distribution becomes approximately normal (see Fig. 2). In the limit $m \to \infty$ or $n \to \infty$, either the exposed or infectious period distribution becomes of fixed duration.

More general distributions can be described using variations of the stage device, for instance by having unequal movement rates or more complicated arrangements of stages, such as stages in parallel as well as in series. Furthermore, the infectiousness of different stages can be allowed to vary, giving a transmission term of the form $\Sigma_i \beta_i S I_i/N$. In some instances, the stages are identified with biologically-defined different stages of an infection, as, for example, in the case of a number of models for HIV [23]. But we emphasize that, in general, the stages are a mathematical device and need not have any biological interpretation.

Linearization of the model (9)–(15) gives the growth rate (of both prevalence and incidence) as the dominant root of the equation

$$\gamma R_0 \left\{ 1 - \left(1 + \frac{r D_I}{n} \right)^{-n} \right\} = r \left(1 + \frac{r D_E}{m} \right)^m . \tag{16}$$

This equation is equivalent to Equation (9) of Anderson and Watson [1], but Lloyd [21] employed this version in which R_0 appears explicitly. Here R_0 is again equal to $\beta D_I = \beta/\gamma$. We remark that in the limit of m approaching infinity, the term $(1 + rD_E/m)^m$ approaches $\exp(rD_E)$, and as n approaches infinity, the term $(1 + rD_I/n)^{-n}$ approaches $\exp(-rD_I)$. Fixed duration latent and/or infectious periods lead to the appearance of exponential terms and a transcendental equation for r in terms of R_0.

Decreasing the variance of the latent period distribution, *i.e.*, increasing m while keeping σ constant, reduces the initial growth rate. This effect can be seen in Fig. 3a, comparing the initial growth of the SEIR model (solid curve) to those seen in the corresponding SE$_5$IR and SE$_{50}$IR models (dotted and dashed curves, respectively). The impact of adding extra stages decreases as the value of m increases: a larger change is seen in the growth rate when m is changed from 1 to 5 than is seen when m is increased from 5 to 50.

Reduction in the variance of the infectious period distribution, *i.e.* increasing n while keeping γ fixed increases the initial growth rate of an outbreak (Fig. 3b).

4 A General Formulation

The stage approach provides a simple way to incorporate gamma-distributed waiting times within the compartmental framework. More general descriptions of the time-course of infection can be accounted for using a number of different approaches, including partial differential equations, delay differential equations, integral equations and integro-differential equations [5–7, 11, 14–16, 18]. As an example, the following integro-differential equation can be used to describe the number of susceptibles

$$\frac{dS}{dt} = -\delta(t) - \frac{S(t)}{N} \int_0^\infty \left(-\frac{dS}{dt} \right)\bigg|_{(t-\tau)} \mathcal{A}(\tau)\,d\tau. \qquad (17)$$

Here $\mathcal{A}(\tau)$ is the infectivity kernel, *i.e.*, the expected infectiousness of an individual τ time units after infection. (In an entirely susceptible population, this would be the rate at which such an individual gives rise to secondary infections.) The delta function depicts the infection of a single individual at the initial time. The integral that appears in this equation depicts the force of infection experienced by susceptibles at time t, while the incidence of infection, which we shall write as $X(t)$, is equal to $-dS/dt$. Notice that, as with all the models we consider in this chapter, we ignore replenishment of the susceptible population.

A number of variants of this formulation appear in the literature. In some instances, the contact rate, c, appears explicitly in Equation (17), with the infectivity kernel being written as $c\mathcal{A}(\tau)$. Several authors write the infectivity kernel as the product $\mathcal{A}(\tau) = A(\tau)\beta(\tau)$, where $A(\tau)$ is the probability that an individual is infectious at time τ and $\beta(\tau)$ is the expected infectiousness of an individual who is infectious at that time. In this formulation, if the duration of the latent period is given by the random variable T_E and the duration of the infectious period by the random variable T_I, then $A(\tau) = \Pr(T_E \leq \tau < T_E + T_I)$.

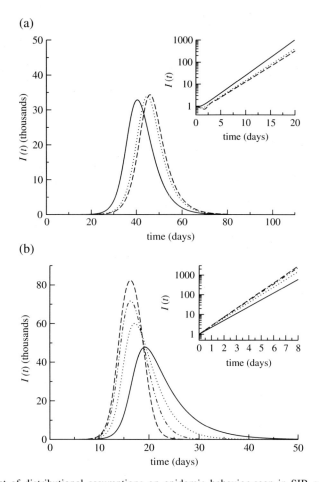

Fig. 3 Impact of distributional assumptions on epidemic behavior seen in SIR and SEIR-type models. Panel (**a**) shows the impact of the latent period distribution in SEIR-type models. In each case the infectious period is exponentially distributed. *Solid curve*: exponentially-distributed latent period (SEIR model). *Dotted and dashed curves*: gamma-distributed latent period, with $m = 5$ and $m = 50$ exposed stages (SE_5IR and $SE_{50}IR$ models), respectively. Panel (**b**) depicts the effect of various descriptions of the infectious period in SIR-type models (no latent period). *Solid curve*: exponentially distributed infectious period (SIR model). *Dotted curve*: gamma-distributed infectious period with $n = 2$ stages. *Dot-dashed curve*: gamma-distributed infectious period with $n = 5$ stages. *Dashed curve*: gamma-distributed infectious period with $n = 50$ stages. For both panels (**a**) and (**b**), the average infectious period D_I is taken to be 5 days, R_0 is 5, and, where relevant, the latent period has an average duration of $D_E = 2$ days. At the initial time, the entire population of $N = 10^6$ is susceptible to the infection, except for one individual who is taken to have just become infectious. The insets focus on the early behavior, including the phase when the behavior can be well approximated by a linear model

The compartmental models described in previous sections can be recast in terms of an infectivity kernel. For the SIR model, the constant level of infectivity over an exponentially distributed infectious period of average duration $1/\gamma$ gives

$$\mathcal{A}(\tau) = \beta e^{-\gamma \tau}, \tag{18}$$

and for the corresponding SEIR model, with average duration of latency D_E equal to $1/\sigma$, we have

$$
A(\tau) = \begin{cases} \beta \dfrac{\sigma}{\gamma - \sigma} \left(e^{-\sigma\tau} - e^{-\gamma\tau} \right) & \text{if } \sigma \neq \gamma \\[2mm] \beta\gamma\tau e^{-\gamma\tau} & \text{if } \sigma = \gamma. \end{cases} \tag{19}
$$

The basic reproductive number for this model is given by

$$
R_0 = \int_0^\infty A(\tau)\, d\tau. \tag{20}
$$

During the early stages of an outbreak, $S(t) \approx N$, and use of the approximation $S(t) = N$ gives the following linear integral equation for the incidence

$$
X(t) = \delta(t) + \int_0^\infty X(t-\tau)A(\tau)\, d\tau. \tag{21}
$$

Substitution of an exponentially growing form for the incidence, $X(t) = X(0)e^{rt}$, for $t \geq 0$ gives the equation

$$
1 = \int_0^\infty e^{-r\tau} A(\tau)\, d\tau, \tag{22}
$$

which can be solved for the rate r at which incidence grows. This equation is the familiar Euler-Lotka formula from demographic theory [see, for example, 30].

The integral that appears in Equation (22) is the Laplace transform of the infectivity kernel. Yan [34] derived a relationship between R_0 and r for a general class of infectivity kernels for which the random variables describing the latent and infectious periods, T_E and T_I, are independent and under the assumption that secondary infections arise at constant rate β over the duration of the infectious period. Assuming that the Laplace transforms of the distributions of both T_E and T_I exist, and writing them as $\mathcal{L}_E(r)$ and $\mathcal{L}_I(r)$, Yan obtained the following general result

$$
R_0 = \frac{D_I}{\mathcal{L}_E(r)\mathcal{L}_I^*(r)}. \tag{23}
$$

Here, $\mathcal{L}_I^*(r) = (1 - \mathcal{L}_I(r))/r$.

All of the relationships between R_0 and r obtained from compartmental models in the earlier sections of this chapter can be obtained as special cases of this result. In particular, the earlier Equation (16) can be seen as a special case of Yan's general result and holds for general gamma distributed latent and infectious periods (*i.e.,* with any positive shape parameters—not just integers).

5 Comparing R_0 Estimates Obtained Using Different Models

The relationships between R_0 and r described in previous sections, obtained from a number of SIR and SEIR-type models, are collected together in Table 1. It is immediately clear that use of the SIR-based formula provides a lower estimate of R_0 than would be obtained using the SEIR-based formula [21, 25, 33]. Ignoring an infection's latent period leads to underestimates of R_0, with the underestimate being more serious for faster growth rates or longer durations of latency (*e.g.*, compare Tables 2, 3 and 4).

The origin of the underestimate is clear from the analysis and simulations presented earlier: given the same values for the transmission parameter and the average

Table 1 Relationships between the initial growth rate r and the basic reproductive number R_0 obtained from various models

Model	Formula
SIR	$R_0 = 1 + r D_I$
$SI_n R$	$R_0 = \dfrac{r D_I}{1 - (1 + r D_I / n)^{-n}}$
$SI_\infty R$	$R_0 = \dfrac{r D_I}{1 - e^{-r D_I}}$
SEIR	$R_0 = (1 + r D_I)(1 + r D_E)$
$SEI_\infty R$	$R_0 = \dfrac{r D_I (1 + r D_E)}{1 - e^{-r D_I}}$
$SE_m IR$	$R_0 = (1 + r D_I)(1 + r D_E / m)^m$
$SE_m I_n R$	$R_0 = \dfrac{r D_I (1 + r D_E / m)^m}{1 - (1 + r D_I / n)^{-n}}$
$SE_\infty IR$	$R_0 = (1 + r D_I) e^{r D_E}$
$SE_\infty I_\infty R$	$R_0 = \dfrac{r D_I e^{r D_E}}{1 - e^{-r D_I}}$

Table 2 R_0 and p_c estimates obtained using various models when $r = 0.04$ day^{-1}, $D_E = 3$ days and $D_I = 8$ days. These parameters were chosen to be similar to those employed in [8] to describe SARS

Model	R_0 estimate	Control fraction p_c
SIR	1.32	0.242
$SI_5 R$	1.20	0.167
$SI_\infty R$	1.17	0.144
SEIR	1.48	0.324
$SEI_\infty R$	1.31	0.236
$SE_5 IR$	1.49	0.327
$SE_5 I_5 R$	1.35	0.260
$SE_\infty IR$	1.49	0.328
$SE_\infty I_\infty R$	1.32	0.241

Table 3 Impact of faster growth rate on R_0 estimates. Here, $r = 0.12$ day^{-1}, while $D_E = 3$ days and $D_I = 8$ days take the same values as in the previous table

Model	R_0 estimate	Control fraction p_c
SIR	1.96	0.490
SI$_5$R	1.64	0.391
SI$_\infty$R	1.56	0.357
SEIR	2.67	0.625
SEI$_\infty$R	2.12	0.527
SE$_5$IR	2.77	0.640
SE$_5$I$_5$R	2.33	0.570
SE$_\infty$IR	2.81	0.644
SE$_\infty$I$_\infty$R	2.23	0.552

duration of infectiousness, the SEIR model would predict a lower growth rate than the corresponding SIR model. Consequently, in order to achieve the same growth rate in this forward problem setting, a higher transmission parameter, and hence R_0, must be used in the SEIR model than in the corresponding SIR model.

Larger estimates of the basic reproductive number are obtained when non-exponential descriptions of the latent period distribution are used. Because the function $(1 + a/x)^x$ is monotonic increasing for $a > 0$, increasing the number of latent stages m (*i.e.*, reducing the variance of the latent period distribution) increases the estimate [21, 27, 33, 34], with the estimate that employs a fixed duration of latency (*i.e.*, $m \to \infty$) providing an upper bound. On the other hand, lower estimates of the basic reproductive number are obtained when the number of infectious stages n is increased [21, 27, 33, 34], with the estimate obtained using a fixed duration of infectiousness (*i.e.*, $n \to \infty$) being a lower bound.

Because estimates of R_0 are often used to determine the severity of measures needed to bring an outbreak under control, assumptions made about the timecourse of infection can have important public health consequences [21, 33]. If the aim of control is to bring the basic reproductive number below one, the transmissibility of the infection must be reduced by a factor of $p_c = 1 - 1/R_0$. Here, we call p_c the control fraction. (In the context of mass vaccination, p_c is called the critical

Table 4 Impact of longer average duration of latency on R_0 estimates. Here, $D_E = 5$ days, while $r = 0.12$ day^{-1} and $D_I = 8$ days, as in the previous table

Model	R_0 estimate	Control fraction p_c
SIR	1.96	0.490
SI$_n$R	1.64	0.391
SI$_\infty$R	1.56	0.357
SEIR	3.14	0.681
SEI$_\infty$R	2.49	0.598
SE$_m$IR	3.45	0.710
SE$_m$I$_n$R	2.89	0.655
SE$_\infty$IR	3.57	0.720
SE$_\infty$I$_\infty$R	2.83	0.647

vaccination fraction.) As we have seen, use of SIR models underestimates the basic reproductive number and hence leads to lower estimates of p_c compared to those obtained using SEIR models. This could be a serious problem as it leads to an overly optimistic prediction of the strength of control needed to curtail an outbreak: a control measure that, on the basis of the incorrect model, is predicted to succeed could, instead, be doomed to failure [21].

We first illustrate these results by providing a few examples using a growth rate and durations of latency and infectiousness based roughly on a SARS modeling study of Chowell et al. [8]. (The study of Chowell et al. accounted for treatment and isolation, using a more complex model than those employed here, so direct comparisons cannot be made.) Table 2 shows estimates obtained for an observed growth rate of 0.04 per day, assuming a three day average duration of latency and an eight day average duration of infectiousness. We imagine that details of how latent and infectious periods are distributed about their means are unknown, and so present estimates based on a number of models. This provides an indication of the degree of uncertainty that arises from incomplete knowledge of these distributions. (Here we ignore the additional complication that the estimate of r would also have some uncertainty.) For this example, comparing the SIR and SEIR-based estimates, we see that ignoring the latent period leads to R_0 being underestimated by about 10%. This translates into a 25% underestimate of the control fraction.

Interestingly, for this set of parameters, the distribution of the latent period (provided that one is used in the first place) has little impact on the estimates, while the infectious period distribution has a more noticeable effect. In this case the latter effect is sufficiently large to offset the differences introduced by ignoring a latent period: the estimates obtained using the SIR and the $SE_\infty I_\infty R$ models are almost identical.

For a more rapidly growing outbreak, in which $r = 0.12$ day^{-1} is three times larger than its previous value, the SIR model underestimates R_0 by a larger amount, roughly 25%, compared to the SEIR estimate (Table 3). This corresponds to a 22% underestimate of the control fraction. We remark that while this underestimate is slightly smaller in percentage terms than that seen under the previous set of parameters, it is larger in absolute terms. Also, given that the required level of control is higher, the increase in effectiveness needed to go from the SIR-based estimate of p_c to the SEIR-based estimate may be much more difficult to achieve. For this set of parameters, the form of the latent period distribution has a more noticeable impact.

If the infection is both more rapidly growing and has a longer duration of latency the underestimate of R_0 is more severe. In the example of Table 4, in which the average duration of latency has been raised from 3 to 5 days, use of the SIR model underestimates R_0 by roughly 38% of the SEIR-based estimate. The two estimates of the control fraction are 0.490 (SIR) and 0.681 (SEIR).

Figure 4 shows how estimates of R_0 obtained using the $SE_m I_n R$ model depend in turn on each of the quantities D_E, D_I, m, n and r for a situation corresponding to Table 4. We take $D_E = 5$ days, $D_I = 8$ days, $r = 0.12$ day^{-1}, $m = 5$ and $n = 5$ as a baseline, and vary just one of these at a time. As discussed above, the estimate of R_0 increases with m, D_E, D_I and r, but decreases with n. We also see that the

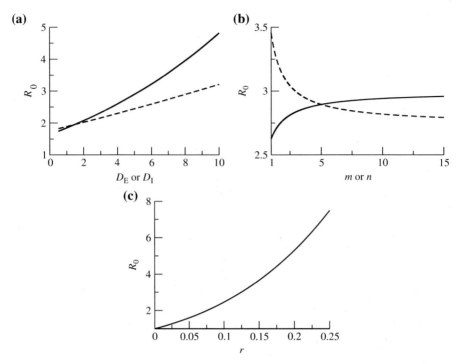

Fig. 4 Sensitivity of the R_0 estimate to variations in single parameter values or the initial growth rate. One of five quantities is varied in turn: Panel (**a**) D_E (*solid curve*) or D_I (*dashed curve*); Panel (**b**) m (*solid curve*) or n (*dashed curve*); Panel (**c**) r. The four other values are taken from the baseline set of $D_E = 5$ days, $D_I = 8$ days, $m = 5$, $n = 5$, and $r = 0.12$ day^{-1}

sensitivity of the estimate varies with these parameters, for instance, the R_0 estimate is less sensitive to m for larger values of m.

A dramatic example of the potential for the underestimation of R_0 was provided by Nowak et al. [25] in a within-host setting that can be modeled using virus dynamics models that are directly analogous to the epidemiological models considered here. The initial growth rate of simian immunodeficiency virus (SIV) in one particular animal in an experimental infection study was found to be 2.2 day^{-1} and the average duration of infectiousness (of SIV infected cells) was 1.35 days. Use of the SIR model gave an estimate of $R_0 = 4.0$, the SEIR model, assuming a one day latent period (*i.e.,* the delay between a cell becoming infected and becoming infectious), gave $R_0 = 13$, while the $SE_\infty IR$ model gave $R_0 = 36$. We remark on the large impact of the distribution of the latent period in this instance. In terms of control fractions, the three models predict values of 0.75 (SIR), 0.92 (SEIR) and 0.97 ($SE_\infty IR$). While there may be hope in achieving a 75% reduction in transmissibility, a 92 or 97% reduction would be much harder to achieve. In this case, use of the SIR model gives a wildly optimistic picture of the effectiveness required of a control measure.

If the latent period in this within-host example was instead assumed to be 0.5 days, the effect would be reduced, with the SEIR and $SE_\infty IR$-based estimates of R_0 falling to 8.3 and 12, respectively. These values are still considerably larger than the SIR-based estimate of 4.0, and the estimate is still highly sensitive to the distribution of the latent period. The corresponding control fractions are 0.88 and 0.92, respectively.

6 Sensitivity Analysis

The numerical examples presented above give an idea of the dependency of R_0 estimates on parameter values in particular settings, but a more systematic exploration can be achieved using sensitivity analysis. It is straightforward to calculate the partial derivatives of the estimated value of R_0 as provided by the $SE_m I_n R$ model (*i.e.*, using Equation 16) with respect to the parameters D_E, D_I, m, n, and the initial growth rate r. The elasticity E_x, which approximates the fractional change in the R_0 estimate that results from a unit fractional change in parameter x (while keeping all other parameters constant), is given by $E_x = (x/R_0) \cdot \partial R_0/\partial x$. The elasticities for the quantities of interest are

$$E_{D_E} = \frac{r D_E}{1 + r D_E/m} \tag{24}$$

$$E_{D_I} = 1 - \frac{r D_I}{(1 + r D_I/n)\left((1 + r D_I/n)^n - 1\right)} \tag{25}$$

$$E_m = m \ln\left(1 + \frac{r D_E}{m}\right) - \frac{r D_E}{1 + r D_E/m} \tag{26}$$

$$E_n = \frac{1}{(1 + r D_I/n)^n - 1}\left(-n \ln(1 + r D_I/n) + \frac{r D_I}{1 + r D_I/n}\right) \tag{27}$$

$$E_r = 1 + \frac{r D_E}{1 + r D_E/m} - \frac{r D_I}{(1 + r D_I/n)\left((1 + r D_I/n)^n - 1\right)}. \tag{28}$$

We remark that if the curves that appear in Fig. 4 were replotted on log-log axes, these elasticities would describe the slopes of these new graphs.

The signs of the elasticities confirm the earlier discussion of how the estimate of R_0 varies as parameter values are changed. Clearly E_{D_E} is positive, meaning that increases in D_E lead to larger estimates of R_0. E_{D_I} is also seen to be positive, since the second term in Equation (25) is smaller than one for positive values of the parameters r, D_I and n: increases in D_I again lead to larger estimates of R_0. E_m is seen to be positive when m, r and D_E are positive because the function $m \ln(1 + x/m) - x/(1 + x/m)$ is monotonic increasing in x and takes the value 0 when x equals zero. A similar argument shows that E_n is negative. Finally, E_r equals the sum of E_{D_E} and E_{D_I} and so is positive, and is greater than either E_{D_E} or E_{D_I}.

A little algebra shows that E_{D_E} is an increasing function of r, D_E or m, $i.e.$, the elasticity of the R_0 estimate with respect to D_E increases with these parameters. E_{D_I} is an increasing function of r or D_I, but parameter sets can be found for which it is non-monotonic as n changes. E_m increases with r or D_E, but can be non-monotonic as m changes. E_n can be non-monotonic as r or D_I changes. As before, E_r inherits the properties of E_{D_E} and E_{D_I}, and so increases with D_E, D_I, m or r, but need not be a monotonic function of n.

For the parameters of Table 2 and when $m = n = 1$ we find that the elasticities are given by $E_{D_E} = 0.107$, $E_{D_I} = 0.242$, $E_m = 0.006$, $E_n = -0.110$, and $E_r = 0.350$. If, instead, we take $m = n = 5$ the elasticities are $E_{D_E} = 0.117$, $E_{D_I} = 0.173$, $E_m = 0.001$, $E_n = -0.026$, and $E_r = 0.290$. In both cases, the R_0 estimate is more sensitive to changes in D_I than to changes in D_E, and here we see that sensitivities to m and n are of smaller magnitude for larger values of m and n, while the sensitivity to D_E increases with increasing m and the sensitivity to D_I decreases with increasing n.

Whether the estimate is more sensitive to changes in D_E or D_I (or to m or n) depends on the values of the parameters. For example, if the parameters of Table 4 are taken, and $m = n = 1$ is assumed, the elasticities are $E_{D_E} = 0.375$, $E_{D_I} = 0.490$, $E_m = 0.095$, $E_n = -0.191$, and $E_r = 0.865$. If, instead, we assumed $m = n = 5$, the estimate of R_0 would be more sensitive to D_E than to D_I ($E_{D_E} = 0.536$ and $E_{D_I} = 0.427$), and if we took $m = 1$ and $n = 5$, the estimate would be more sensitive to m than to n ($E_m = 0.095$ and $E_n = -0.052$).

One important question that the elasticities discussed in this section do not address is the impact of neglecting the latent period entirely. Having said this, they are useful in understanding how uncertainties in the average duration of the latent or infectious period, the dispersions of these distributions, as described by m or n, or the initial growth rate impact the estimation of R_0 in the $SE_m I_n R$ model framework.

7 Discussion

The importance of non-exponential infectious periods and time-varying infectiousness has long been appreciated for chronic infections, such as HIV, for which a constant recovery rate assumption is clearly untenable [5–7, 16, 23, 24]. Even in the setting of models of acute infections, there is a surprisingly long history of the use of more complex models: Kermack and McKendrick's groundbreaking paper of 1927 [18] contains an integral equation formulation along the lines of Equation (17), and Bailey [3] used the stage approach and the resulting $SE_m I_n R$ model. The importance of distributional assumptions has typically been viewed in terms of their impact on the behavior of a model for a given set of parameters ($i.e.$, the forward problem): effects such as the slower growth of epidemics for infections with latency have long been appreciated.

The impact of distributional assumptions on the inverse problem, ($i.e.$, the estimation of parameters given the observed behavior), however, appears to have only recently become fully appreciated. Nowak et al. [25] showed that the SIR-based estimates of the within-host basic reproductive number of SIV (simian immunodeficiency virus) severely underestimated R_0 when compared to estimates obtained using more realistic SEIR models. Little et al. [20] carried out a similar analysis in the setting of HIV infection. Much of the theory and results discussed in this chapter were laid out by Lloyd [21], in the setting of within-host infections, although, because of the obvious correspondence between within-host and between-host models, the application to estimation in the epidemiological setting was highlighted [see also the discussion of 22]. Wearing et al. [33] further illustrated these results in an epidemiological setting, and broadened consideration to include estimation of R_0 based on data from the entire outbreak, as discussed below. A complementary approach was taken by Wallinga and Lipsitch [31] and Roberts and Heesterbeek [27], who examined the relationship between R_0 and r in terms of the generation interval of the infection (*i.e.*, the time between an individual becoming infected and the secondary infections that they cause). Both of these studies considered gamma distributed latent and infectious periods, including the exponential and fixed duration cases, giving equivalent results to those discussed here. Additional families of distributions were also considered, including trapezoidal infectivity kernels [27] and normally distributed generation intervals [31]. Yan [34] provided a comprehensive analysis that encompassed and unified most of these earlier studies, deriving general results in terms of Laplace transforms of the latent and infectious period distributions.

The results presented here demonstrate that estimates of the basic reproductive number obtained from the initial growth rate of a disease outbreak can be sensitive to the details of the timing of secondary infection events (*i.e.*, to the distribution of infectious and latent periods). Such details, while clearly important, are often difficult to obtain. Data that identifies when an individual was exposed to infection and when their secondary transmissions occurred, such as family-based transmission studies or contact tracing data—even if incomplete—can be highly informative in this regard [2, 4, 12, 13]. It is important to realize that models are often framed in terms of transmission status, *e.g.* whether an individual is infectious, while data may reflect disease status, *e.g.* whether an individual is symptomatic or not. This distinction is important in the interpretation of the most commonly available distributional data, namely the incubation period distribution [28], because the incubation period of an infection may not, and often does not, correspond to its latent period [see, for example, 29].

In this chapter we only considered the estimation of R_0 from initial growth data, but similar results are obtained if models are instead fitted to data obtained over the entirety of an outbreak [33]. This makes sense given the observation that distributional assumptions affect not only the initial growth rate but the whole time course of an outbreak in the forward problem (see Figs. 1 and 3). Whole-outbreak data is considerably more informative than initial growth data, for instance Wearing et al. [33] used a least-squares approach to estimate β, D_E and D_I as well as the shape parameters m and n of the gamma distributions describing latency and infectiousness. Initial growth rate data, on the other hand, does not even allow β and γ to be independently estimated. Capaldi et al. (manuscript in preparation) examine the types of data that allow for the estimation of different parameters in more detail.

Wearing et al. [33] also make the important observation that different estimates of R_0 can, in some instances, be obtained if initial data is used rather than data from an entire outbreak [see also 9].

If detailed information on the distribution of latent and infectious periods is absent, caution should be taken in basing an estimate of R_0 by fitting a single model. The use of a number of models can provide bounds on the estimate, giving an indication of the uncertainty arising from our incomplete knowledge of the transmission process. Any model-based uncertainty is in addition to that which arises from noise in the data—an issue that we have not discussed in this chapter—and so the most informative uncertainty estimate would account for both sources of error. (Sensitivity calculations, such as those discussed above, can be informative in this regard.) In some instances, however, model-based uncertainty may place a much greater limit on our ability to estimate parameters. As in the within-host example of Nowak et al. [25], this uncertainty can be so large as to render the estimates almost uninformative—but at least the deficiency is exposed by the approach advocated here.

References

1. Anderson DA, Watson RK (1980) On the spread of disease with gamma distributed latent and infectious periods. *Biometrika* 67:191–198.
2. Bailey NTJ (1954) A statistical method for estimating the periods of incubation and infection of an infectious disease. *Nature* 174:139–140.
3. Bailey NTJ (1964) Some stochastic models for small epidemics in large populations. *Appl. Stat.* 13:9–19.
4. Bailey NTJ (1975) *The Mathematical Theory of Infectious Diseases*. Griffin, London.
5. Blythe SP, Anderson RM (1988) Variable infectiousness in HIV transmission models. *IMA J. Math. Appl. Med. Biol.* 5:181–200.
6. Blythe SP, Anderson RM (1988) Distributed incubation and infectious periods in models of the transmission dynamics of the human immunodeficiency virus (HIV). *IMA J. Math. Appl. Med. Biol.* 5:1–19.
7. Castillo-Chavez C, Cooke K, Huang W, Levin SA (1989) On the role of long incubation periods in the dynamics of HIV/AIDS, Part 1: Single population models. *J. Math. Biol.* 27: 373–398.
8. Chowell G, Fenimore PW, Castillo-Garsow MA, Castillo-Chavez C (2003) SARS outbreaks in Ontario, Hong Kong and Singapore: the role of diagnosis and isolation as a control mechanism. *J. Theor. Biol.* 224:1–8.
9. Chowell G, Nishiura H, Bettencourt LMA (2007) Comparative estimation of the reproduction number for pandemic influenza from daily case notification data. *J. R. Soc. Interface* 4: 155–166.
10. Cox DR, Miller HD (1965) *The Theory of Stochastic Processes*. Methuen, London.
11. Diekmann O, Heesterbeek JAP (2000) *Mathematical Epidemiology of Infectious Diseases*. John Wiley & Son, Chichester.
12. Donnelly CA, Ghani AC, Leung GM, Hedley AJ, Fraser C, Riley S, Abu-Raddad LJ, Ho L-M, Thach T-Q, Chau P, Chan K-P, Lam T-H, Tse L-Y, Tsang T, Liu S-H, Kong JHB, Lau EMC, Ferguson NM, Anderson RM (2003) Epidemiological determinants of spread of causal agent of severe acute respiratory syndrome in Hong Kong. *Lancet* 361:1761–1766.

13. Haydon DT, Chase-Topping M, Shaw DJ, Matthews L, Friar JK, Wilesmith J, Woolhouse MEJ (2003) The construction and analysis of epidemic trees with reference to the 2001 UK foot-and-mouth outbreak. *Proc. R. Soc. Lond. B* 269:121–127.
14. Hethcote HW, Tudor DW (1980) Integral equation models for endemic infectious diseases. *J. Math. Biol.* 9:37–47.
15. Hoppensteadt F (1974) An age dependent epidemic model. *J. Franklin Inst.* 297:325–333.
16. Hyman JM, Stanley EA (1988) Using mathematical models to understand the AIDS epidemic. *Math. Biosci.* 90:415–473.
17. Jensen A (1948) An elucidation of Erlang's statistical works through the theory of stochastic processes. In E. Brockmeyer, H. L. Halstrøm, and A. Jensen, editors, *The Life and Works of A. K. Erlang*, pages 23–100. The Copenhagen Telephone Company, Copenhagen.
18. Kermack WO, McKendrick AG (1927) A contribution to the mathematical theory of epidemics. *Proc. R. Soc. Lond. A* 115:700–721.
19. Lipsitch M, Cohen T, Cooper B, Robins JM, Ma S, James L, Gopalakrishna G, Chew SK, Tan CC, Samore MH, Fisman D, Murray M (2003) Transmission dynamics and control of severe acute respiratory syndrome. *Science* 300:1966–1970.
20. Little SJ, McLean AR, Spina CA, Richman DD, Havlir DV (1999) Viral dynamics of acute HIV-1 infection. *J. Exp. Med.* 190:841–850.
21. Lloyd AL (2001) The dependence of viral parameter estimates on the assumed viral life cycle: Limitations of studies of viral load data. *Proc. R. Soc. Lond. B* 268:847–854.
22. Lloyd AL (2001) Destabilization of epidemic models with the inclusion of realistic distributions of infections periods. *Proc. R. Soc. Lond. B* 268:985–993.
23. Longini IM, Clark WS, Byers RH, Ward JW, Darrow WW, Lemp GF, Hethcote HW (1989) Statistical analysis of the stages of HIV infection using a Markov model. *Stat. Med.* 8: 831–843.
24. Malice M-P, Kryscio RJ (1989) On the role of variable incubation periods in simple epidemic models. *IMA J. Math. Appl. Med. Biol.* 6:233–242.
25. Nowak MA, Lloyd AL, Vasquez GM, Wiltrout TA, Wahl LM, Bischofberger N, Williams J, Kinter A, Fauci AS, Hirsch VM, Lifson JD (1997) Viral dynamics of primary viremia and antiretroviral therapy in simian immunodeficiency virus infection. *J. Virol.* 71:7518–25.
26. Riley S, Fraser C, Donnelly CA, Ghani AC, Abu-Raddad LJ, Hedley AJ, Leung GM, Ho L-M, Lam T-H, Thach T-Q, Chau P, Chan K-P, Lo S-V, Leung P-Y,Tsang T, Ho W, Lee K-H, Lau EMC, Ferguson NM, Anderson RM (2003) Transmission dynamics of the etiological agent of SARS in Hong Kong: Impact of public health interventions. *Science* 300:1961–1966.
27. Roberts MG, Heesterbeek JAP (2007) Model-consistent estimation of the basic reproduction number from the incidence of an emerging infection. *J. Math. Biol.* 55:803–816.
28. Sartwell PE (1950) The distribution of incubation periods of infectious disease. *Am. J. Hygiene* 51:310–318.
29. Sartwell PE (1966) The incubation period and the dynamics of infectious disease. *Am. J. Epidemiol.* 83:204–216.
30. Smith D, Keyfitz N (1977) *Mathematical Demography. Selected Papers.* Biomathematics, Volume 6. Springer-Verlag, Berlin.
31. Wallinga J, Lipsitch M (2007) How generation intervals shape the relationship between growth rates and reproductive numbers. *Proc. R. Soc. Lond. B* 274:599–604.
32. Wallinga J, Teunis P (2004) Different epidemic curves for severe acute respiratory syndrome reveal similar impacts of control measures. *Am. J. Epidemiol.* 160:509–516.
33. Wearing HJ, Rohani P, Keeling M (2005) Appropriate models for the management of infectious diseases. *PLoS Medicine* 2(7):e174.
34. Yan P (2008) Separate roles of the latent and infectious periods in shaping the relation between the basic reproduction number and the intrinsic growth rate of infectious disease outbreaks. *J. Theor. Biol.* 251:238–252.

An Ensemble Trajectory Method for Real-Time Modeling and Prediction of Unfolding Epidemics: Analysis of the 2005 Marburg Fever Outbreak in Angola

Luís M. A. Bettencourt

Abstract We propose a new methodology for the modeling and real time prediction of the course of unfolding epidemic outbreaks. The method posits a class of standard epidemic models and explores uncertainty in empirical data to set up a family of possible outbreak trajectories that span the probability distribution of models parameters and initial conditions. A genetic algorithm is used to estimate likely trajectories consistent with the data and reconstruct the probability distribution of model parameters. In this way the ensemble of trajectories allows for temporal extrapolation to produce estimates of future cases and deaths, with quantified levels of uncertainty. We apply this methodology to an outbreak of Marburg hemorrhagic fever in Angola during 2005 in order to estimate disease epidemiological parameters and assess the effects of interventions. Data for cases and deaths was compiled from World Health Organization as the epidemic unfolded. We describe the outbreak through a standard epidemic model used in the past for Ebola, a closely related viral pathogen. The application of our method allows us to make quantitative prognostics as the outbreak unfolds for the expected time to the end of the epidemic and final numbers of cases and fatalities, which were eventually confirmed. We provided a real time analysis of the effects of intervention and possible under reporting and place bounds on population movements necessary to guarantee that the epidemic did not regain momentum.

Keywords Epidemic models · Real time estimation · Marburg-like viruses · Measurements epidemiologic · Projections and predictions

1 Introduction

Over the last few years mathematical epidemiology [1, 4] has taken an increasing interest in the quantitative study and prediction of unfolding epidemic outbreaks [2, 3, 5, 6, 21]. This is both motivated by the spectacular progress in information

L.M.A. Bettencourt (✉)
Los Alamos National Laboratory, Theoretical Division, MS B284, Los Alamos, NM 87545, USA;
Santa Fe Institute, 1399 Hyde Park Road, Santa Fe, NM 87501, USA
e-mail: lmbett@lanl.gov

G. Chowell et al. (eds.), *Mathematical and Statistical Estimation Approaches in Epidemiology*, DOI 10.1007/978-90-481-2313-1_7,
© Springer Science+Business Media B.V. 2009

technologies, which allow for the spread of epidemiological information worldwide in real time, but also to the increased monitoring of emerging infectious diseases [9, 12, 14, 22, 24–26] such as H5N1 influenza, as well as of potentially engineered biological threats [10].

The well-established tools of mathematical epidemiology built primarily for a posteriori analysis of outbreaks [1, 4] are however in several respects inadequate to measure and predict the course of unfolding epidemics. The main challenge arises from the necessary confrontation of model predictions to future data, which must be probabilistic.

Standard epidemic models, such as SIR or SEIR [1, 4], are deterministic and make a prediction for the average number of cases or deaths incurred during an outbreak. It is expected that data for large outbreaks is representative of that mean and a trajectory that fits well these data in terms of a goodness of fit measure is well accepted as the canonical procedure to estimate average epidemiological parameters.

The situation is murkier when outbreaks are small or, more to the point, when predictions from the models are to be confronted with new observations. Then the probabilistic nature of contagion becomes manifest in that no number of actual cases or deaths will usually match the predicted mean value. Thus to assess whether a model is representative of the epidemic under way it is necessary to add to this type of prediction a measure of quantified uncertainty [2, 3], e.g. in the form of a confidence interval. At that level of confidence we can then reject a model if future predictions fall outside the predicted interval (through a simple p-test), or otherwise accept the model as predictive.

This article introduces a methodology to do just this. It starts from the standard mean field models of epidemics and takes them, as specified by their initial conditions and parameter values, which we collectively denote Γ, as a possible trajectory of the outbreak. Many such trajectories are proposed via a stochastic update rule (a variant genetic algorithm) and weighted in terms of their agreement with the data at a prescribed level of uncertainty. This allows us in turn to reconstruct a probability distribution on Γ and estimate epidemiological parameters and any of their correlations with quantified uncertainty.

The remaining of this paper introduces the mathematical ensemble trajectory method and the associated estimation procedure, and then proceeds to apply it to an outbreak of a poorly known disease: Marburg hemorrhagic fever in 2005 in Angola, for which it was developed. The method made early accurate predictions of the final toll of the epidemic and its termination time and revealed erroneous trends in late reporting.

2 Uncertainty Quantification and Model Parameter Estimation

In this section we give a general description of the stochastic parameter estimation procedure. We start from the observation that simple (homogeneous mixing) population models, cannot be expected to give perfect descriptions of any actual data set. This always results in a minimum level of discrepancy between the best model output and the data. We parameterize this discrepancy by the absolute value deviation between the best model prediction and each data point, per point. This is called the least deviation per datum (ldpd)

$$ldpp(\Gamma) = \frac{1}{N_X N_O} \sum_{i=1}^{N_X} \sum_{j=1}^{N_O} \left| X_i^M(t_j) - X_i^O(t_j) \right| \tag{A1}$$

where $X_i^M(t_j)$ is the ith state variable (e.g. deaths D, or number of cases C, see below), as an output of the model (a function of a parameter set Γ) at observation time t_j. N_X is the number of variables constrained by data and N_O is the number of observation points.

This measure allows us to discuss and compare how good models are at describing a specific data set, i.e. their goodness of fit. Secondly, we expect in general that data contain errors, e.g. due to under reporting, false positives, accounting errors, *etc.* An allowable level of uncertainty in the data will then translate into an ensemble of acceptable model of solutions or trajectories, which correspond in turn to a set of initial conditions and model parameters, which we write $\{\Gamma\}$. Each Γ in this set can then be weighted by their goodness of fit in a way that generates an estimate of the probability distribution function for the ensemble of model parameters that is compatible with the data. As a whole this is a stochastic optimization problem (see, e.g. [19] for a general discussion). Based on this idea we perform an estimation of the joint parameter distribution of model parameters $P(\Gamma)$, conditional on a set of allowable deviations per datum.

To be more specific we write that the unknown *exact* data point $X^E(t_j)$, can be expressed in terms of the observed datum $X^O(t_j)$ and an error $\xi(t_j)$ as

$$X^E(t_j) = X^O(t_j) + \xi(t_j). \tag{1}$$

The error $\xi(t_j)$ is only known statistically so that in order to proceed we need to specify a model for ξ. Because we expect the variance of the error to be bounded we assumed a Gaussian distribution for ξ, such that

$$P[\xi(t_j)] = P[X^E(t_j) - X^O(t_j)] \propto \exp\left[-\frac{\xi^2(t_j)}{2\sigma^2(t_j)} \right], \tag{2}$$

where the standard deviation $\sigma(t_j)$ parameterizes the allowed discrepancy between model outputs and data and is to be specified through general expectations on the data.

This expectation for the errors defines implicitly an objective function that can be minimized to produce optimal parameter estimates through a search procedure. For example, for each model realization in terms of a set of parameters in a SEIR model $\Gamma=[S(t_0), E(t_0), I(t_0), D(t_0), R(t_0), \beta,\varepsilon,\gamma,p]$ we take this function to be

$$A(\Gamma) = \frac{1}{N_X N_O} \sum_{i=1}^{N_X} \sum_{j=1}^{N_O} \frac{\left| X_i^M(t_j) - X_i^O(t_j) \right|^2}{2\sigma^2(t_j)}, \tag{3}$$

which is an implicit function of Γ. If the model could generate exact results we could then make the natural association $X^E(t_j) \rightarrow X^M(t_j)$. This is usually not the case, since a residual minimal deviation always persists, the minimum *ldpd*. To account for this we normalize this function to zero by taking $H(\Gamma) = A(\Gamma) - A(\text{best } \Gamma)$, i.e. by subtracting the minimal value of $A(\Gamma)$, obtained for the best parameter set.

Given this choice of H we can produce, in analogy with standard procedures in statistical physics, a joint probability distribution for model parameters. Since we only have expectations on $A(\Gamma)$ (and not higher moments A^2, A^3, etc) the maximum entropy distribution in

$$P[\Gamma|\{X_i^O\}] \propto e^{-H}. \tag{4}$$

We can now see how this distribution can be reconstituted from sampling many realizations of the model in terms of different Γ. Note that the probability of each trajectory $w(\Gamma)$ is

$$w(\Gamma) = \frac{1}{N_w} e^{-H(\Gamma)}, \ N_w = Tr[w_s]. \tag{5}$$

Then $P[\Gamma|\{X_i^O\}]$ can be estimated from many trajectories N_t as

$$P[\Gamma|\{X_i^O\}] \sim \sum_{i=1}^{N_t} \delta(\Gamma - \Gamma_i)w(\Gamma_i) \tag{6}$$

Figure 1 illustrates an ensemble of trajectories with variable degree of goodness of fit; trajectories with large deviations to the data points are exponentially suppressed in their contributions to the parameter distribution.

This joint probability distribution can then be used to compute any moment of any set of parameters in Γ,

$$\langle F \rangle = Tr\left[P[\Gamma|\{X_i^O\}]F(\Gamma) \right] \rightarrow \sum_{i=1}^{N_s} F(s)w(\Gamma_i) \tag{7}$$

including single parameter distribution functions, and cross-parameter correlations, such as covariances, but also any higher moments. The prediction of future observations can now be obtained by convolving the model with the parameter probability distribution estimated to that point as

$$P[X_{i+1}^O] = Tr_\Gamma\left[P[X_{i+1}^O|\Gamma, \{X_i^O\}]P[\Gamma|\{X_i^O\}] \right], \tag{8}$$

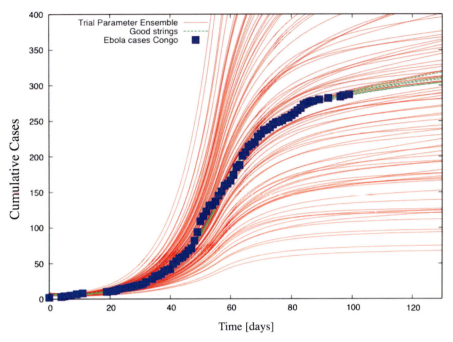

Fig. 1 Example of SEIR trajectories with varying degrees of goodness of fit for data for an outbreak of Ebola (data courtesy of Gerardo Chowell). Green trajectories fit the data (*blue squares*) well

where $P[X_{i+1}^O | \Gamma, \{X_i^O\}]$ is the model taken for a specific trajectory specified by a particular Γ.

In practice the estimation procedure via trajectories, each corresponding to a parameter set, is potentially difficult because we are dealing with an inverse problem in which, given a trial set of parameters, comparison with the data is performed only after the non-linear model dynamical equations have been solved. Fortunately for models that consist of small numbers of ordinary differential equations the computational effort is relatively trivial on a modern computer.

In every case discussed below, we used an ensemble of trial solutions, from which we select a number of best sets Γ, according to a standard Monte Carlo procedure, weighted by Eq. (5), to generate the next generation of the ensemble. In order to do this we introduce a mutation implemented in terms of random Gaussian noise around the previous best parameter set. This mutation, followed by the selection of minima, yields an effective downhill search method, capable of exploring large regions of parameter space. It also creates as a byproduct an ensemble of good strings with small deviations to the data. For small enough deviations from the best string we can sample parameter space in an unbiased manner. It is this ensemble, and its best string, that is then used to estimate Eq. (6). Results given in the manuscript involve ensembles with several million realizations and a choice of σ, common to all data points, corresponding the 20% of the *ldpd*. The standard deviation σ can be made to vary from point to point if more information about the quality of the datum is available. In this sense the procedure is able to incorporate variable expectations of uncertainty as the data are collected.

3 Real Time Analysis of Outbreak of Marburg Fever in Angola

We now proceed to describe the application of the method to estimate in real time the course of an outbreak of the rare Marburg hemorrhagic fever in Uige, Angola during 2005. This example posed many of the challenges that lead to the development of the present methodology. The pathogen is rare and its epidemiological parameters were largely unknown beyond the observation of the apparent incubation time and time from incidence of symptoms to death in a handful of cases. The mortality was also extremely high and took the lives of many of the medical care providers that intervened early in this remote African region. Because the disease affected dispro-portionally children under five the implementation of isolation control measures was also extremely difficult, and their results uncertain at the time according to reports by the World Health Organization and journalists on the ground. Nevertheless even with very scant information, model predictions were accurate from one case report to the next and detected successfully the over-counting of cases and deaths that characterized late stage reports.

The current work uses data from WHO reports, freely available online or via email, together with basic epidemiological modeling to generate a characterization and outlook for the outbreak. As sparse as the data are, we hoped that our results would help quantify the progression of the disease and assess the efficacy of inter-vention efforts necessary to stop the epidemic. Section 3.1 gives general background information on the disease and the anatomy of the outbreak as far as it was reported at the time in medical journals and the general media. Section 3.2 describes the specific model and parameter estimation procedure. Section 3.3 analyses the sce-narios of progression for the disease, taking into account the data points and some qualitative information in WHO reports. In this way we were able to estimate the effect of the interventions started shortly after March 23, in lowering contact rates, and discuss here the effects of under reporting and place bounds on population movement restrictions, so as not to reignite the epidemic. We also estimated the time horizon at which the spread would cease, as well as the final number of cases and fatalities.

3.1 Brief Anatomy of the Outbreak

The 2005 outbreak of Marburg hemorrhagic fever in Angola [13, 15–18, 27] has highlighted the direst need for fast and creative intervention in the face of the most severe infrastructure constraints imaginable. Intervention measures, which are the only way to stop the progression of the disease in the absence of a cure, were met with significant levels of noncompliance from the population. Due to the extremely high mortality and lack of adequate preparation initially, health workers took a large toll of the early deaths, eroding confidence in their effectiveness. Furthermore the viral strand attacked primarily children under five, making it extremely difficult for families to entrust them to the healthcare system under the knowledge of very probable fatality.

Under these circumstances it was paramount to provide the best quantitative guidance and prognosis for the outbreak in real time so that limited resources can be allocated optimally. This is now starting to be possible, thanks to several outbreak surveillance and news systems, provided by the World Health Organization (WHO) [27], Pro-Med mail [15], CDC [17] and others. We used these reports to generate a data series, analyze the outbreak, and at each time elaborate scenarios for the future course of the outbreak. These can also be used to help gauge the effectiveness of the current levels of intervention and establish quantitative goals for new and/or increased measures aiming at stopping the epidemic.

The 2005 outbreak of the Marburg fever in Angola was uncommon in several respects [13, 15, 20, 27]. It was the largest of the disease to date in a general population, it had an extremely high case fatality rate (88%, compared with 23% and 70% in previous smaller outbreaks) and attacked disproportionately children under five (75% of the cases). Marburg fever symptoms in their earliest stages are non-specific. The condition can be easily confused with other more common endemic diseases in the region such as malaria, yellow fever and typhoid fever, an issue that lead to biases in reporting, especially once awareness was raised after the identification of several hundred cases and deaths. Estimates for several of the outbreak's relevant rates are [27], an incubation period of about 3–9 days, a time to death (2005 outbreak) of 3–7 days after onset of symptoms, and a high proportion of cases develop hemorrhagic symptoms within 5–7 days.

The Marburg virus is a member of the family *Filoviridae*, which also includes Ebola. Marburg however is much rarer. The reservoir of the disease remains unknown (some clues point to bats or other cave dwelling animals [11, 20]). Primates can carry the virus but also contract the disease and manifest symptoms.

Uíge is a tropical province in the interior North West of Angola, bordering the Democratic Republic of Congo. The total population of the province is estimated at about half a million people and is mostly rural. In 2005 Uíge's province two largest cities were Uíge, with about 170,000 people, and Negage with about 25,000 people. These cities' hospitals serve most of the province's population. The population of Angola is young (43.5% under 14) and with high fertility rate (6.33 children/woman), creating conditions for very high and effective transmission of the Marburg virus.

Intervention efforts by the Government and the World Health Organization started in earnest in March 23, 2005 (judging from WHO reports), a few days after the identification of the virus by the US Centers for Disease Control, Special Pathogens Branch [17, 27]. Significant efforts were also developed by nongovernmental organizations such as *Medicins sans Frontiers* (Belgium, France,

Holland and Spain). Additional efforts by other international organizations are described in the WHO outbreak news reports, especially that of March 29 [27].

3.2 Homogeneously Mixing SEIR Population Model

We use a simple modification of the standard SEIR epidemic model, in order to account for the high mortality rate of the present outbreak. The model applies to homogeneously mixing population and thus does not distinguish individuals by e.g. age, a factor that is important in the current outbreak. The data necessary to draw such distinctions, if it exists at all, is not available in the public domain. Because most cases have occurred in Uíge, or are thought to have originated through contagion incurred there, we will take the total number of cases and the total number of fatalities as the targets for parameter estimation.

The SEIR model [1, 4] has been shown to describe well the outbreak dynamics of the related Ebola virus [7]. Specifically our model is:

$$\frac{dS}{dt} = -\beta \frac{SI}{N}, \quad \frac{dE}{dt} = \beta \frac{SI}{N} - \varepsilon E,$$
$$\frac{dI}{dt} = \varepsilon E - \gamma I, \quad \frac{dD}{dt} = p\gamma I, \quad \frac{dR}{dt} = (1 - p)\gamma I. \tag{9}$$

Here, as usual, S(t) are the number of susceptibles at time t, E(t) the number of exposed, which naturally progress to manifest the disease as Infective I(t). D(t) is the number of fatalities at time t, whereas R(t) is the number of recovered.

With these choices the population, summed over all classes, is fixed. The total number of cases, tallied at time t, is the sum of the presently infected, deceased and recovered. The incubation time is parameterized by ε^{-1}, β is the contact rate, which is the product of the (assumed independent) probability of a contact between an infected and a susceptible and the effectiveness of that contact. Lowering the value of β is the target of intervention [7]. The mean time spent in the infective class is γ^{-1}, after which an individual transits to the recovered class with probability (1-p) and dies with complementary probability p.

The set of parameters $\Gamma=\{S(t_0), E(t_0), I(t_0), D(t_0), R(t_0), \beta,\varepsilon,\gamma,p\}$, i.e. the initial conditions for each of the state variables and the dynamical parameters, is the target of our estimation procedure, as described in Section 2.

Parameter estimations will be bound within intervals dictated by knowledge of the outbreak [27]. These intervals are summarized in Table 1 below:

3.3 Parameter Estimation and Outbreak Prediction

We started tracking the outbreak in the beginning of April shortly after it was first identified on March 23. Our first predictions were made on April 26. At that time there were two possible viable scenarios for the history of the outbreak: one where it had started soon before March 23 (which we will call the simplest scenario)

Table 1 Model parameters and their allowed ranges (see text). Some of the ranges are not known and absolute maxima or minima are used

Name	Symbol	Minimum value	Maximum value
Initial Susceptibles	$S(t_0)$	10	500,000
Initial Exposed	$E(t_0)$	0	500
Initial Infective	$I(t_0)$	0	100
Initial Deceased	$D(t_0)$	0	500
Initial Recovered	$R(t_0)$	0	500
Contact rate	β	0	10
Incubation time	ε^{-1}	3 days	9 days
Lifetime infective	γ^{-1}	3 days	7 days
Case mortality	p	0	0.95

and another where it would have started sometime during October 2004. The latter was supported by retrospective analysis [27], and was eventually confirmed by our estimation procedure. We proceed to tell a brief history of our prognosis as it happened.

3.3.1 April 27: Simplest Scenario

In the simplest scenario we constrain the model by the estimated number of cases and deaths as reported by WHO, without any other further constraints. Below we consider the fact that the epidemic is though to have started in October 2004 as an additional qualitative constraint. The best fit trajectories for cases and fatalities are shown in Fig. 1, together with the data points, while parameters are displayed in Table 2.

These estimates predict an incubation time and lifetime of the infective state to be on the shorter end of their allowed ranges and mortality at the higher end. The contact rate is high leading to a large basic reproductive number, which measures the expected number of new cases caused by the introduction of an infective individual in a population of susceptibles. Given the population conditions, the high infant mortality due to the disease, and cultural practices of care for the ill and deceased we believe these numbers could not be excluded.

Table 2 Estimates for model parameters corresponding to the trajectories of Figs. 1 and 2. The initial time t_0 for parameter estimation is arbitrarily taken to be March 1

Name	Symbol	Best fit	95% CL interval
Initial Susceptibles	$S(t_0)$	200	[190, 218]
Initial Exposed	$E(t_0)$	0.2	[0.1, 0.3]
Initial Infective	$I(t_0)$	0.	[0, 1]
Initial Deceased	$D(t_0)$	87.7	[84, 90]
Initial Recovered	$R(t_0)$	0	[0, 1]
Contact rate	β	1.43	[1.18, 1.56]
Incubation time	ε^{-1}	4 days	[3.5, 5]
Lifetime infective	γ^{-1}	3 days	[3, 4]
Mortality	P	0.92	[0.91, 0.93]
Basic reproductive number	$R_0 = \beta/\gamma$	4.29	[3.58, 4.69]

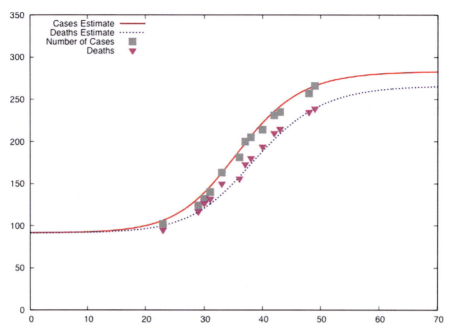

Fig. 2 Estimated best trajectories for total number of cases and deaths constrained to data from WHO surveillance reports. The least deviation per datum (ldpd) is 5.22. The curves asymptote to about 276 total cases and 261 deceased at around May 9, 2005 (the origin is the beginning of March)

This estimate predicted that the outbreak was then nearly over. The number of new infected cases was dropping in time. Its final state would be reached around May 9, with a total number of cases of 276 and 261 deaths. The upper end of the 95% confidence level intervals, shown in Fig. 2, would take these numbers up to 304 cases and 287 deaths by May 9–10. We show below that this scenario could be rejected as more data eventually came in.

Figure 3 shows the 95% confidence level intervals for number of cases and deaths. This is drawn from an ensemble of about 100,000 realizations of the model that fit the data within 20% of the best fit shown in Fig. 2.

3.3.2 Estimating Effectiveness of Intervention

The effectiveness of intervention can be assessed by allowing the contact rate β to vary in time. This strategy was used by Chowell et al. [7] to model intervention in recent Ebola epidemic outbreaks in Uganda and the Democratic Republic of Congo. The varying contact rate can be parametrized as [7]

$$\beta = \begin{cases} \beta_0, & t \leq t_{\text{int}} \\ \beta_1 + (\beta_0 - \beta_1)e^{-\kappa(t-t_{\text{int}})}, & t > t_{\text{int}} \end{cases} \tag{10}$$

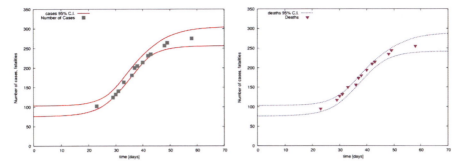

Fig. 3 95% confidence level intervals estimated from fitting the model to the data within 20% of the best fit shown in Fig. 2, for the number of cases, between *red lines* (*left*) and for number of deaths, between *blue lines* (*right*)

where t_{int} is the time at which intervention starts. κ is the time for the intervention to set in and β_0 and β_1 are the asymptotic contact rates before and after. We chose t_{int} to be March 23, when WHO reported for the first time to be "supporting efforts by the Ministry of Health in Angola to strengthen infection control in hospitals, to intensify case detection and contact tracing, and to improve public understanding of the disease and its modes of transmission" [27] (March 23 report).

We find a modest but significant change in contact rates from β_0=1.534 ± 0.013 to β_1=1.401 ± 0.010 over a period of just over 10 days. i.e. a decrease in the contact rate of about 8.7%. This gives the best fit to the data of all scenarios with ldpd=4.51. This change in contact rate highlights both the monumental efforts on the ground to contain the spread of the disease and the amply reported [8, 13] resistance they encountered, due, in large extent to the unkind characteristics of the disease.

3.3.3 Population Movements and Possible Epidemic Restart

Although the model estimated that the epidemic was then contained there can still be population movements that escape health care intervention, so that more people can enter the susceptible class. These effects can be monitored in real time via the estimation of the critical number of additional susceptibles that will cause the epidemic to regain momentum.

The simplest estimate follows from asking what number of susceptibles will reignite the growth of infected (i.e. make dI/dt>0). From Eqs. (1) this is

$$\frac{S^*}{N} = \frac{\gamma}{\beta} \tag{11}$$

For S>S* the number of new infections will grow. We can further write $S^* = S_{now} + \Delta S$ and similarly N=N_{now} + ΔS, where S_{now}, N_{now} are the present numbers of susceptible and of the population participating in the epidemic (i.e. the sum of numbers over all classes) and ΔS is the critical number of additional susceptibles. Given best parameter estimates for the simple scenario on April 27 this resulted in

$\Delta S \approx 70$ individuals, which is clearly a very small fraction of the general population. We repeat this procedure in other scenarios below.

3.3.4 Impact of Possible Under Reporting and Parameter Estimation

In discussing the results of parameter estimation in this simplest scenario we found that both the case fatality rate and γ appeared at the higher end of their allowed ranges. In this section we discuss how this may be the result of case under reporting. Under reporting is probable given the remoteness of the region and the initial resistance to intervention efforts amply reported in the news [8].

To estimate the effects of under reporting we assume that number of infected reported cases I(t) is in fact a (assumed fixed) fraction λ of the real number of total cases $I^{tot}(t)$, so that

$$I(t) \rightarrow \lambda I(t) = I^{tot}(t), \qquad \lambda > 1. \tag{12}$$

We also assume that the fraction of under reporting in deaths is much smaller, so that effectively $D(t) \approx D^{tot}(t)$. We can therefore ask for the transformation in parameters that leave the dynamics of deaths invariant under the rescaling of infected. The equation become

$$\frac{dD'}{dt} = p'\gamma'I' = p'\gamma'\lambda I = \frac{dD}{dt} = p\gamma I \Rightarrow p'\gamma'\lambda = p\gamma \tag{13}$$

Thus, since $\lambda > 1$, this implies that the actual mortality is lower than estimated, and/or that the lifetime of the infectious state γ^{-1} is longer.

If we ask e.g. that $\gamma^{-1} = 5$ days and that the mortality is similar to that observed in the previous outbreak of Marburg fever in the Democratic Republic of Congo (about 70%), we would obtain

$$\lambda = \frac{p\gamma}{p'\gamma'} \cong 2.2, \tag{14}$$

suggesting that less than half of infected cases may have been reported. This was at the time most probably an overestimate. If we allow the mortality to remain above 90% then $\lambda \approx 5/3 = 1.67$, which still suggests a large fraction of unaccounted cases if the simplest scenario was to hold. This transformation has also implications for the evolution of E and S, but as these states are unconstrained by the data we shall not discuss such features here. Whether case underreporting was an explanation of the high estimates for p and γ or the modeling of the progression of the infective state was too simple in this scenario, was an issue that required more data. It was resolved by the release of the next two data points, see below.

3.3.5 April 27: Enforcing the Start of the Epidemic in October 2004

There is evidence, based on retrospective analysis [27] (March 23 report), that the epidemic started in October 2004. This section enforces such constraint in the parameter estimation procedure, analyses resulting parameter ranges and uses them to make prognoses for the development of the epidemic.

There are two caveats in performing parameter estimates under these circumstances. First, the start of the epidemic in October 2004 introduces a constraint, 4–5 months (158–121 days taking the beginning and end of the month as bounds) before the first number of cases was announced. Estimating epidemic parameters under such distant constraint is delicate and tends to lead to high sensitivity in the parameter search. As such it is intrinsically more difficult to guarantee a fair sampling of all possible solutions consistent with the data, at some error level. Second, in the very early stages of the epidemic a stochastic model is probably more appropriate than (9), which makes a number of assumptions about a homogeneously mixing population, and the applicability of averages to single instance data.

As such the results of the present estimation should be considered more susceptible to systematic error than those given above. With these caveats in mind we proceed with the estimate. Results are shown in Table 3 and in Fig. 4.

The essential qualitative consequence of enforcing that the epidemic started in October 2004 is to make the derivative in the solution for the total number of cases be positive, if small, when the virus started being tracked on March 23. Because the model (9) is monotonic in the total number of cases and deaths this necessarily generates a solution with a larger positive derivative at those first few data points. Taken at face value this constraint had two consequences: (i) it suggests that initial reported number of cases (until about March 31) were underestimates of the real numbers, (although the number of deaths is well fit by the model, and may thus not have been itself underestimated) and (ii) it led to a higher estimate – relative to the simplest scenario above – of the eventual number of cases and deaths.

Without further intervention (which was then on the way), in the absence of population movements, or any other significant external event, the epidemic was

Table 3 Estimates for model parameters corresponding to the trajectories of Figs. 4 and 5. The initial time is October 1, 2004. The estimated value of the basic reproductive number is roughly similar to that computed for recent Ebola outbreaks in Uganda and the Democratic republic of Congo [7]

Name	Symbol	Best fit	95% CL interval
Initial Susceptibles	$S(t_0)$	763	[760, 765]
Initial Exposed	$E(t_0)$	0	[0, 0.1]
Initial Infective	$I(t_0)$	0	[0, 1]
Initial Deceased	$D(t_0)$	0.5	[0, 1]
Initial Recovered	$R(t_0)$	0.35	[0, 1]
Contact rate	β	0.54	[1.18, 1.56]
Incubation time	ε^{-1}	6.5 days	[6, 7]
Lifetime infective	γ^{-1}	3 days	[3, 4]
Mortality	P	0.91	[0.90, 0.92]
Basic reproductive number	R_0	1.62	[1.60, 1.64]

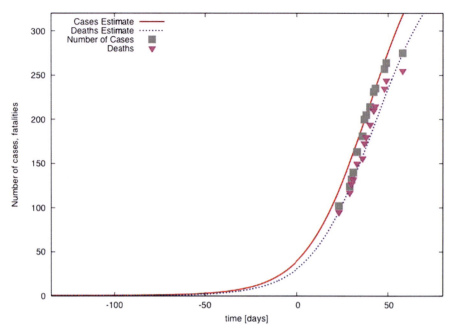

Fig. 4 Best estimated trajectories for total number of cases and deaths, under the constraint that the outbreak started October 1, 2004, without taking into account interventions. The deviation per datum is 11.15. The curves eventually asymptote to about 495 total cases, with 451 deceased by the last week of July

then expected to be extinguished only by the last week of July, with a total number of cases around 495, and 451deceased. These numbers should be taken as upper bounds. The upper end of the 95% confidence level intervals gave 519 cases and 471 deaths, whereas the lower estimated 486 cases and 440 deaths. The epidemic would

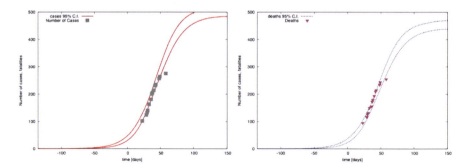

Fig. 5 The 95% confidence level intervals estimated from fitting the model to the data within 20% of the best fit shown in Fig. 4, for the number of cases, between *red lines* (*left*) and for number of deaths, between *blue lines* (*right*). The last point, reported April 27, suggests that this scenario is ruled out at 95% confidence level. This was due to interventions, see below

then need a number greater than about 180 people becoming new susceptibles, in the days after April 26, to regain growth in the number of new infectious.

Changing this constraint for the start of the epidemic from the first of October 2004 to the last generates similar, if slightly higher, estimates. This is the result of forcing the solution to be steeper, as it has to rise from zero to the case numbers reported in March over a smaller period of time. Specifically this change predicted a final number of 502 cases with 456 deaths, again by the end of July, which again would be the results in the absence of interventions. The 95% confidence level intervals are [495, 529] and [446, 480] for cases and deaths, respectively.

3.3.6 May 19: Accounting for Interventions and Distinguishing Scenarios the Beginning and End of the Outbreak

The next two data points released by the WHO in the first half of May permitted the clear distinction between the two scenarios for the beginning of the outbreak and a clear estimate of the impact of the intervention on the further development of the outbreak. Only the scenario where the outbreak started in October 2004 remained viable.

The results show that intervention – modeled by allowing β to vary according to (10), holding other parameters to the values of Table 3 – had by then managed to curb the growth rate of the outbreak, but not stop it altogether. The pool of susceptibles was estimated not to have grown over the weeks before May 9, although a small growth could not be completely excluded and was suggested by news reports, see below. The mean trajectory would eventually asymptote to an expected number of 356 total cases, with 331 deaths. This compares to the estimates (done before April 27) for 497 cases and 452 deaths, in the absence of intervention (black lines, Fig. 6). Intervention cut contact rates by a factor of about 40% and is estimated to have taken effect starting April 4, 2005 and taking about 12 days to be implemented (Fig. 7).

3.3.7 May 26: Statistical Anomalies and Over Reporting

Interestingly, as the outbreak seemed to be simmering down, the next few data points indicated a dramatic re-start of the epidemic. Results up to May 9 showed that intervention was curbing the growth rate of the outbreak, but had not succeeded at stopping it altogether. The new data released by the Angolan Government and WHO on May 26 showed a dramatic reversal of that trend. Many new cases have been registered: 399 from 337 a week before, accompanied by a sharp increase in the number of deaths to 355 from 311.

These numbers were statistical anomalies, lying far above the upper end of the 95% confidence for cases and deaths estimated on May 9. Thus they required a change in qualitative events on the ground. In the context of the model these new data points could only be accounted for in two very different scenarios. First, the new numbers could simply be wrong, attributing cases and deaths due to other causes to Marburg. Alternatively, the new data could indicate that a large number of

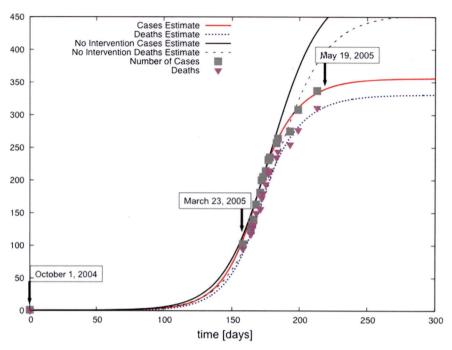

Fig. 6 Best trajectories for total number of cases and deaths, under the constraint that the outbreak started October 1, 2004 (day 0). The deviation per datum (a measure of goodness of fit) is 14.11. The color lines show the average solution under the effects of intervention and compare favorably with the trajectories estimated on April 27 (*black lines*), where this was not taken into account

new individuals (several hundred) had entered the susceptible population over the preceding few weeks and that the contact rate incurred by them had also increased, possibly up to pre-intervention levels. Clearly such a dramatic expansion of the susceptible pool should have qualitative signatures on the ground. To be true, the new data and model estimates under this scenario suggested that the epidemic threshold

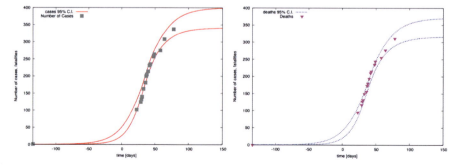

Fig. 7 95% Confidence level intervals for the number of deaths (*left*) and cases (*right*), under the constraint that the outbreak started October 1, 2004 (day 0)

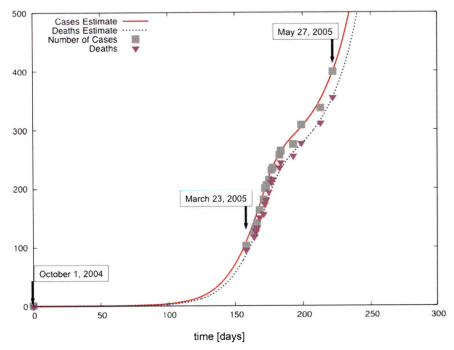

Fig. 8 Best trajectories for total number of cases and deaths, under the constraint that the outbreak started October 1, 2004 (day 0). The deviation per datum (a measure of goodness of fit) is 13.20. The new data of May 27 was an anomaly, far exceeding the upper bound of the 95% confidence level intervals for cases and deaths, estimated up to May 9. The new best fit trajectories allow β to vary upwards and require an linear inflow of people into the susceptible class at a rate of 68 persons a day

had been crossed again and that the number of new infected would subsequently grow at an accelerated pace.

In fact we could estimate that the susceptible population would have to be growing then, after the very end of April, at a rate up to 68 individuals per day. This was tantamount to an epidemic restart, visible in Fig. 8, as the average trajectories changed curvature. Needless to say, under such conditions the outlook for the development of the outbreak was rather bleak, with hundreds more cases and deaths predicted to follow.

These data points were eventually revised down, after a long hiatus in reporting between June 17 and July 13, confirming the prognosis of May 9.

3.3.8 Epilogue

The outbreak of Marburg hemorrhagic fever in Uige, Angola was officially declared over on November 7, 2005 by the Angolan Ministry of Health [23], with its last laboratory confirmed case reported July 22. The outbreak claimed a total of 329 lives out of 374 identified cases, a case fatality rate of 88%. These numbers were correctly predicted on May 9, 2005, amid much uncertainty in WHO reports and in the news about the future development of the outbreak.

4 Discussion and Conclusions

The principal objective of the present study was to investigate the possibility of modeling in real time the spread of a new epidemic of a rare emerging disease, with very sparse data available. We have used standard outbreak reports available online from the WHO [27] and Pro-med mail [15] to construct a small data set, which we then employed to estimate epidemiological parameters and future case and death numbers with quantified uncertainty. The output of the model was used to provide guidance for the outlook of the epidemic under given qualitative scenarios and construct quantitative goals for intervention policy on the ground, creating the potential for helping optimize quantitatively severe logistical constraints.

Among other quantities our approach allows for the quantitative estimate of epidemiological parameters with quantified uncertainty, and to the projection for the total number of cases and deaths at the also predicted time for the end of the outbreak. These estimates can then be used to test qualitative scenarios about the outbreak, such as the time for the occurrence of the index case, and to quantify in real time the effects of interventions and estimate population movements. This approach, much like any general epidemiological mathematical modeling [1, 4] makes certain general simplifying assumptions about the nature of the outbreak. While these may be suspect to practitioners on the ground, it has been amply demonstrated that models retain substantial predictive power, which tends to trump projections for case numbers and deaths generated by expert opinion.

We believe that even if not perfect this type of "real time" epidemiological modeling is now feasible [2, 3, 5, 6, 21] and could become an essential tool useful in providing quantitative scenarios and targets for limited resource allocation on the ground. It should also be used to inform the scientific community and the public, as well as public health officials, of rational expectations and choices under unfolding new outbreaks.

References

1. Anderson RM, May RM (1995) Infectious Diseases of Humans. Oxford: Oxford University Press.
2. Bettencourt LMA, Ribeiro RM (2008) Real Time Bayesian Estimation of the Epidemic Potential of Emerging Infectious Diseases. PLoS ONE 3(5): e2185. doi:10.1371/journal.pone.0002185
3. Bettencourt LMA, Ribeiro RM, Chowell G, Lant T, Castillo-Chavez C. Towards real time epidemiology: Data assimilation, modeling and anomaly detection of health surveillance data streams. In: Zeng D, Gotham I, Komatsu K, Lynch C, editors. Lecture Notes in Computer Science; 2007; New Brunswick, NJ: Springer-Verlag. pp. 79–90.
4. Brauer F, Castillo-Chavez C (2001) Mathematical Models in Population Biology and Epidemiology. New York: Springer-Verlag.

5. Cauchemez S, Boelle P-Y, Donnelly CA, Ferguson NM, Thomas G, et al. (2006) Real-time estimates in early detection of SARS. Emerging Infectious Diseases 12: 110–113.
6. Cauchemez S, Boelle P-Y, Thomas G, Valleron A-J (2006) Estimating in real time the efficacy of measures to control emerging communicable diseases. American Journal of Epidemiology 164: 591–597.
7. Chowell G, Hengartner NW, Castillo-Chavez C, Fenimore PW, Hyman JM (2004) The reproductive number of ebola and the effects of public health measures: The cases of Congo and Uganda. Journal of Theoretical Biology 229(1):119326.
8. Denise Grady (2005) "Mysterious Viruses as Bad as They Get", New York Times April 26.
9. Fauci AS (2005) Race against time. Nature 435: 423–424.
10. Lawson AB, Kleinman K, editors (2005) Spatial and Syndromic Surveillance for Public Health. Chichester: John Wiley & Sons.
11. Leroy EM, Kumulungui B et al. (2005) Fruit bats as reservoirs of Ebola virus. Nature 438: 575–576.
12. Morens DM, Folkers GK, Fauci AS (2004) The challenge of emerging and re-emerging infectious diseases. Nature 430: 242–249.
13. Nature News http://www.nature.com/news/2005/050404/full/050404-12.html
14. Osterholm MT (2005) Preparing for the next pandemic. New England Journal of Medicine 352: 1839–1842.
15. Pro-Med mail reports http://www.promedmail.org.
16. Schou S, Hansen AK (2000) Marburg and ebola virus infections in laboratory non-human primates: A literature review. Comparative Medicine 50(2):108.
17. See Center for Disease Control briefings http://www.cdc.gov/ncidod/dvrd/spb/mnpages/dispages/marburg.htm
18. See Virginia Bioinformatics Institute Pathport site for general background http://pathport.vbi.vt.edu/pathinfo/pathogens/Marburg_virus_Info.shtml
19. Spall JC (2003) Introduction to Stochastic Search and Optimization. Hoboken NJ: Wiley.
20. Swanepoel R, Smit SB, Rollin PE, Formenty P, Leman PA, Kemp A, et al. (2007) Studies of reservoir hosts for Marburg virus. Emerging Infectious Diseases 13: 1847–1851.
21. Wallinga J, Teunis P (2004) Different epidemic curves for severe acute respiratory syndrome reveal similar impacts of control measures. American Journal of Epidemiology 160: 509–516.
22. Webby RJ, Webster RG (2003) Are we ready for pandemic influenza? Science 302: 1519–1522.
23. WHO (2005) Marburg hemorrhagic fever: Angola 2005 outbreak. Action Against Infection. 4(6).
24. Wolfe ND, Dunavan CP, Diamond J (2007) Origins of major human infectious diseases. Nature 447: 279–283.
25. Woolhouse ME, Gowtage-Sequeria S (2005) Host range and emerging and reemerging pathogens. Emerging Infectious Diseases 11: 1842–1847.
26. Woolhouse ME, Haydon DT, Antia R (2005) Emerging pathogens: the epidemiology and evolution of species jumps. Trends in Ecology & Evolution 20: 238–244.
27. World Health Organization Outbreak updates, http://www.who.int/csr/don/archive/disease/marburg_virus_disease/en/index.html

Statistical Challenges in BioSurveillance

Tom Burr, Sarah Michalak, and Rick Picard

Abstract One goal in biosurveillance is to detect patterns in disease rates, such as temporal and/or geographic clustering. Traditionally, disease rates are available by geographic unit over weekly, monthly, or yearly time bins, and covariates such as age, gender, and socio-economic status can be used to adjust predicted rates prior to testing for clustering. Recently, more timely pre-diagnostic data including emergency department visits have been used in "syndromic surveillance" in order to more rapidly detect either natural or bioterrorist-related outbreaks. Typically, such data are categorized by chief complaint into one of several syndromes such as gastro-intestinal or respiratory.

This chapter describes outbreak detection using either traditional diagnosed case rates or syndromic surveillance data. Outbreak detection involves many issues; our focus is the associated statistical challenges, including: (1) approaches to characterizing the natural background; (2) algorithms for detecting abnormal increases above background disease rates, (3) methods for adjusting for covariates such as gender, age, etc.; (4) detecting spatial-temporal clusters, and (5) methods for protecting data confidentiality.

1 Introduction

Our topic is statistical aspects of detecting disease outbreaks. The definition of disease "outbreak" depends on the context and analysis goals. In many cases, the goal is to detect an outbreak in near real time, using, for example, daily counts of a specific illness or perhaps of a less-specific syndrome. In other cases, purported disease clusters are identified retrospectively. Although outbreak detection is too broad a topic to fully cover in this chapter, we will focus on a few specific examples that illustrate many of the statistical issues.

T. Burr (✉)
Statistical Sciences Group, Los Alamos National Laboratory, Los Alamos NM 87545, USA
e-mail: tburr@lanl.gov

G. Chowell et al. (eds.), *Mathematical and Statistical Estimation Approaches in Epidemiology*, DOI 10.1007/978-90-481-2313-1_8,
© Springer Science+Business Media B.V. 2009

In some contexts, various types of disease clusters (Section 2) are considered to be outbreaks. Throughout this chapter, a disease outbreak will be defined as any abnormal increase in disease rate. An effective definition of what is meant by "abnormal" depends on the situation. Some diseases such as flu have roughly annual peaks due to seasonal effects. Such annual peaks could be considered to be part of the ordinary background of disease frequency and then would not be considered to be an outbreak. In other applications, rapid detection of the beginning of the annual peak might be the main goal and the annual peak would be regarded as an outbreak. Even in the case of flu, epidemiologists are unlikely to agree on exactly when a given year's flu outbreak began in a particular region of the country. An arbitrary but reasonable definition is that the starting day of the flu season is the day on which the number of new flu cases exceeds some threshold defined on the basis of the recent daily background case rate, and the numbers of new cases for each of the following days are also above the recent background for at least some specified number of days.

Although people often associate the word "outbreak" with a rapid increase in disease frequency, we define a disease outbreak as any abnormal increase in disease rate. Therefore, the example "outbreaks" discussed below include any elevation in disease rate, which could occur as a subtle increase over multiple years, and thus would not be a rapid increase in disease frequency. Note that if the normal background is nearly zero, such as anthrax cases in humans or relatively rare cancers in humans, then the increase could be a small number of cases. If the normal background is substantial, such as with flu-like illnesses, then an abnormal increase in frequency would be a relatively large number of cases.

Any of several types of public health outcome surveillance data such as yearly cancer rates by geographic region or daily counts of patient chief complaints in emergency departments (EDs) can be used, with varying levels of success, to monitor for outbreaks. Roughly speaking, there is a tradeoff between timeliness and quality of information. For example, in syndromic surveillance (SS), the chief complaint of each patient visiting an ED is typically categorized into a syndrome category, such as respiratory or gastro-intestinal. This is relatively low-quality count data because of the coarseness and overlap of categories; however, it is available in near real time. In practice, there are several challenges in using SS data that we will describe, such as assessing the non-outbreak background rate of cases in each syndrome category. An example of higher quality, less timely data is disease rates by geographic region, perhaps available by week, month, or year, but even these will suffer from misdiagnosis, and under reporting, for example, which we will discuss.

Outbreak detection is challenging in many ways; our focus is the associated statistical challenges, including: (1) approaches to characterizing the natural background; (2) algorithms for detecting abnormal increases above background in disease rates, (3) methods for adjusting for covariates such as gender, age, etc.; (4) detecting spatial-temporal clusters; and (5) methods for protecting data confidentiality.

Following sections include background and discussion of the five issues above for public health outcome surveillance and for syndromic surveillance.

2 Background

The background disease rate is the expected risk of disease in the absence of other information about an individual or group of individuals.

We will consider three types of elevated disease rates:

- a temporal cluster is an elevated disease rate for a period of time that is less than the study period;
- a spatial cluster is an elevated disease rate throughout the study period in a specific geographic region; and
- a spatio-temporal cluster is an elevated disease rate in a region of space for a period of time less than the study period.

A temporal cluster that does not persist over the full study region is difficult to detect. Because data from the full study region is used in searching for evidence of temporal clustering, if the study region is too large, it might be difficult to detect a temporal cluster. Similarly, if the period is too long, it might be difficult to detect a spatial cluster (Chapter 14, [27]). Therefore, the study region and temporal period are important. This chapter assumes that both have been well chosen and describes methods to monitor for clusters of elevated risk.

There are other types of elevated risk not discussed here. For example, a goal in some contexts is to detect elevated risk by demographic group or by individual-level variables such as indicators of overall health.

3 Public Health Outcome Surveillance

Public Health Outcome Surveillance relies on diagnosed case rates, often by home address, perhaps aggregated to zip code. A common example is spatial analysis of small area health data where population and disease counts are available over various time periods, such as by week, month, or year for each spatial unit.

Assume the study region is divided into N subregions or cells. Assume disease rate data are available by cell, where a cell could, for example, be a zip code region or census tract.

Denote the number of cases in cell i as x_i and the expected number of cases as E_i, where E_i could depend on covariates. Assume that x_i has a Poisson distribution with mean $r_i E_i$, denoted $x_i \sim \text{Poisson}(r_i E_i)$, where r_i captures departures from E_i and is called the standardized incidence ratio.

Statistical challenges in Public Health Outcome Surveillance to be described here include:

(1) Adjusting for covariates, and
(2) Issues involving maximally selected measures of evidence of clustering associated with data mining.

3.1 Adjusting for Covariates

Adjusting for covariates involves building a statistical model for cell i such as

$$E(x_i) = f(r_i, g_i, a_i, n_i | \beta) + e_i, \tag{1}$$

where $E(x_i)$ denotes the expected value of the number of disease cases in cell i, f is a function, linear in the parameters β or not, and linear in the predictors or not, and the vertical line indicates we are conditioning on values for the parameters β (which will in practice be estimated). The predictor r_i depicts racial information (perhaps vector-valued) for cell i, g_i denotes gender information for cell i (such as the percent female), a_i depicts age information for cell i (perhaps vector-valued), n_i is the number of individuals at risk for the disease in cell i, and e captures all error sources. Other common predictors include smoking status, socio-economic indicators, and body mass index. There is a large literature on fitting such models and performing diagnostic tests of their goodness of fit. See for example Venables and Ripley [40] and Hastie et al. [16].

Here our focus is observational data, which implies that spurious associations could exist. For example, suppose we have gender data by county and a fit to Equation (1) suggests that Caucasians have a higher rate of the monitored disease than non-Caucasians. If the Caucasian population is predominantly male and the non-Caucasian is predominantly female, but we are unaware of this demographic information, then the disease rate could be higher in males, but we falsely attribute the higher rate to something associated with being Caucasian. This could lead to wrong conclusions in establishing causality, but does not necessarily harm our analysis because we could still successfully apply Equation (1) to adjust correctly for elevated rates in a numerical sense, albeit for the wrong reason. Therefore, although there are major distinctions between observational and experimental studies, they will not be discussed. Note also that in some contexts not considered here, one goal is to identify subgroups, such as Caucasians, for which disease rates are higher (or lower).

We also point out that adjusting for covariates prior to testing for clustering implicitly assumes there is no masking of covariates with the spatial and/or temporal clustering we are trying to detect. For example, assume a study area consisting of coal mining areas and non mining areas and that more males than females of working age live and work in the coal mining areas. Assume that, due to exposure to carcinogenic coal dust, cancer rates are higher among coal miners. If the relative population sizes are such that an apparent gender effect is present, once that effect is corrected for using Equation (1), we could fail to notice the spatial clustering of cases associated with mining.

3.2 Maximally Selected Measures of Evidence

Example 1 gives an example of "maximally selected" measure of evidence. Suppose a researcher hypothesizes a reason for spatio-temporal clustering of a disease. Reasons could be that the disease is contagious or that some environmental effect

Table 1 Reproduction of one table from Knox [24] on clustering of childhood leukemia

	Close in residence	Not close in residence
Close in time	$a = 5$	$b = 147$
Not close in time	$c = 20$	$d = 4388$

impacted a small region over a short time period. For example, some have proposed that childhood leukemia can be caused by an infection. If so, this would help explain purported clusters of cases [24]. Here we simply examine the evidence for clustering, without speculating why clustering might occur.

Example 1 (Knox Statistic). This example develops and then extends the example provided in Knox [24], in which the onset times and residences for 96 childhood leukemia cases were analyzed by partitioning the cases as either being "close in time" or "close in residence" or both or neither, as shown in Table 1. Note that the total number of Table 1 entries is $N = \binom{96}{2} = 4,560$. We do not know how the "close in time" or "close in residence" thresholds were chosen. Therefore, later in this example we will consider how to adjust for the possibility that the evidence for clustering was quantified using each of several possible thresholds, as an example of what we refer to as "maximally selected measure of evidence."

The main goal for the Knox statistic is to identify spatio-temporal clustering if it is present. Spatio-temporal clustering is defined here to occur if the probability of cases being close in time is higher if they are close in space than if they are not close in space. This would imply that the probability of two cases being close in space is not independent of their time separation. In other contexts, if the joint probability of being both close in time and close in space is high, this would be evidence of clustering.

A commonly-used statistic to evaluate whether the two categories in a two-way table are independent is $S_1 = \sum_{i,j} \frac{(O_{ij} - E_{ij})^2}{E_{ij}}$, where O_{ij} is the observed count in cell i, j and $E_{ij} = N \frac{N_{i \cdot}}{N} \frac{N_{\cdot j}}{N} = \frac{N_{i \cdot} N_{\cdot j}}{N}$ is the estimated expected cell count assuming the categories are independent. Here, N is the total number of table entries, $N_{i \cdot}$ is the sum of counts in row i, $N_{\cdot j}$ is the sum of counts in column j, and by "independent" in this context, we mean that knowing two cases are close in space does not impact whether they are likely to be close in time. More formally, independence in space and time means here that the joint probability of being close in time and close in space is the marginal probability of being close in space multiplied by the marginal probability of being close in time. If the two categories are independent, then this S_1 statistic is approximately distributed as a χ_1^2 random variable (a chi-squared random variable with one degree of freedom).

Exercise 1a. Compute S_1 for Table 1 and evaluate the "p"-value, defined as $p = \text{Prob}(S_1 \geq S_{1,\text{observed}})$ assuming that $S_1 \sim \chi_1^2$. Next, compare S_1 to the 0.99 quantile of the χ_1^2, which is 6.63. A common statistical approach to evaluate whether data contradicts a model assumption, such as the independence of "close in time" and "close in space," is to compare the value of an observed statistic such as the $S_{1,\text{observed}}$ value to an appropriate reference distribution such as the χ_1^2 in this case. If the observed S_1 value is extreme (large rather than small in this case) compared to the reference distribution, that is evidence against the modeling assumption such as the independence of "close in time" and "close in space." Does $S_{1,\text{observed}}$ for Table 1 indicate a lack of fit to the "independent categories" assumption? To summarize this exercise, the model assumes the two categories are independent, and if so, then S_1 should have approximately a χ_1^2 distribution, which then serves as a reference distribution against which to compare $S_{1,\text{observed}}$. Here, $S_{1,\text{observed}}$ could be large because a was larger or smaller than its expected value, and therefore, the test based on S_1 is two-sided.

Exercise 1b. Use the entries a, b, c, and d in Table 1 to compute the conditional probability that a given pair is close in space given that it is close in time, and the conditional probability that a given pair is close in space given that it is not close in time.

Knox [24] further assumed that $a \sim \text{Poisson}(\frac{N_i.N_{.j}}{N})$, and the corresponding Knox statistic uses the observed value of a to test for nonindependence. Note that $\frac{a}{a+b} = 0.033$ and $\frac{c}{c+d} = 0.0045$ so the conditional probability $\frac{a}{a+b}$ that a given pair is close in space given that it is close in time is much larger than $\frac{c}{c+d}$, the conditional probability that a given pair that is close in space is not close in time. Also note that the expected count in the close in time and space cell is $\frac{N_i.N_{.j}}{N} = 0.833$, which is considerably less than the observed count of 5, thus providing some evidence against the null hypothesis of independence between "close in space" and "close in time."

Exercise 1c. Compute the "p"-value of Knox's statistic, where the "p"-value is defined as $p = \text{Prob}(a \geq a_{\text{observed}}$ assuming that $a \sim \text{Poisson}(\frac{N_i.N_{.j}}{N}))$. Compare this result to the "p"-value for the S_1 from Exercise 1a. Caution: statistical analyses depend on modeling assumptions, including distributional assumptions. It is not unusual to reach different conclusions (such as different "p"-values) depending on how the data are analyzed.

Recall that the S_1 could be large because a was larger or smaller than its expected value, and therefore, the test based on S_1 in Exercise 1a is two-sided. The test based on $a \sim \text{Poisson}(\frac{N_i.N_{.j}}{N})$ in Exercise 1c is one-sided. Therefore, the tests rely on different distributions, and one test is one-sided while the other test is two-sided.

A conceptually simple alternative to the χ_1^2 test and the Poisson test just described is a randomization test. The randomization test can be motivated by assuming that the "close in time" and/or "close in residence" labels are merely labels, having nothing to do with the actual times and locations. Suppose then that we randomly permuted the time labels among the 96 cases, and reordered the cases according to the sorted "incorrect" time labels. We could then recompute each of the four cell counts in Table 1 and we could repeat the random permutation step many times. Either the S_1 statistic or Knox's statistic could be recorded for each permutation to produce a reference distribution of values, and the observed S_1 value could be compared to this reference distribution. Alternately, the space labels could be permuted, or both the time and space labels could be permuted. It is statistically appropriate to permute either the time or space labels, but is also acceptable to permute both to perform this type of randomization test.

Exercise 1d. How many permutations of the 96 onset times are possible? Is it likely that the randomization test would actually compute this many values of the chosen test statistic?

Note that because 96! is a huge number of distinct orderings, in practice, we would typically randomly select 1,000 to 10,000 orderings, compute the chosen statistic for each, and the resulting distribution is the randomization test distribution against which the observed value of the statistic can be compared, as illustrated above for the χ_1^2 test and the Poisson test.

Table 1 appears to be a standard 2-by-2 table suited for a standard test for association between space and time; however, the 4,560 pairs of cases are not independent pairs. The non-independence arises because of the multiple triangle inequalities among the pairs of time distances and among the pairs of spatial distances. For example, $d(t_1, t_3) \leq d(t_1, t_2) + d(t_2, t_3)$, so these three pairs of distances are not mutually independent because $d(t_2, t_3)$ and $d(t_1, t_2)$ jointly provide information about $d(t_1, t_3)$. Therefore, neither the χ_1^2 distribution for the S_1 statistic nor the Poisson distribution for a can hold exactly. Barbour and Eagleson [1] used the Stein-Chen method to show that Knox's Poisson assumption was very accurate for the sample size Knox used. Although the technical details are beyond our scope here, the Stein-Chen method provides tight bounds on approximation errors when assumptions such as the independence assumption in this case are violated.

Before assuming that the Stein-Chen method justifies the use of the Knox statistic for analysis of the Table 1 data, it is important to consider how "close in time" and "close in space" were defined. For example, it is possible that the arbitrary definitions of "close" were chosen while analyzing the data. Burr [6] uses simulation to show that if both "close in time" and "close in space" were defined while analyzing the data to maximize the evidence for clustering, and that if adjustments are made to penalize for maximizing the evidence for clustering, then the p-values for the S_1 statistic and for Knox's statistic are revised upward considerably. The simulation in Burr [6] to adjust for maximally selecting a measure of evidence leads to a reference distribution that combines the randomization approach described above with a search over definitions of "close in time" and "close in space" that maximize the evidence for spatio-temporal clustering. A few similar versions of this type of approach are described in Example 2.

If the search for a maximally selected measure of evidence involves only one of the "close in time" and "close in space" definitions, then an approach based on the Wiener process [6, 35] provides a suitable analytical approximation to adjust for maximally selecting the evidence for clustering. Alternatively, a simulation-based reference distribution is of course also available as shown in Burr [6]. The Wiener process is a well-known continuous time stochastic process having stationary (constant over time) independent increments and satisfying the conditions $W(t = 0) = 0$, $W(t)$ is almost surely continuous ("almost surely" continuous means that it is continuous except perhaps for a set having probability 0), and $W(t) - W(s)$

has independent increments with distribution $N(0, t - s)$ for $0 \leq s < t$, where $N(\mu, \sigma^2)$ denotes the normal distribution with mean μ and variance σ^2. The condition that it has independent increments means that if $0 \leq s_1 \leq t_1 \leq s_2 \leq t_2$, then $W(t_1) - W(s_1)$ and $W(t_2) - W(s_2)$ are independent random variables.

Using the standardized Wiener process (which is forced to start and end at 0, and is called the "Brownian Bridge"), Miller and Seigmund [35] showed in another setting that the statistic $S_2 = \sup_{0 < x_1 \leq x \leq x_2 < 1} (\chi_1^2)^{(1/2)}$ satisfies

$$P(S_2 \geq w) = \frac{4\phi(w)}{w} + \phi(w)\left(w - \frac{1}{w}\right) \log 10 \left(\frac{\tau_2}{\tau_1}\right) + o\left(\frac{\phi(w)}{w}\right), \quad (2)$$

where the supremum is taken over the time or space threshold x to define close in time or space, ϕ is the standard normal density $(2\pi)^{-1/2} \exp^{(-w^2/2)}$, the "little oh" notation $o(\frac{\phi(w)}{w})$ denotes a small term compared to $\frac{\phi(w)}{w}$, and x_1 and x_2 are values not too close to 0 or 1, respectively. If x_1 is very close to 0 and/or x_2 is very close to 1, then the approximation is not very accurate.

Miller and Siegmund [35] did not provide any simulation results to determine what sample sizes are needed for Equation (2) to be a good approximation, and their context allowed them to assume the two rows sums in their tables that correspond to Table 1 here were nearly equal. Therefore, Burr [6] provided simulation results to evaluate the quality of the Wiener approximation under various conditions. Generally, the quality is acceptably good, but in this application, the table is typically unbalanced, having more observations "not close in time" than "close in time," and more observations "not close in space" than "close in space," because the search for a threshold to define close in space or time is typically restricted to a narrow range, such as between the 0.005 and 0.01 quantiles of the space or time distance values. Because of this unbalance, the Equation (2) approximation will be acceptably good, within approximately ± 0.02 of the correct value, only if there are at least 100 observations that are close in space and at least 100 observations that are close in time. This is a relatively strong requirement, and therefore, the accuracy of p-values from Equation (2) is unlikely to be within ± 0.02 of the correct value for the data in Table 1, because only 25 observations are close in space.

Another complication related to testing for spatio-temporal clustering involves population shift bias. Mantel [30] showed that if population growth rates differ among spatial regions, then this population shift bias creates spatio-temporal interaction among any random sample of individuals, thus tending to lead to spurious evidence for clustering. Kulldorff and Hjalmers [25] illustrated how to include the effect of population shifts in a simulated reference distribution.

Although Example 1 is a retrospective application of Knox's statistic, Marshall et al. [31] apply a local Knox statistic in a simulated real-time setting similar to syndromic surveillance (Section 4).

Example 2 (Spatio-Temporal Scan Statistic). This example is based on Kulldorff et al. [26], who applied a spatio-temporal scan statistic, which scans spatially and temporally for maximal clustering as described below.

A purported cancer cluster involved 10 brain cancer cases during the years 1986–1990 in Los Alamos, New Mexico. The expected number of brain cancer cases was 3.7, or 3.9 when adjusted for population shift bias as mentioned above [26]. At the time of the study, the state of NM had brain cancer records by year for each of its 32 counties from 1973 to 1991. Demographics including age, gender, and race are available by county each year to make adjustments if appropriate. The analysis presented here does not adjust for covariates.

Exercise 2a. Assume the number of brain cancer cases X in Los Alamos, NM from 1986 to 1990 is distributed as a Poisson variate having mean 3.7. Compute Prob($X \geq 10|\mu_X = 3.7$), where μ_X is the mean or expected value of X.

Assume that a spatial-temporal scan statistic was used to find maximal evidence of clustering [26]. There are many varieties of scan statistic, but the general idea is to scan for regions in search of relatively large (or small in some contexts) numbers of events. We will describe this statistic in terms of how it is typically implemented in the context of disease rate surveillance. There are a few other options available, for example, at www.satscan.org.

A spatial-temporal scan statistic can be implemented using circular scanning regions in space, using a particular county seat location as the center of a candidate circle, varying the radius of the circle to include varying numbers of neighboring counties, and simultaneously also scanning over blocks of 1, 2, 3, or more successive years. This can be repeated allowing each county seat to be the center of the scanning circle, and the maximum evidence found for clustering can be reported. Kulldorff suggests that the time windows could be any number of years ranging from 1 year to one-half of the total study period.

To adjust for this type of "maximally selected measure of evidence," Kulldorff [26] suggests a simulation-based reference distribution obtained by simulating case rates by county and year according to a Poisson distribution having a mean that is estimated using the historical state-wide case rate, adjusting for demographics if appropriate. Because the number of simulated cases will not typically exactly equal the number of actual cases, this option is sometimes called the "unconditional" option. Another alternative, particularly when extensive historical data is not available, is to constrain the number of simulated cases to equal the number of observed cases ("conditional"), but to permute the time and/or spatial labels of the cases during each repetition of the scan statistic.

Exercise 2b. Describe how to compute a simulation-based reference distribution that accounts for the spatial-temporal scanning described.

The solution to Exercise 2b involves making decisions such as whether to constrain the number of simulated cases to equal the number of observed cases. Suppose we do not enforce this constraint. Then, the solution can be described as follows. Simulate one realization of cases according to a Poisson distribution, adjusting for covariates if necessary. Implement the search of space and time regions to produce a large number of specific regions. For example, one specific region could be "the space-time region centered at county A with a 100 mile radius and spanning

1980–1990." For each region in the search over space and time regions, the numbers of simulated cases inside and outside the region are counted and the expected number of cases is calculated using the population at risk, adjusting for covariate if necessary. Find and save the smallest p-value over all such regions. Repeat for many (1000 or more) simulated realizations, saving the smallest p-value from each realization. The archived smallest p-values from each realization are the simulation-based reference distribution against which to compare the p value computed in Exercise 2a. The small p-value found in Exercise 2a is then revised upward considerably [26], because it is compared to the p-values in the reference distribution of smallest p-values, which tend to be quite small, again reflecting the fact that maximal evidence for clustering was used. For example, if the original unadjusted p-value is 0.01, then 0.01 might be at the 25th percentile in the simulated reference distribution, thus revising the p-value upward from 0.01 to 0.25.

Los Alamos, NM is a small rural community of approximately 20,000 residents. In 1991, a community resident voiced concern over what appeared to be a neighborhood brain cancer cluster. So, it is likely that the geographic region and time window were not actually chosen by the maximal selection process assumed by the simulation-based reference distribution. It is almost impossible to quantify the selection process (what temporal window and what spatial region) that was actually used. Therefore, choosing the most appropriate reference distribution to be used to estimate the p-value for evidence of clustering is a difficult issue to resolve.

Health officials are often asked to evaluate what appears to be a local disease cluster, as they were in this case. After agreeing on a case definition (what type of brain cancer, whether it must be the primary cancer, etc.), in addition to the maximal selection process over space and time described above, a related challenge not often considered involves whether many other diseases were also evaluated (another type of "selection of maximal evidence") for clustering.

3.3 Other Statistical Issues

There are many other statistical issues in public health outcome surveillance, including:

1. In order to apply the scan statistic as described, there must be a model for the expected number of cases. Given such a model, summarized perhaps by the expected number of cases in each cell in each time period, the observed number of cases in cell i at time t, $O_{i,t}$ can be compared to the expected number of cases $E_{i,t}$, and a residual or forecast error, such as $e_{i,t} = (O_{i,t} - E_{i,t})/E_{i,t}$ can be computed. These errors $e_{i,t}$ can be monitored using standard methods quality control, including sequential tests (see, for example, the description of Page's test in Section 4.6.3) that search over time and/or space for regions of elevated observed numbers of cases [6, 40] and scan statistics (such as in Example 2).

2. Misdiagnosis and under or over reporting of diseases are related issues and both lead to error sources that should be considered. Misdiagnosis includes both types of error – labeling an individual as having the disease (as a "case") when the

individual does not, or labeling an individual as not having the disease when the individual does have it. Under reporting occurs when not all cases are identified for various reasons, other than from misdiagnosis. If the under reporting is approximately constant in all regions, it does not necessarily lead to spurious conclusions, although prevalence estimates would be too low. On the other hand, if a particular region has a much higher rate of reporting than other regions, then it "over" reports, and especially for rare diseases, this could easily lead to spurious evidence of a disease cluster.

3. The suitability of using home address as the "location" of a new case should be considered. Whether the home address of each infected is suitable or adequate will be case specific. For example, the work address could easily be more relevant, depending on disease etiology. Also, binning cases by county and assigning them to the county seat in location is done for convenience. Inference quality can be impacted by choice of spatial and/or temporal scale.

4. Lack of effective training data having, for example, outbreaks with clearly defined start and stop times, is a common problem in monitoring for disease outbreaks. There is a general lack of well-established disease outbreak data that can be used to test and compare methods for disease monitoring. Generally, all methods of monitoring for disease outbreaks involve fitting a model that allows the expected number of cases E_i to be computed for spatial region i for a specified time period, adjusting for covariates if appropriate and feasible. Having computed each E_i, regions of elevated count rates can be detected as described above.

5. Disease rates based on small population sizes, particularly for rare diseases, are notorious for having relatively large variances. Disease mapping using hierarchical Bayesian methods [29] can mitigate the effect of large variability in small regional disease rate estimates. In MacNab et al. [29], the log-transformed regional disease rates are assumed to arise from a Gaussian prior. Under reasonable assumptions, this leads to "shrinkage to the mean" in which the estimated local disease rates are smoothed by two effects: the estimated disease rate in region i is modified by using the average rate among region i neighbors (local averaging) and also by using the average rate over the entire study region (global averaging). Such smoothing attempts to greatly reduce the relatively large variance of regional disease rate estimates in exchange for what should be an acceptably small increase in bias due to pooling all of the data (more heavily weighting data from neighboring regions) to estimate each region's disease rate. Hierarchical Bayesian methods are described further in Section 4.1 in the context of inconsistent seasonal effects.

4 Syndromic Surveillance

We focus on frequent (usually daily) monitoring of counts of patient visits categorized into syndromes, which is one particular type of syndromic surveillance (SS). Categorization arises upon mapping patient chief complaint and/or diagnosis data to syndrome categories such as respiratory, neurological, or gastro-intestinal. A broader definition of SS also includes non-clinical data sources such as pharmacy sales, absenteeism, nurse hotline calls, etc. Although we focus on syndrome counts, seasonal patterns are sometimes present in these and other SS data sources. For overviews of SS, see reports from the 2004 National SS Conference in the Morbidity and Mortality Weekly Report (see, e.g., [28]) or publications available from the International Society for Disease Surveillance [20].

Although SS appears promising, there are concerns regarding signal-to-noise ratios, costs, data confidentiality, system maintainability, etc. Some of these concerns involve statistical issues. The statistical challenges in SS to be described here include:

(1) Inconsistent seasonal effects: some syndrome counts (such as respiratory) vary with season in a manner that is not consistent from year to year. This implies that modeling the ordinary background, which includes seasonal increases, is difficult.
(2) Reporting delays: real systems tend to experience reporting delays, which must be adjusted for in real time if the timeliness goals for SS are to be met.
(3) System population coverage: it is necessary to relate outbreak size in the covered population to additional counts in a SS data source. It is difficult to estimate the system's population coverage, which is needed in order to estimate the expected number of extra counts in a SS data source (patient visits, medicine sales, etc.) corresponding to an outbreak of a particular size in a particular demographic subset. In other words, although it is simple to inject synthetic counts into a real SS data source, it is difficult to estimate the corresponding number of extra counts in the covered population. Therefore, the system alarm probability (the probability that a decision threshold is exceeded, i.e., that a small p-value is obtained, and an outbreak is detected) for a given outbreak size in the covered population is also difficult to estimate.
(4) Lack of effective training data: in general there is a lack of training data that includes real outbreaks having clearly defined start and stop times. Therefore, most studies rely on injecting simulated counts into real background data to estimate outbreak detection probabilities.
(5) Data confidentiality: some data such as personal information included in ED visits must be protected as confidential.

4.1 Inconsistent Seasonal Effects

Some syndrome counts (such as respiratory) vary with season in a manner that is not consistent from year to year. This implies that monitoring the ordinary background, which includes seasonal increases, is difficult. See, for example, Fig. 1, which uses weekly counts of new deaths due to pneumonia and influenza (P & I) to illustrate the differences in three flu seasons in Albuquerque, NM. We assume here as others have, that P & I deaths provide a surrogate or indicator for influenza case rates. The

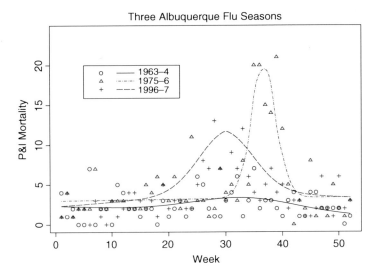

Fig. 1 Illustration of inconsistent seasonal effects using three Albuquerque flu seasons that are assumed to correspond to the annual P & I deaths

three smooth curves fit to the weekly counts show that the three flu seasons showed considerably variability in onset time, duration, and magnitude.

To accommodate inconsistent seasonal effects, Burr et al. [7, 8] develop and apply a hierarchical model by extending a non hierarchical "one-season-fits-all" model [22] similar to

$$C_d \sim \text{Poisson}\left(\sum_{i=1}^{7} c_i I_i(d) + c_8 + c_9 d + c_{10} \times \cos\left(\frac{2\pi d}{365.25} \right) + c_{11} \times \sin\left(\frac{2\pi d}{365.25} \right) \right).$$

(3)

In Equation (3), C_d is the day d counts, $\sum_{i=1}^{7} c_i I_i(d)$ captures day-of-week effects and $I_i(d)$ denotes the indicator function for day d, i.e., $I_i(d) = 1$ when day d is the i-th day of the week and $I_i(d) = 0$ otherwise (and the seven model coefficients c_i are constrained to sum to zero), $c_8 + c_9 d$ captures a long-term linear effect, and $c_{10} \times \cos(\frac{2\pi d}{365.25}) + c_{11} \times \sin(\frac{2\pi d}{365.25})$ captures the seasonal component, where the average number of days per year is 365.25, and the coefficients c_{10} and c_{11} determine the time and amplitude of the seasonal effect.

Bayesian hierarchical modeling in this context is a generalization of linear modeling in which model parameters such as the seasonal and day-of-week coefficients and other parameters follow a probability distribution whose parameters may be estimated from the data [13]. The hierarchical model in Equation (4) is similar to Equation (3), except the seasonal peak is modeled using a scalable Gaussian function, instead of the fixed-width and fixed-location sine and cosine functions. Also, the baseline is allowed to change linearly within a year as opposed to varying linearly over a longer time period. With this model,

$$E(C_d) = b_y(d) + \frac{a_y}{\sigma_y} \phi \left(\frac{d - \delta_y}{\sigma_y} \right) + \sum_{i=1}^{7} c_i I_i(d), \qquad (4)$$

where $E(C_d)$ is the expected value of the day d count, and variance$(C_d|E(C_d)) = \frac{1+\psi}{\psi}$, and as $\psi \to \infty$, the variance to mean ratio approaches 1, as in the Poisson distribution. The term $b_y(d) = b_{y-1} + \frac{d}{365}(b_y - b_{y-1})$ models changing baseline by linearly interpolating between the current (b_y) and the previous (b_{y-1}) year's off-peak baseline, a_y is the scaled peak amplitude for year y, ϕ is the probability density for a standard normal variable as above, δ_y denotes the time of the peak for year y, and σ_y corresponds to the duration of the peak in year y, and day-of-week effects are as in Equation (3). Note that letting variance$(C_d|E(C_d)) = \frac{1+\psi}{\psi}$ allows for overdispersion (larger than Poisson variance), which has been observed in many data sets.

The parameters such as ψ, δ_y, and σ_y in Equation (4) are not fixed, but instead are assigned a prior distribution (the "hyperprior" in this context) having parameters that are estimated from the data. For example, ψ is assigned a vague (large variance) prior, and as with the other parameters, the data is used to update its prior. The hyperprior for each parameter is in the hierarchy of modeling assumptions ("Bayesian hierarchical modeling") relating data and parameters, and the hyperprior is updated, resulting in a posterior distribution, by using the available data.

Graves and Picard [15] applied a hierarchical model to pneumonia and influenza mortality data using Markov Chain Monte Carlo to generate observations from the posterior distribution of the parameters (in a Bayesian setting suitable for hierarchical models) in a model similar to Equation (4), and the approach was also used in Burr et al. [7, 8]. Burr et al. [7, 8] showed that outbreak detection probability estimates are improved if based on data simulated from the hierarchical model rather than the corresponding non hierarchical model.

Exercise 3. Choose values for the model parameters in Equation (3) and then simulate data from Equation (3) for two years and plot it. It might be necessary to use trial-and-error to find reasonable parameter values. Is it likely that real data could be this repeatable? If not, a hierarchical model might be more appropriate.

4.2 Reporting Delays

Some systems experience unfortunate reporting delays. For example, on a given Monday, perhaps 60% of Monday's final total count data are available by the end of that particular day, with the remaining 40% trickling in over the next one to five days. Of course such delays defeat the purpose of using timely pre diagnostic data. If the 60/40 percentage were highly repeatable, it would be reasonable to adjust each day's counts by multiplying by 1/0.6. Of course, the delay distribution is not necessarily highly repeatable and in practice leads either to an undercount, an analysis delay, or to an increase in the system noise if an adjustment is attempted. The BioSense initiative [28] is pursuing methods to adjust for such reporting delays. For example, see the task description at www.cdc.gov/Biosense/extramuralprojects.

4.3 System Population Coverage

In order to estimate the probability that a given data stream will exhibit elevated counts when an outbreak of a specified size occurs in the population, it is necessary to estimate the fraction of the population that is served by the entity associated with a given data stream, such as a nurse hot line or ED.

Human behavioral issues such as the propensity of those having the disease to go to the ED, as opposed, say, to simply staying home or continuing to go to work or school must be considered. There has been some research on this issue, such as in New York City [34], which estimates that each ED visit for flu-like illness represents approximately 60 such illnesses in the metropolitan area. Patient demographics and socioeconomic factors are relevant; for example, the New York City study showed that females are more likely to go to a hospital with flu-like symptoms than are males and, not surprisingly, those with health insurance are far more likely to go than are those without it. A similar study in Canada [33] found, in contrast, that each respiratory visit represented only 7 upper respiratory infections in the population, indicating that considerable study-to-study uncertainty exists in quantifying behavior in this regard.

4.4 Lack of Effective Training Data

As with traditional public health outcome surveillance, there is a general lack of training data having known start and stop times of outbreaks. Therefore, SS studies typically rely on injecting synthetic counts into background data, although in a few instances (e.g., [4, 23]) real outbreaks were identified retrospectively using other data sources.

When injecting synthetic counts into real background data, relating the number of injected counts to the number of cases in the population is very difficult. Some SS studies have used models for the shape of an outbreak curve in a population [21], with separate models used, for example, for an airborne biological weapon [5], a point-source, and for community transmission. Such models together with a model for population coverage of the data sources being used for SS guide the choice for features (shape and magnitude) of simulated outbreaks to be superimposed on background counts in order to assess the detection probability of various monitoring schemes. However, there remains a general inability to verify that modeled outbreak curves are sufficiently close to real outbreak curves for performance claims based on modeled curves to be relevant.

Airborne releases are usually modeled using plume dispersion models. Plume dispersion modeling is a large topic, and not surprisingly, there is a wide range in model quality. For community transmission models, a large literature in classical epidemiology involves disease etiology and associated model fitting once it is established that an outbreak has occurred. An example is the well-known S-E-I-R (susceptible, exposed, infected, recovered) model that partitions the at-risk population into susceptible, exposed, infected, and recovered subgroups. Many statistical challenges are involved in fitting and interpreting such models [9] and the associated temporal shape of the corresponding disease outbreak. One goal is to estimate the basic reproductive number R_0 (the expected number of secondary cases per primary case in a completely susceptible population) using the shape of the outbreak curve. Estimates of R_0 can be used in real time to predict the cumulative number of infected individuals ("outbreak size"). S-E-I-R type models can include mitigation effects such as isolation and vaccination, and an active area of research is to predict the impact on R_0 and thus on final outbreak size resulting when various mitigation strategies are applied [10].

One method of producing synthetic training data, and perhaps assisting with estimation of population coverage, is agent-based epidemiological models such as EpiSims [11]. EpiSims combines estimates of population mobility in social networks using census and land-use data with models for simulating disease progression within a host. Such an approach would have to be modified to model the data stream(s) of interest such as ED visits or nurse hot-line calls.

4.5 Data Confidentiality

Modern health-care-related patient confidentiality rules inhibit the widespread sharing of SS data. For example, regulations resulting from the Health Insurance Portability and Accountability Act (HIPAA) refer to the need for a statistical expert to assist in applying statistical and scientific principles to render information not individually identifiable [14]. Statistical approaches attempt to balance the competing goals of effective analysis and patient confidentiality [12].

Two types of information disclosure are considered: exact and inferential. Exact disclosure means that the identity of an individual respondent or participant is revealed. Participant identity could be used to link records and maliciously exploit the revealed identify. Identity or attributes are said to be inferred if the probability of the inference being correct is less than one, but large enough that correct inference is likely. Much effort continues to be directed toward developing tools to limit disclosure while providing usable statistical tables or databases. For example, data swapping and perturbation can enable effective statistical inference while limiting disclosure [12].

4.6 Two SS Systems

The next two subsections briefly describe two SS systems.

4.6.1 BSafer

Features in the BSafer SS system [4] are common to many SS systems. The BSafer dictionary for mapping chief complaints to syndromes such as respiratory, gastrointestinal, neurologic, skin, lymphatic, and undifferentiated infection is provided in Brillman et al. [4], and Equation (3) is fit to daily counts from each syndrome. The detection probability for Page's sequential test [36] and a one-day-at-a-time test is estimated for each of many randomly generated outbreaks that inject additional counts into eight years of background data at random onset times for random durations. Page's sequential test monitors for sequences of large (or perhaps small in some contexts) counts; a one-day-at-a-time test monitors for a large count on a single day. The inconsistent seasonal effects led Burr et al. [7, 8] to apply the hierarchical model previously described. However, this hierarchical model has not yet been implemented in any real SS system, and it is currently unknown to what extent a hierarchical model can help identify outbreak regions in a timely manner.

4.6.2 BioSense

Oversimplifying somewhat, raw data for BioSense [28] include daily, zipcode-specific counts for approximately 10 syndromic categories from various regions, such as the southwestern United States. There are three sources for these data streams: the Veteran's Administration, the Department of Defense, and laboratory test orders. Other sources such as civilian ED visits are anticipated.

To analyze count-level data, BioSense uses two analytic methods that are supplemented by visual displays. It is important to realize that BioSense, like most SS systems, is used primarily by non statisticians who may prefer relatively simple analyses. The extent to which more elaborate methods would outperform the simple methods described next is currently unknown.

The first method is based on Shewhart scores and cumulative sum (cusum) monitoring, similar to standard quality control applications. The second method is a regression-based approach as in Equation (3) that is designed to predict counts for each day and, if the actual count differs sufficiently from the predicted count, produce an alarm, indicating a potential outbreak.

4.6.3 Cusums

There are three cusum procedures implemented in BioSense, denoted $C1$, $C2$, and $C3$ [17, 18]. These cusums are intended to be sensitive to different types of disease outbreaks. The first, $C1$, uses a seven-day moving average with a one-day lag, with the lag included to avoid problems related to delayed reporting and to effects of rapidly increasing counts. More formally, for $C(d)$ denoting the syndromic count for a given syndrome on day d, the seven-day moving average with a one-day lag $MA(1)$ is

$$MA(1) = \sum_{t=d-7}^{d-1} C(t) / 7$$

and the seven-day moving average with a three-day lag $MA(3)$ is

$$MA(3) = \sum_{t=d-9}^{d-3} C(t) / 7.$$

Similarly, standard deviations for the respective seven-day periods are

$$\hat{\sigma}(1) = \sqrt{\sum_{t=d-7}^{d-1} [C(t) - MA(1)]^2 / 6}$$

and

$$\hat{\sigma}(3) = \sqrt{\sum_{t=d-9}^{d-3} [C(t) - MA(3)]^2 / 6}.$$

Using these estimates, conventional cusum statistics [36] are recursively computed as

$$S_d(1) = max \left\{ 0, \ S_{d-1}(1) + \frac{C(d) - MA(1)}{\hat{\sigma}(1)} - 1 \right\}$$

and

$$S_d(3) = max \left\{ 0, \ S_{d-1}(3) + \frac{C(d) - MA(3)}{\hat{\sigma}(3)} - 1 \right\}.$$

That is, excess counts (normalized by the standard deviations) are accumulated and compared to a decision threshold. A single day having a sufficiently large count could trigger an alarm, as could a string of days of smaller but nonetheless larger-than-anticipated counts.

The statistics $C1$, $C2$, and $C3$ as implemented in BioSense, however, are not traditional cusums. Instead, $C1$ and $C2$ are Shewhart scores, defined as

$$C1 \equiv C_d(1) \equiv \frac{C(d) - MA(1)}{\hat{\sigma}(1)} - 1$$

and

$$C2 \equiv C_d(2) \equiv \frac{C(d) - MA(3)}{\hat{\sigma}(3)} - 1,$$

where values less than 0 are set to 0. The statistic $C3$ is a type of cumulative sum, defined on day d as the sum $C_d(2) + C_{d-1}(2) + C_{d-2}(2)$ where $C_{d-1}(2)$ and $C_{d-2}(2)$ are set to 0 if they exceed a threshold. Cusums $C1$, $C2$, and $C3$ can be plotted in control charts and visually inspected. The underlying philosophy is virtually identical to that in statistical process control.

[The above description is not quite complete. One minor complication involves adjusting for the fact that counts are typically higher for weekdays than weekends. Therefore, separate cusums are computed for weekdays only and weekend-days only. A second minor complication is introduced by "bad dates" for which the daily counts are deemed anomalous for various reasons. Counts from such dates are excluded from the cusum calculation. Also, holiday or day-after-holiday effects can be seen, although it is unclear whether it is helpful to adjust for holiday effects.]

4.6.4 Small Area Regression Testing Procedure

In addition to the above cusums, Small Area Regression Testing (SMART) scores are computed using a model that is similar to Equation (3). A generalized linear model (GLM) [32] is fit to the zipcode-specific, syndrome-specific daily counts, incorporating seasonal and day-of-the-week effects. Using past data up through the previous Friday, the regression predicts counts for the current week.

The SMART regression for the southwestern US, for example, involves over 150 parameters, including 1 offset parameter, 140 zipcode parameters, 6 day-of-week parameters, 2 seasonal parameters, 1 holiday parameter, and 1 day-after holiday parameter. SMART parameter estimation is carried out via a GLM using a log link function. Once the model fitting on the log scale is completed, a predicted value is then exponentiated to give a predicted count. That predicted count is then treated as being the (known) mean for a Poisson distribution, and the p-value for the day's actual count is computed relative to that known mean.

The SMART model parameter estimates are updated each Saturday. That is, parameter estimates are re-computed weekly upon incorporating the most recent week's data so that the effects of extrapolation on the predicted values are minimized. This mitigates somewhat the impact of inconsistent seasonal effects; however Burr et al. [7, 8] applied weekly updating for BioSense data, and inconsistent seasonal effects were still shown to have an important impact on outbreak detection probabilities.

The cusum and SMART testing procedures are one-sided. That is, they alarm only when counts are too large. Counts that are anomalously small relative to their predictions, which might reflect modeling shortcomings, are ignored. Moreover, although each procedure is sensitive to large counts in its own way, there is a partial redundancy among the test statistics. Generally, we have focused on detecting clusters of high rather than low disease rates. Clusters of low disease rate are certainly also of interest because they could lead to ways to improve health (such as avoiding certain fats, which may explain why some nations have lower cancer rates than others).

5 Discussion

Although our focus is statistical challenges in detecting disease clusters, there are many practical considerations that make cluster detection difficult, some of which we describe below.

5.1 Data Quality

Data quality is a key issue in surveillance for outbreaks using diagnosed case rates and in SS. Therefore, the availability of timely and useful data is an ongoing concern for many reasons, including the following.

(1) Few surveillance systems are specifically designed for the early detection of disease outbreaks. Virtually all data sets used for disease surveillance are *not* collected for purposes of timely detection of outbreaks. Instead, health care facilities already collect data for other reasons, including billing, staffing, planning, and so on. Consequently, the effectiveness of surveillance activities has been questioned [2–5]).

For example, as in Section 3.3, use of home address as the "location" for a new case can be problematic – in some cases, a work or (for children) a school address could easily be more relevant, depending on disease etiology. Subsequent binning of cases by county and assigning them the county seat as their location is often done for reporting purposes, and the choice of spatial and/or temporal scale may be done more for convenience than for optimal surveillance.

(2) The quality (or lack thereof as measured by mistake rates) of demographic and other predictor variables, disease rates, home and/or work address, etc., can easily overwhelm the signal of interest.

(3) There is little financial incentive for health care facilities to improve SS data quality. Data quality therefore suffers from typing errors, inconsistency across different facilities in terms used, procedure codes that change when billing rules change, inadvertent duplication of records, etc. In light of the ongoing debate regarding how to finance health care in the U.S., we do not see a clear path to improve this situation, because it would require ongoing dedicated funding that would not arise from pure market forces.

The bottom line regarding the use of (nearly) freely available data streams, but which are collected for other purposes, is that "you get what you pay for." Thus, data cleansing is an essential precursor to good statistical analysis.

(4) In surveillance for outbreaks using diagnosed case rates, it is important to establish the case definition prior to monitoring for clusters. Consider the Los Alamos brain cancer example. Some almost unexplainable selection process among all possible cancer types occurred by the local resident who noticed several brain cancer cases in Los Alamos. Under- or over-reporting as mentioned in Section 3.3 is another important consideration, particularly for small case rates.

5.2 Background Assessment

Another issue with SS is that assessing the background is difficult for several reasons. Most facilities (such as EDs or pharmacies) have only tracked syndromic counts for a short time, and have possibly modified the dictionary that maps chief complaints to syndromes. Background levels also change as the result of changing population and/or demographic groups being served by the facility. Also, some major events, such as a large SARS (severe acute respiratory syndrome) outbreak in Toronto or the sarin gas release in Tokyo cause perturbations in the background (including the effect of panic-related increases in health care usage) that should be removed to obtain event-free background. Pooling data over multiple EDs in an area, where each ED is likely to have its own dictionary is problematic. Even at a given ED, the recording systems change periodically because of changes in insurance rules which tend to cause coding changes that favor adequate or better reimbursement. For example, if an ED cannot bill insurance for allowing the patient to sleep off a state of inebriation, the ED is unlikely to code the chief complaint as inebriation. Similarly, another type of coding change occurred in 1999 regarding how the Centers for Disease Control collects pneumonia and influenza mortality data, which can be used to monitor for outbreaks. The change arose because of a revision to how death certificate information was used to categorize pneumonia and influenza deaths. For more detail regarding this change, see Morbidity and Mortality Weekly Report 49(09):173–177, available at www.cdc.gov/mmwr.

For data streams such as over-the-counter medicine sales, it is necessary to account for effects such as advertising promotions leading to increased medicine sales. Finally, in real time situations such as in EDs, data are often manually entered, with many errors, misspellings, and abbreviations for lengthy disease names. Considering only the issues mentioned above, it is clear that obtaining good background data is itself a challenge.

5.3 Complications Arising From Monitoring
   Multiple Data Sources

In surveillance for outbreaks using SS, Stoto et al. [37] mention concerns about the wide net being cast over multiple syndromes, data streams, and regions. Such a wide net implies that there are many opportunities for false alarms, and therefore requires that each monitored stream have very wide alarm limits in to avoid high false alarm rates. Stoto et al. [37] presented a simple simulation study by injecting various outbreaks onto "influenza-like illness" cases at the George Washington ED from 1998 to 2001, which varied from approximate 3 per day to 20 per day during the annual peak. Page's cusum was one of the four statistical algorithms used to monitor for outbreaks and the detection times and probabilities for small, medium, and large outbreaks were evaluated, but with many uncertainties omitted, such as the population coverage mentioned in Section 4.

Because SS is currently treated as a research topic, the importance of integrating SS into public health systems was stressed. However, many facilities will continue SS only if federal funds continue to support it.

5.4 Creating Synthetic Outbreak Data

The lack of effective training data was mentioned in Section 4.4, and one option for producing realistic training data is agent-based epidemiological models such as EpiSims. This would require considerable effort to implement because creating synthetic outbreak data for assessing the merits of SS (e.g., [37]) requires understanding how disease outbreaks are manifested in observed surveillance data. For BioSense data streams, for example, one description of this process is:

(a) Certain people are infected immediately as a result of the exposure;
(b) The contagious disease propagates through the general public, possibly to locations beyond the geographic area where the outbreak occurred;
(c) Of the people affected, some portion of them are among the BioSense patient populations (e.g., they are eligible to go to hospitals/clinics within the domain of BioSense monitoring);
(d) Of those eligible to go to BioSense-related facilities, some number of them actually do, and their counts appear in the BioSense data streams; and
(e) The syndrome counts from those affected by the outbreak are combined with the corresponding baseline counts.

Clearly it is time- and labor-intensive to develop realistic training data.

6 Open Challenges

Outbreak detection is a large topic and we have presented only a few subtopics, focusing on statistical challenges. The topics discussed raise open challenges, some of which we now describe.

Whether used retrospectively or not, in order to correct for maximal selection over time and space, the only current approach is simulation. An example was given in Burr [6], and free software is available at www.statscan.org. Is an approximate analytical method possible, perhaps following the "selection over time" or "selection over space" approximation based on the Wiener process described in Section 3.2?

Data in SS systems have exhibited more than Poisson variability. One approach to model extra-variability is to use a hierarchical model such as that presented in Section 4.1. Another approach is presented in Wieland et al. [39] who used one regression for the mean count and a separate regression for the variance of the count. Both regressions were similar to Equation (3). Neither approach has been thoroughly tested with real data.

With respect to the hierarchical model in Section 4.1, it is currently unknown to what extent a hierarchical model can improve outbreak detection in near real time. An inherent performance limit involves the fact that in near real time, an outbreak can have the same shape as the start of the annual peak, thus tending to modify the current estimate of the onset time of the current year's peak.

Another issue in SS is the inherent noise due to the nonspecific and overlapping nature of the syndromes. A possible improvement (CADDY, computer aided differential diagnosis) described in Burr et al. [7, 8] tracks disease probabilities that are estimated using each patient's recorded symptoms. A forward model relating each of approximately 250 diseases (including rare diseases such as anthrax) to probable symptoms, allowing for probabilities of symptom combinations that are not based on an independence assumption, is used to estimate the probability of the most likely diseases given a test patient with observed measurements such as heart rate, blood pressure, etc. The CADDY approach has the potential to detect diseases having very low background levels, unlike SS, which suffers due to the nonspecific nature of the syndromes.

7 Summary

We have described some of the statistical challenges in public health outcome surveillance and in syndromic surveillance. Both types of surveillance require a model for the background disease rate and a method of detecting departure from that background. Performance assessments usually involve the injection of counts corresponding to simulated outbreaks into the background data.

Although statistical analysis is a component of monitoring for disease outbreaks, it cannot always recover signal from data having poor quality. Concerns about data quality were discussed in Section 5. Typically, statistical analysis forces researchers and users to consider limitations due to data quality. In some cases, poor data quality simply translates into a reduction in the signal to noise ratio and commensurate reduction in outbreak detection probability. In other cases, data quality can be too poor to adequately assess outbreak detection probabilities.

References

1. Barbour A, Eagleson G (1983) Poisson approximation for some statistics based on exchangeable trials. Advances in Applied Probability 15:585–600.
2. Bradley C, Rolka H, Walker D, Loonsk J (2005) BioSense: implementation of a national early event detection and situational awareness system. Morbidity and Mortality Weekly Report (MMWR) 54(Suppl): 11–19.

3. Bravata D, McDonald K, Smith W, et al. (2004) Systematic review: surveillance systems for early detection of bioterrorism-related diseases. Annals of Internal Medicine 140: 910–922.
4. Brillman J, Burr T, Forslund D, Joyce E, Picard R, Umland E (2005) Modeling emergency department visit patterns for infectious disease complaints: results and application to disease surveillance. BMC Medical Informatics and Decision Making 5(4).
5. Buckeridge D, Burkom H, Moore A, Pavlin J, Cutchis P, Hogan W (2004) Evaluation of syndromic surveillance systems–design of an epidemic simulation model. Morbidity and Mortality Weekly Report 53(Suppl):137–143.
6. Burr T (2001) Maximally selected measures of evidence of disease clusters. Statistics in Medicine 20:1443–1460.
7. Burr T, Graves T, Klamann R, Michalak S, Picard R, Hengartner N (2007) Accounting for seasonal patterns in syndromic surveillance data for outbreak detection, BMC Medical Informatics and Decision Making 6(40).
8. Burr T, Koster F, Picard R, Forslund D, Wokoun D, Joyce E, Brillman J, Froman P, Lee J (2007) Computer-aided diagnosis with potential application to rapid detection of disease outbreaks. Statistics in Medicine 26: 1857–1874.
9. Burr T, Chowell G (2008) Signatures of non-homogeneous mixing in disease outbreaks. Mathematical and Computer Modeling 48:122–140.
10. Chowell G, Ammon C, Hengartner NW, Hyman J (2006) Transmission dynamics of the great influenza pandemic of 1918 in Geneva, Switzerland: assessing the effects of hypothetical interventions. Journal of Theoretical Biology 241(2), 193–204.
11. Eubank S, Guclu H, Kumar V, Marathe M, Srinivasan A, Toroczkal Z, Wang N (2004) Modelling disease outbreaks in realistic urban social networks, Nature 429: 180–184.
12. Fienberg S (2001) Statistical perspective on confidentiality and data access in public health, Statistics in Medicine 20:1347–1356.
13. Gelman A, Carline J, Stern H, Rubin D (1995) Bayesian Data Analysis, Boca Raton, FL: Chapman & Hall/CRC.
14. Gibson J, Hodge J (2004), Health information privacy and syndromic surveillance systems. Morbidity and Mortality Weekly Report 53(Suppl): 221–225.
15. Graves T, Picard R (2002) Predicting the evolution of pneumonia and influenza mortality during a flu season. Los Alamos National Laboratory Report LA-UR-02-4717.
16. Hastie T, Tibshirani R, Friedman J (2001) The Elements of Statistical Learning. Springer: New York.
17. Hutwagner L, Browne T, Seeman G, Fletcher A (2005a) Comparing aberration detection methods with simulated data. Emerging Infectious Diseases 11: 314–316.
18. Hutwagner L, Thompson W, Seeman G, Treadwell T (2005b) A simulation model for assessing aberration detection methods used in public health surveillance for systems with limited baselines. Statistics in Medicine 24: 543–550.
19. Influenza activity in the US, 1999–2000 season, Morbidity and Mortality Weekly Report 49(09): 173–177.
20. International society for disease surveillance [http:www.syndromic.org].
21. Jackson M, Baer A, Painter I, Duchin J (2007) A simulation study comparing aberration detection algorithms for syndromic surveillance. BMC Medical Informatics and Decision Making 7:6.
22. Kleinman K, Lazarus R, Platt R (2004) A generalized linear mixed models approach for detecting incident clusters of disease in small areas with an application to biological terrorism. American Journal of Epidemiology 159(3) 217–224.
23. Kleinman K, Abrama A, Yih W, Platt R, Kulldorff M (2006) Evaluating spatial surveillance: detection of known outbreaks in real data. Statistics in Medicine 25:755–769.
24. Knox G (1964) Epidemiology of childhood leukaemia in Northumberland and Durham. British Journal of Preventive Social Medicine 18:17–24.
25. Kulldorff M, Hjalmers U (1999) The Knox method and other tests for space-time interaction. Biometrics 55:544–552.

26. Kulldorff M, Athas W, Feuer E, Miller B, Key C (1998) Evaluating cluster alarms: a space and time scan statistic and brain cancer in Los Alamos, New Mexico. American Journal of Public Health 88:1377–1380.

27. Lawson L, Denison D (2002) Spatial Cluster Modeling. Chapman and Hall: New York.

28. Loonsk J (2004) BioSense–a national initiative for early detection and quantification of public health emergencies. Morbidity and Mortality Weekly Report 53(Suppl): 53–55, available at www.cdc.gov/mmwr.

29. MacNab Y, Farrell P, Gustafson P, Wen S (2004), Estimation in Bayesian disease mapping. Biometrics 60: 865–873.

30. Mantel N (1967) The detection of disease clustering and a generalized regression approach. Cancer Research 27:209–220.

31. Marshall J, Spitzner D, Woodall W (2007) Use of the local Knox statistic for the prospective monitoring of disease occurrences in space and time. Statistics in Medicine 26: 1579–1593.

32. McCullagh P, Nelder J (1990) Generalized Linear Models. Chapman and Hall: New York.

33. McIsaac WJ, Levine N, Goel V (1998) Visits by adults to family physicians for the common cold. Journal of Family Practice 47 366–369.

34. Metzger K, Hajat A, Crawford M, Mostashari F (2004) How many illnesses does one emergency department visit represent? Using a population-based telephone survey to estimate the syndromic multiplier. Morbidity and Mortality Weekly Report 53(Suppl) 106–111, available at www.cdc.gov/mmwr.

35. Miller R, Siegmund D (1982) Maximally selected chi square statistics. Biometrics 38: 1011–1016.

36. Page E (1954) Continuous inspection schemes. Biometrika 41:100–115.

37. Stoto M, Schonlau M, Mariano L (2004) Syndromic surveillance: is it worth the effort? Chance 17(1): 19–24.

38. Venables W, Ripley B (1999) Modern Applied Statistics with Splus. Springer: New York.

39. Wieland S, Brownstein J, Berger B, Mandl K (2007) Automated real time constant-specificity surveillance for disease outbreaks. BMC Medical Informatics and Decision Making 7:15.

40. Woodall W (2006) Use of control charts in health care monitoring and public health surveillance. Journal of Quality Technology, 38:89–104.

Death Records from Historical Archives: A Valuable Source of Epidemiological Information

Rodolfo Acuna-Soto

Abstract In almost every geographic location around the world, historic archives store a wealth of valuable epidemiological information. Mostly scrutinized by social scientists, historic information has an enormous potential for epidemiologic research, yet this information remains largely forgotten. This situation is starting to change. A renewed interest in historic data has flourished as recent reports, based on the information retrieved from historic records, have demonstrated that the information stored in historic archives is of an exceptional quality. Initially studied by a few intrepid epidemiologists, the field is growing vigorously. The application of quantitative methods and geographic information systems to historical data is producing a more detailed picture of the dynamics of human disease in space and time.

Keywords Historical epidemiology · Historic data · Epidemics · Excess mortality · Mortality

1 Introduction

Today, reports on the analysis of epidemiological events based on historical data are infrequent, despite the fact that there are massive amounts of information available around the world. The reluctance of many epidemiologists to consider working with historical data is not because they had previous unhelpful or bad experiences with historical data, but rather because of the weight of tradition. Avoiding history can be explained by the way modern epidemiology emerged as a renovated science in the second half of the 20th century. As it relied on innovative concepts and methods, modern epidemiology required also reliable data. Almost naturally, old archives were the first victims of this new trend. Without laboratory confirmation, and with too many ill-defined concepts and different diseases grouped under the

R. Acuna-Soto (✉)
Departamento de Microbiología y Parasitología, Facultad de Medicina, Universidad Nacional Autónoma de México, Delegación Coyoacán, México, DF 04510, México
e-mail: yvonne@ibt.unam.mx

G. Chowell et al. (eds.), *Mathematical and Statistical Estimation Approaches in Epidemiology*, DOI 10.1007/978-90-481-2313-1_9,
© Springer Science+Business Media B.V. 2009

same diagnosis, old archives turned into unsuitable sources of information for modern epidemiology. This concept was incorporated to every epidemiology course and taught to generations of students.

Recently, two major events indirectly re-opened the interest in historical data. The first was the possible use of smallpox virus or other highly pathogenic infectious microorganisms of the past as agents of bioterrorism and the second was the emergence of the H5N1 avian influenza virus and its possible recombination to become a human pandemic strain, similar to the Spanish influenza of 1918. The possibility that episodes comparable to past catastrophic events may arise has had a strong influence on the usage and the analysis of the epidemiological information stored in historic archives. When properly used, this information has proved to be of an exceptional quality.

2 The Nature of Historical Death Records

For hundreds of years, different institutions in countries around the world have recorded the birth and death of almost every person. Church and civil archives commonly keep the information indefinitely and therefore their archives enclose an immense source of epidemiological information. Frequently, the researcher is confronted with the decision of choosing among numerous archives with potential useful information. To help in the decision-making process, I recommend consulting historians with expertise in the area and the period of time of interest. A primary survey and comparison of several possible sources will rapidly give a good estimate of the quality of the information as well as of the amount of work required for data extraction. In general, retrieving long-term epidemiological data from historical archives requires a rather large investment of time and effort. It is advisable to keep the original nomenclature as this allows clarifying and extending the meaning of the original data. To have a more complete picture of the general health situation for the period under study, it is also very important to recover additional original information: census, maps, routes of transportation, health practices, published historical data, newspapers, and as many descriptions as possible of eyewitnesses. Needless to say that historic material is very fragile and must be handled with extreme care. In general, the custodians of the archives, civil and religious, are very protective about the material. This is because the records are unique and contain important historic documents projected to last for centuries.

Records from cemeteries are a very rich and valuable source of information on the mortality trends of a given population over a long period of time. For hundred of years Towns and cities had only one main cemetery, generally associated to the local Church. In almost every case these records were kept in the Church's office for a certain period of time, after which most records were transferred to centralized municipal or state archives; some of them remain in their original places. Fortunately for us, most of those large collections of data remain organized and available for research. In recent years, major efforts have been done to preserve these complete records and to make then available on the Internet in Canada, United States,

Germany, England, and other countries. Some of those are continuous series of causes of death at individual level, dating from the sixteenth century to the present. This is indeed a great opportunity for epidemiologists. Thus, data collection on the historic trends of mortality can be performed in almost any part of the world [13]. I will present the examples of Quebec, United States and Mexico City.

In Quebec, Canada all the provincial burial records have been copied and concentrated in the *Bibliothèque et Archives Nationales du Québec* in Montreal. This material is extremely interesting since the information of a long period of time for a large area is concentrated in one place. Much of this information is also available on line today. With the information stored in those archives, epidemics of smallpox, measles, influenza, polio and other infectious diseases can be followed day by day, throughout the entire region.

In the United States, over the last two decades, local historical societies as well as genealogical and religious organizations have taken the lead in organizing and preserving historic archives. The result is an increasing number of valuable databases available for research; many of them are already online.

In Mexico the situation is different; burial records from the sixteenth-century to 1861 were transferred to state Cathedrals or major Churches, where most of them remain available for research. Almost all records dating from the sixteen century to today include the cause of death. The records after 1861 are in the offices of cemeteries or in municipal archives and most of them include date, age, sex, and address in addition to the cause of death. Results built with information retrieved from municipal archives and cemeteries produce long-term records on the causes of death of specific communities. With few exceptions, almost all records remain on paper; therefore to retrieve information from those records, a big investment of time and effort is required.

Many infectious diseases can be identified easily in historical records (smallpox, measles, syphilis, rabies, tuberculosis, cholera, whooping cough, diphtheria, yellow fever, influenza, plague, polio, typhus, dengue and malaria). Other diseases are hidden under different names, but the information is still very reliable. However, some specific diseases are impossible to identify since they are grouped under common clinical manifestations. For example, the terms "intestinal infection", "acute diarrhea" etc. include all the etiological causes of diarrhea. In any case, it is absolutely necessary to be familiar with the medical terminology for the region and period of time under study. Some common examples of old English medical terms for some infectious diseases are presented in Table 1.

3 Uses of Historical Data

Although the analysis of historical trends of mortality is a relatively new field for modern epidemiologists, this theme has been extensively investigated by demographers and other social scientists. Indeed, historic demography embraces a variety of themes, methodologies and theories with many of the studies being centered

Table 1 Old english medical terms for some important infectious diseases

Cholera	Cholera Asiatica, Algid Cholera, Cholera Maligna
Croup	Angina suffocata, Angina Trachealis, Roup
Dengue	Dunga, Dingee, Breakbone Fever, Broken-wing Fever, Aden Fever, Bouquet Fever, Bucket fever, Colorado Fever, Dandy Fever
Diphtheria	White throat, Cyanche Maligna, Dyphtherits, Angina Diphterica, Hogkin Angina
Erysipela	Hell's Fire, Saint Anthony's Fire
Malaria	Ague, Intermittent Fever, Febris Intermittans, Jungle Fever, Marsh Fever, Paludal Fever, Congestive Chills, Tertian Fevers, Chills and Fevers
Mumps	Angina Parotidea, Antiades, Gissa, Cynanche Parotidea
Pulmonary tuberculosis	Phthisis, Pulmonary Consumption, Consumption, White Plague
Rabies	St. Hubert Disease
Rubella	Bastard Measles, False Measles, French Measles, German Measles, Hard Measles, Hybrid Measles
Syphilis	Plague of Venus, Mal-Venerea, Lues Venerea, French Distemper, Canton Disease, Russian Disease, Polish Disease, Neapolitan Disease, Christian Disease, Italian Disease, Pox, Great Pox
Typhus (*Rickettsia prowasekii*)	Ship Fever, Gaol Fever, Irish Ague, Spotted Ague, Petechial Fever, Jail Fever, Famine Fever, Hunger Typhus, Typhus Gravior, Ataxic Fever, Maculated Fever
Variola minor	Milkpox, Cottonpox
Whooping cough	Blue Cough, Dog Bark, Chin Cough, Kink Cough
Yellow fever	Yellow Jack, Black Vomit, American Plague, Bronze John (Texas)

on analyses of the history, the social response, and the impact of epidemics. The epidemiological analysis of historical material is currently expanding our understanding of the epidemic process. This has been demonstrated recently for almost every aspect of human disease for which historical data have been used. Some of the most relevant features are: transmission dynamics [3, 6, 14, 24, 25, 29], effect of climate [1, 26], epidemic events [2, 5, 15], effects of public health interventions [4, 18, 22] and spread geographic distribution [12, 16, 21].

Ever since Hippocrates wrote his classic text "Airs, water and Places" [19], there has been an interest to understand how epidemic diseases originate and evolve in human societies. For centuries, this initial work has been followed by numerous studies. Among them, Noah Webster in the United States wrote a seminal work "A Brief History of Epidemic and Pestilential Diseases" published in 1799 [28]. This trend of recapitulation of epidemics culminate in the monumental work of August Hirsch [20] published between 1860 and 1864. In this book Hirsch unified all the information available to his days in the field of historic epidemiology. Recent history started with the interest of the world's disease distribution and transmission dynamics during and after World War II. After the war, Hope-Simpson and others initiated a new trend in the quantitative approach of disease transmission. This beginning was followed by Andrew D. Cliff, Peter Haggett, Matthew Smallman-Raynor, Klaus Dietz, Niels Becker, Bryan Grenfell among others [7–12, 15, 17, 23, 27].

Today Hippocrates's intention remains intact: understanding the paths by which epidemics spread through human communities. Today's geographic epidemiology incorporates a synergetic combination of historic information, Geographic Information Systems, and refined quantitative analysis. As a result, data provided by these new and old disciplines have significantly contributed to improve the resolution of epidemiologic analysis. The field of historic epidemiology is growing vigorously, feeding in part from historic records. This should not be surprising since those records are the written record of our biological co- evolution with infectious agents.

References

1. Acuna-Soto R, Stahle DW, Cleaveland MK et al (2002) Megadrought and megadeath in 16th century Mexico. Emerg Infect Dis 8(4):360–2.
2. Andreasen V, Viboud C, Simonsen L (2008) Epidemiologic characterization of the 1918 influenza pandemic summer wave in Copenhagen: Implications for pandemic control strategies. J Infect Dis 197:270–8.
3. Barry JM, Viboud C, Simonsen L (2008) Cross-protection between successive waves of the 1918–1919 influenza pandemic: Epidemiological evidence from US army camps and from Britain. J Infect Dis 198(10):1427–34.
4. Bootsma MC, Ferguson NM (2007) The effect of public health measures on the 1918 influenza pandemic in US cities. Proc Natl Acad Sci USA 104(18):7588–93.
5. Chowell G, Ammon CE, Hengartner NW et al. (2007) Estimating the reproduction number from the initial phase of the Spanish flu pandemic waves in Geneva, Switzerland. Math Biosci Eng 4(3):457–70.
6. Chowell G, Bettencourt LM, Johnson N et al. (2008) The 1918–1919 influenza pandemic in England and Wales: Spatial patterns in transmissibility and mortality impact. Proc Biol Sci 275(1634):501–9.
7. Cliff A (1995) Incorporating spatial components into models of epidemic spread in: Epidemic Models: Their Structure and Relation to Data, ed. Denis Mollison, Series: Publications of the Newton Institute (No. 5). Heriot-Watt University, Edinburgh.
8. Cliff A, Haggett P (2004) Time, travel and infection. Brit Med Bull 69:87–99.
9. Cliff AD, Peter Haggett J, Ord K (1986) Spatial Aspects of Influenza Epidemics. London, Routledge.
10. Cliff AD, Haggett P, Smallman-Raynor M (1998) Deciphering Global Epidemics: Analytical Approaches to the Disease Records of World Cities, 1888–1912. Cambridge, Cambridge University Press.
11. Cliff AD, Haggett P, Smallman-Raynor MR (2000) Island Epidemics, Oxford, Oxford University Press.
12. Cliff AD, Haggett P, Smallman-Raynor M (2008) An exploratory method for estimating the changing speed of epidemic waves from historical data. Int J Epidemiol 37(1):106–12.
13. Covarrubias D, Van Emburgh M, Naqvi HR et al. (2008) To know or not to know: archiving and the under-appreciated historical value of data. Mol Cancer 7:18.
14. Eichner M (2003) Analysis of historical data suggests long-lasting protective effects of smallpox vaccination. Am J Epidemiol 158(8):717–23.
15. Eichner M, Dietz K (2003) Transmission potential of smallpox: Estimates based on detailed data from an outbreak. Am J Epidemiol 158(2):110–7

16. Gottfredsson M, Halldórsson BV, Jónsson S et al. (2008) Lessons from the past: familial aggregation analysis of fatal pandemic influenza (Spanish flu) in Iceland in 1918. Proc Natl Acad Sci USA 105(4):1303–8.
17. Haggett P (2000) The Geographical Structure of Epidemics. Oxford, Oxford University Press.
18. Hatchett RJ, Mecher CE, Lipsitch M (2007) Public health interventions and epidemic intensity during the 1918 influenza pandemic. Proc Natl Acad Sci USA 104(18):7582–7.
19. Hippocrates (1948) Airs, water and places. Cambridge, Harvard University Press.
20. Hirsch A. Handbuch der Historish-geographischen Patologie, 1860–1864. Translated into English by Charles Creighton and published as: Handbook of Geographical and Historical Pathology, The New Sydenham Society, 3 vols, London 1883–6.
21. Hope-Simpson RE (1952) Infectiousness of communicable diseases in the household. Lancet 2(6734):549–54.
22. Markel H, Lipman HB, Navarro JA et al. (2007) Nonpharmaceutical interventions implemented by US cities during the 1918–1919 influenza pandemic JAMA. 298(6):644–54. Erratum in: JAMA. 298(19):2264.
23. Matt J, Keeling MJ, Grenfell BT (2002) Understanding the persistence of measles: Reconciling theory, simulation and observation. Proc Biol Sci 269: 335–43.
24. Nishiura H (2006) Epidemiology of a primary pneumonic plague in Kantoshu, Manchuria, from 1910 to 1911: statistical analysis of individual records collected by the Japanese Empire. Int J Epidemiol 35(4):1059–65.
25. Nishiura H, Brockmann SO, Eichner M (2008) Extracting key information from historical data to quantify the transmission dynamics of smallpox. Theor Biol Med Model 5:20.
26. Stenseth NC, Samia NI, Viljugrein et al. (2006) Plague dynamics are driven by climate variation. PNAS 103:13110–5.
27. Trevelyan B, Smallman-Raynor M, Cliff AD (2005) The spatial dynamics of poliomyelitis in the United States: From epidemic emergence to vaccine-induced retreat, 1910–1971. Annals of the Association of American Geographers 95(2):269–93
28. Webster N (1800) A Brief History of Epidemic and Pestilential Diseases. Connecticut, Hudson and Goodwin Hartford.
29. White LF, Pagano M (2008) Transmissibility of the influenza virus in the 1918 pandemic. PLoS ONE 3(1):e1498.

Sensitivity Analysis for Uncertainty Quantification in Mathematical Models

Leon Arriola and James M. Hyman

Abstract All mathematical models are approximate and their usefulness depends on our understanding the uncertainty inherent in the predictions. Uncertainties can affect the reliability of the results at every stage of computation; they may grow or even shrink as the solution of the model evolves. Often these inherent uncertainties cannot be made arbitrarily small by a more complex model or additional computation and we must understand how the uncertainty in the model parameters, the initial conditions, and the model itself, lead to uncertainties in the model predictions. This chapter is an introductory survey of sensitivity analysis and illustrates how to define the derivative of the model solution as a function of the model input and determine the relative importance of the model parameters on the model predictions.

1 Introduction and Overview

Sensitivity analysis (SA) can be used to quantify the effects of uncertainties on a model's input parameters and the subsequent effect on the model's output [2, 5–10, 13, 16, 19, 21–23, 27–30, 32]. That is, SA can determine how variability of the inputs causes variability in the outputs. The purpose of SA is to quantify this relationship through the ubiquitous derivative of the output as a function of the input. We provide an introductory survey of SA, how it's is done, what can go wrong, and apply SA to examples from epidemiology, illustrating how these tools can be used to improve mathematical models by quantitatively identifying key aspects that lead to strategies for reducing the spread of a disease.

1.1 Sensitivity Analysis: Forward and Adjoint Sensitivity

Consider a mathematical model consisting of user specified inputs, which are subsequently utilized by the model to create output solutions. Variations in the input parameters create variations in the output. The primary objective of SA is to

L. Arriola (✉)
Department of Mathematical and Computer Sciences, University of Wisconsin–Whitewater, Whitewater, WI 53190, USA
e-mail: arriolal@uww.edu

G. Chowell et al. (eds.), *Mathematical and Statistical Estimation Approaches in Epidemiology*, DOI 10.1007/978-90-481-2313-1_10,
© Springer Science+Business Media B.V. 2009

precisely quantify the ratio of output perturbations with respect to the input perturbations. That is, SA provides an approach to determine which parameters have
the most/least effect on the output solution. For example, if u denotes the output
solution to a mathematical model and p denotes any of the input parameters, the
primary objective of SA is to efficiently calculate $\partial u/\partial p$.

We introduce and apply the concepts and methodology of SA to three types of
mathematical models:

- static problems
- dynamical systems
- optimization problems

Although static problems do not change in time, they can include complex
relationships between parameters and the solution. As a typical example, consider solving a system of linear equations $\mathbf{Au} = \mathbf{b}$. SA can determine how the
solution $\mathbf{u}$ depends on perturbations to the coefficients a_{ij} or the right-hand side
terms b_i. Perturbations to these input parameters will directly affect the solution
and raises the question: Which of these parameters has the most effect on the
solution? To answer this question, we calculate the derivative expression $\partial u/\partial p$,
where p represents any of the a_{ij} or b_i by introducing an auxiliary problem-the
adjoint problem. This adjoint problem will allow us to efficiently find the desired
derivative.

The same type of situation occurs for the common eigenvalue problem $\mathbf{Au} =
\lambda\mathbf{u}$ that arises, for example, in determining the reproductive number in epidemic
models. Since the eigenstructure of this linear operator depends on the underlying parameter space, uncertainty in the a_{ij} produces uncertainty in the eigenvalues and eigenvectors of $\mathbf{A}$. SA is an approach that can define how λ or $\mathbf{u}$
will change if the elements of the matrix $\mathbf{A}$ change as measured by: $\partial\lambda/\partial a_{ij}$
and $\partial\mathbf{u}/\partial a_{ij}$. We will use the adjoint SA methodology to derive explicit formula
for the derivatives of the eigenvalue and eigenvector. In epidemic models, the
elements of $\mathbf{A}$ are often functions of the parameters, such as the infectivity or population size, in the underlying mathematical model and SA is used to determine
how the eigenvalues change as a function of, say, a change in the transmission
rate.

Epidemiological phenomena are often modeled by time dependent ordinary
differential equations (ODEs), or if there is spatial, age, or other relational depen-
dences, by partial differential equations (PDEs). If the time or spatial dependence
is formulated on a lattice structure, then difference equations can be used as the
mathematical model. Often the parameters or initial conditions (IC's) are not known
exactly. Again, SA is an approach that can quantify how the uncertainty in input
values is related to uncertainty in the model output $\mathbf{u} = \mathbf{u}(t)$. As in the static
case, we will introduce an appropriate auxiliary problem, the adjoint problem. When
chosen properly, the adjoint formation can reduce the computational complexity to
answer targeted questions when the full SA is not needed, or is not computationally
feasible.

1.2 Parameter Estimation

Parameter estimation is needed:

- when there is observational data with significant errors,
- when there are unknown or unspecified parameters, in the model that must be estimated (parameter estimation (PE)),
- to quantify the inevitable effects of uncertainty, in the observed data set and on the specification of parameter values, which ultimately leads to uncertainty in the model prediction (forward sensitivity analysis (FSA)), and
- to determine which regions in time or parameter space have the most effect on the model prediction (adjoint sensitivity analysis (ASA)).

Consider the graphical representation in Fig. 1 of the overall structure of the FSA problem, where **ODS** represents observational data set, **PS** denotes the parameter space, and **MP** represents the set of model predictions. Notice that the PS is partitioned into two disjoint sets; one containing those parameters for which we currently do not have specified values: $\{p_1, \ldots, p_k\}$, and the other set of parameters which do have assigned values $\{p_{k+1}, \ldots, p_{k+l}\}$. The application of a computational algorithm whereby one uses the incomplete ODS and obtains specific values for the unknown parameters can be viewed as the mapping $F : ODS \mapsto \{p_1, \ldots, p_k\}$. This is the objective of data assimilation. Once the unknown parameters are specified, the mathematical model can be evaluated providing the MP, that is, $G : PS \mapsto MP$.

Measurement errors in the ODS (shown as the dashed curves in Fig. 2) introduce uncertainties produce uncertainty in the PS, and hence uncertainty in the MP.

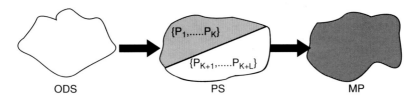

Fig. 1 Using the observational data set (ODS) to obtain values for unspecified parameters $\{p_1, \ldots, p_k\}$ in the parameter space (PS), which allows evaluation of the epidemiological model to obtain the model prediction (MP)

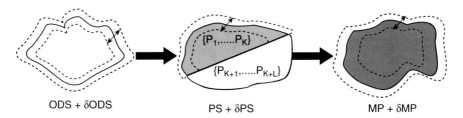

Fig. 2 Uncertainty in the ODS, (shown as *dashed curves*), produces uncertainty in the PS, which leads to uncertainty in the MP of the epidemiological model

We will describe local SA approaches to estimating the change in the solution resulting from small changes in nominal fixed values of the defining parameters. This introduction to SA will not discuss in detail the methodology of data assimilation, as applied to parameter estimation in epidemiology. However, we will provide the basic tools needed for parameter estimation. Furthermore, global SA (uncertainty quantification) [28] issues such as the sensitivity of bifurcation points, critical/degenerate points, extrema, variance-based methods such as Monte Carlo methods or the Fourier Amplitude Sensitivity Tests, Latin Hypercube or Fractional Factorial sampling, or Bayesian SA.

2 Sensitivity Analysis

2.1 Normalized Sensitivity Index

The fundamental objective of SA is to quantitatively estimate how uncertainty of inputs gives rise to uncertainties of the model outputs. In particular, we describe FSA and ASA for deterministic (non-stochastic) mathematical models.

FSA quantitatively determines how the output solution u, to our mathematical model, or some response function(al) $J(u)$, changes as small perturbations are made to a model parameter p, as is shown in Fig. 3. If the solution and functional are differentiable wrt. a parameter p, then in FSA we calculate the derivatives $\partial u/\partial p$ and $\partial J(u)/\partial p$ and define the *normalized sensitivity indexes* (SI):

$$S_{u_p} := \lim_{\delta p \to 0} \left(\frac{\delta u}{u}\right)\left(\frac{\delta p}{p}\right)^{-1} = \left(\frac{p}{u}\right)\frac{\partial u}{\partial p} \tag{1}$$

$$S_{J_p} := \lim_{\delta p \to 0} \frac{\delta J}{J}\left(\frac{\delta p}{p}\right)^{-1} = \left(\frac{J}{p}\right)\frac{\partial u}{\partial p}. \tag{2}$$

The normalized SI [13, 28–30] measure the relative change in the output $\delta u/u$ or $\delta J/J$, wrt. a small relative change to the input $\delta p/p$.

Fig. 3 The forward problem (FP-*top figure*) takes nominal input parameters p and produces the associated output solution u. Forward sensitivity analysis (FSA-*bottom figure*) introduces perturbations to the input parameters, via δp and quantifies the subsequent perturbations to the output solution via δu

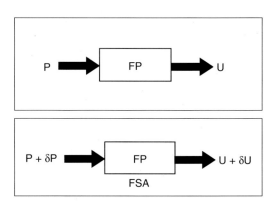

Fig. 4 Adjoint sensitivity
analysis (ASA) introduces
perturbations to the output
solution, via δu and
quantifies how these changes
are related to perturbations in
the input parameters via δp

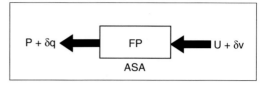

One of the pitfalls in applying the results of SA is in not paying close attention to the relationships between the signs of S, u, δu, p, and δp. Often the output variable u is nonnegative, such as the infected population in an epidemic model and, without loss of generality, we will assume that the parameters and output variables in this article are all positive. When this is not the case, then the analysis must pay close attention to signs of the variables.

If the mathematical model is a dynamical system, then the SI can depend on time and the relative importance of the parameters can also depend on time. For example, for $t \leq t_c$, the parameter p_1 might have more affect on the solution than the parameter p_2, whereas for $t > t_c$ the roles of importance might reverse. This often occurs when comparing the relative importance of model parameters in early and late stages of an epidemic.

Whereas, for dynamical systems, FSA measures the future change in the solution caused by small changes in the parameters, ASA [12, 21–23] looks back in time, as shown in Fig. 4.

2.2 Motivation for Sensitivity Analysis

Consider the two species symbiotic population model [26] given by

$$\frac{du_1}{dt} = u_1(1 - u_1 - au_2) \tag{3}$$

$$\frac{du_2}{dt} = bu_2(1 - u_2 - cu_1), \tag{4}$$

where the parameters a, b, and c are nonnegative, ac is constant, and we are given the initial population of the two species as $u_1(0)$ and $u_2(0)$. For physical reasons, we require that the parameters satisfy the conditions $0 < a, c < 1$.

Some typical questions one might ask are

- Which of the parameters has the most influence on the value (not stability) of the equilibrium point(s)?
- Which of the parameters has the most influence on the stability/instability of the equilibrium points?
- Which of the parameters has the most influence on the time dependent solutions u_1 and u_2?

For more sophisticated models [1], numerous other relevant questions could easily come to mind. We will study this problem in more detail in the following sections.

3 Linear System of Equations and Eigenvalue Problem

3.1 Linear System of Equations: Symbiotic Population

For the two species symbiotic population model given above, let us determine which of the three parameters has the most influence on the value (not stability) of the equilibrium point(s) $(\bar{u}_1, \bar{u}_2)$ of Equations (3, 4). In other words, we would like to know how the solutions $(\bar{u}_1, \bar{u}_2)$ of the steady state system

$$\bar{u}_1(1 - \bar{u}_1 - a\bar{u}_2) = 0$$
$$b\bar{u}_2(1 - \bar{u}_2 - c\bar{u}_1) = 0$$

are affected by changes to the two parameters a or c.

Solving this nonlinear system, we find the four equilibrium points

$$(\bar{u}_1, \bar{u}_2) = \left\{ (0, 0), (0, 1), (1, 0), \left(\frac{1 - a}{1 - ac}, \frac{1 - c}{1 - ac} \right) \right\}.$$

Notice that the extinct and single species equilibrium points $(0, 0)$, $(0, 1)$, and $(1, 0)$ are independent of the a or c and therefore are unaffected by perturbations to these parameters. The two species equilibrium point however does depend on these parameters in which case we find the normalized relative sensitivity indices to be

$$\frac{a}{\bar{u}_1} \frac{\partial \bar{u}_1}{\partial a} = -\frac{a(1 - c)}{(1 - a)(1 - ac)}, \qquad \frac{a}{\bar{u}_2} \frac{\partial \bar{u}_2}{\partial a} = \frac{ac}{1 - ac},$$

$$\frac{c}{\bar{u}_1} \frac{\partial \bar{u}_1}{\partial c} = \frac{ac}{1 - ac}, \quad \text{and} \quad \frac{c}{\bar{u}_2} \frac{\partial \bar{u}_2}{\partial c} = -\frac{c(1 - a)}{(1 - c)(1 - ac)}.$$

Notice that the sensitivity of u_1 wrt. c is the same as it is for u_2 wrt. a.

The relative importance, as measured by the sensitivity indices, may be different in different regions of the parameter space. For this example, consider the sensitivity of u_1 wrt. a and u_2 wrt. c, where we want to know what the ordering is;

$$\frac{a}{\bar{u}_1} \frac{\partial \bar{u}_1}{\partial a} \boxed{?} \frac{c}{\bar{u}_2} \frac{\partial \bar{u}_1}{\partial c}$$

$$-\frac{a(1 - c)}{(1 - a)(1 - ac)} \boxed{?} -\frac{c(1 - a)}{(1 - c)(1 - ac)}$$

$$\frac{1 - c}{\sqrt{c}} \boxed{?} \frac{1 - a}{\sqrt{a}}.$$

Here the symbol $\boxed{?}$ is an inequality symbol, such as $<$ or $>$. Since the function $f(x) := (1 - x)/\sqrt{x}$, for $x \in (0, 1)$ is a strictly decreasing function, if $x_1 < x_2$, then

$f(x_1) > f(x_2)$. In other words, the relative importance, via the sensitivity indices, depends on whether $c > a$ or $c < a$.

Although we now have a methodology for determining the sensitivity of the equilibrium points, even more information can be gleaned by using SA for the evolution of the solution. In simpler examples the closed form solution is easily found and elementary calculus can be applied to find the associated sensitivity indices.

Let us restate and reformulate the problem of interest, that is to obtain the derivatives $\partial \bar{u}_1 / \partial p$ and $\partial \bar{u}_2 / \partial p$, where p represents any of the three parameters a, b or c. Even when the closed form solutions for the equilibrium points is not known, then we can directly construct the FSA by differentiating the equilibrium problem. The associated forward sensitivity equations (FSE) containing these derivatives are found by taking the partial derivatives $\partial / \partial p$ of both equilibrium equations, and applying the standard chain rule, to get the linear system

$$\mathbf{D_u} \frac{\partial \mathbf{u}}{\partial p} = -\nabla_p F,$$

where, the notation we use will become apparent shortly,

$$\mathbf{D_u} = \begin{pmatrix} 1 - 2\bar{u}_1 - a\bar{u}_2 & -a\bar{u}_1 \\ -bc\bar{u}_2 & b(1 - 2\bar{u}_2 - c\bar{u}_1) \end{pmatrix}, \quad \frac{\partial \mathbf{u}}{\partial p} = \begin{pmatrix} \dfrac{\partial \bar{u}_1}{\partial p} \\ \dfrac{\partial \bar{u}_2}{\partial p} \end{pmatrix},$$

$$\nabla_p F = \begin{pmatrix} -\bar{u}_1 \bar{u}_2 \dfrac{\partial a}{\partial p} \\ -\bar{u}_1 \bar{u}_2 \dfrac{\partial c}{\partial p} \end{pmatrix}.$$

One could calculate $\mathbf{D_u}^{-1}$ directly, however for large systems of equations this procedure is both analytically difficult or computationally expensive. Direct inversion of the linear operator should always be avoided, except in very small systems. Instead for large systems, we obtain $\mathbf{D_u}^{-1} \nabla_p F$ by introducing an auxiliary problem called the adjoint problem.

Before describing the adjoint problem, we make the important observation that the system of equations defining the derivative $d\mathbf{u}/dp$ is *always* a linear system, even though the original system was nonlinear. This particular example suggests that although the equilibrium point(s) could be solutions to nonlinear equations, the FSE's are linear in the derivative terms. To see this is true in general, consider the 2-D system

$$\frac{du_1}{dt} = f_1(u_1, u_2; p)$$

$$\frac{du_2}{dt} = f_2(u_1, u_2; p)$$

where f_1 and f_2 are differentiable in u_1, u_2 and p. Since the equilibrium points are solutions of the nonlinear system

$$f_1(\bar{u}_1, \bar{u}_2; p) = 0$$
$$f_2(\bar{u}_1, \bar{u}_2; p) = 0$$

then the associated FSE's is the linear system

$$\mathbf{D_u} \frac{\partial \mathbf{u}}{\partial p} = -\nabla_p F, \tag{5}$$

where

$$\mathbf{D_u} = \begin{pmatrix} \dfrac{\partial f_1}{\partial \bar{u}_1} & \dfrac{\partial f_1}{\partial \bar{u}_2} \\[2ex] \dfrac{\partial f_2}{\partial \bar{u}_1} & \dfrac{\partial f_2}{\partial \bar{u}_2} \end{pmatrix}, \quad \frac{\partial \mathbf{u}}{\partial p} = \begin{pmatrix} \dfrac{\partial \bar{u}_1}{\partial p} \\[2ex] \dfrac{\partial \bar{u}_2}{\partial p} \end{pmatrix}, \quad \nabla_p F = \begin{pmatrix} \dfrac{\partial f_1}{\partial p} \\[2ex] \dfrac{\partial f_2}{\partial p} \end{pmatrix}.$$

The notation chosen is suggestive: $\mathbf{D_u}$ denotes the Jacobian wrt. the variables $\mathbf{u}$ and $\nabla_p F$ denotes the gradient wrt. the parameters $\mathbf{p}$.

Thus, the FSE for the equilibrium solutions of the IVP can be written in the general form

$$\mathbf{A}\mathbf{w} = \mathbf{b}, \tag{6}$$

where $\mathbf{A}$ is a real $N \times N$ nonsymmetric and nonsingular matrix, which in this example is the Jacobian matrix. Let p denote any of the parameters a_{ij} or b_i and assume that for the specified values of p, the forward solution $\mathbf{w}$ is a differentiable function of the parameters and is sufficiently far away from any singularities in the parameter space, then the FSE are given by

$$\mathbf{A} \frac{\partial \mathbf{w}}{\partial p} = \frac{\partial \mathbf{b}}{\partial p} - \frac{\partial \mathbf{A}}{\partial p} \mathbf{w}. \tag{7}$$

Since perturbations to the parameter p produces perturbations in the forward solution $\mathbf{w}$, FSA requires the calculation of the derivative $\partial \mathbf{w}/\partial p$. This FSE equation could be solved by premultiplying by the matrix inverse $\mathbf{A}^{-1}$, however, for larger systems, this procedure is computationally expensive, often numerically unstable, and should be avoided if at all possible.

The ASA accomplishes the same goal, while avoiding computing $\mathbf{A}^{-1}$, by introducing an auxiliary problem which isolates how the solution depends on the parameters; that is, $\partial \mathbf{w}/\partial p$. This is accomplished by defining an appropriate inner product and cleverly choosing conditions so as to isolate the desired quantity. For this simple case, we use the usual vector inner product for standard Euclidean space and premultiply the FSE by some, as of yet unspecified, nontrivial vector $\mathbf{v}^T$

$$\mathbf{v}^T \mathbf{A} \frac{\partial \mathbf{w}}{\partial p} = \mathbf{v}^T \left(\frac{\partial \mathbf{b}}{\partial p} - \frac{\partial \mathbf{A}}{\partial p} \mathbf{w} \right). \tag{8}$$

Now consider the $1 \times N$ vector $\mathbf{c}^T := \mathbf{v}^T \mathbf{A}$, or written as the associated adjoint problem

$$\mathbf{A}^T \mathbf{v} = \mathbf{c}. \tag{9}$$

Since we wish to isolate the derivative term $\partial \mathbf{w}/\partial p$, choose N forcing vectors of the form $\mathbf{c}_i^T = \begin{pmatrix} 0 \cdots 0 \ 1 \ 0 \cdots 0 \end{pmatrix}$, where the 1 is located in the ith column. This forces the product $\mathbf{v}^T \mathbf{A}$ to project out the desired components $\partial w_i/\partial p$, for $i = 1, \ldots, N$, in which case

$$\frac{\partial w_i}{\partial p} = \mathbf{v}_i^T \left(\frac{\partial \mathbf{b}}{\partial p} - \frac{\partial \mathbf{A}}{\partial p} \mathbf{w} \right). \tag{10}$$

This particular choice for the adjoint problem leads to an intimate relationship between the inverse matrix $\mathbf{A}^{-1}$ and the matrix of adjoint vectors $\mathbf{V} := \begin{pmatrix} \mathbf{v}_1 \ \mathbf{v}_2 \cdots \mathbf{v}_N \end{pmatrix}$, namely $\mathbf{V}^T = \mathbf{A}^{-1}$. The relationships between the forward and adjoint problems and sensitivity equations, in this example, shown in Fig. 5, illustrates connections between the forward and adjoint problem.

3.2 Stability of the Equilibrium Solution: The Eigenvalue Problem

The stability of the equilibrium solution of (3) and (4) depends upon the eigenvalues of the Jacobian of the linearized system at the equilibrium. These eigenvalues are functions of the parameters p. Therefore, we can use sensitivity analysis to

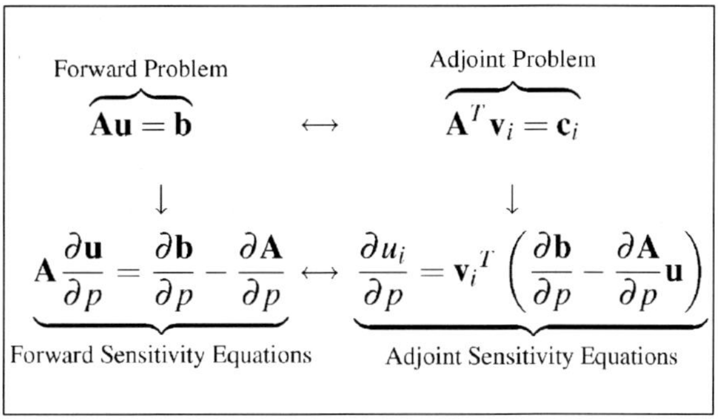

Fig. 5 The relationships between the forward sensitivity and associated adjoint problems creates a self-consistant framework for sensitivity analysis

Forward Problem $\qquad$ Adjoint Problem

$$\underbrace{\mathbf{A}\mathbf{u} = \mathbf{b}}_{} \qquad \longleftrightarrow \qquad \underbrace{\mathbf{A}^T \mathbf{v}_i = \mathbf{c}_i}_{}$$

$$\downarrow \qquad\qquad\qquad \downarrow$$

$$\underbrace{\mathbf{A}\frac{\partial \mathbf{u}}{\partial p} = \frac{\partial \mathbf{b}}{\partial p} - \frac{\partial \mathbf{A}}{\partial p}}_{\text{Forward Sensitivity Equations}} \longleftrightarrow \underbrace{\frac{\partial u_i}{\partial p} = \mathbf{v}_i^T \left(\frac{\partial \mathbf{b}}{\partial p} - \frac{\partial \mathbf{A}}{\partial p} \mathbf{u} \right)}_{\text{Adjoint Sensitivity Equations}}$$

determine how the stability of an equilibrium point is affected by changes to the parameters. The eigenvalues λ of the Jacobian

$$A = \begin{pmatrix} 1 - 2\bar{u}_1 - a\bar{u}_2 & -a\bar{u}_1 \\ -bc\bar{u}_2 & b\left(1 - 2\bar{u}_2 - c\bar{u}_1\right) \end{pmatrix} \tag{11}$$

could be found by constructing the characteristic polynomial and solving the associated characteristic equation

$$p(\lambda) = \lambda^2 - (1 - 2\bar{u}_1 - a\bar{u}_2 + b(1 - c\bar{u}_1 - 2\bar{u}_2))\lambda - abc\bar{u}_1\bar{u}_2 \quad \text{and} \quad p(\lambda) = 0.$$

For this simple problem, the eigenvalues can be explicitly found, and subsequently the derivatives $\partial\lambda/\partial p$ can be calculated. However, as the system of differential equations increases, so does the degree of the associated characteristic polynomial and this approach becomes impracticable. The roots of high degree polynomials cannot be defined analytically, and the numerical methods for finding these roots often suffer from numerical instabilities.

As was done in the previous example of finding the sensitivity of a linear system of equations, we proceed to find the sensitivity of the right eigenvalue problem[1]

$$\mathbf{Au} = \lambda\mathbf{u} \tag{12}$$

where $\mathbf{A}$ is an $N \times N$ nonsymmetric matrix with distinct eigenvalues and an associated complete, nonorthonormal set of eigenvectors, which span $\mathbb{R}^N$. This particular example will shed light on a significant inherent limitation of ASE that is rarely discussed, much less emphasized.

Since the eigenvalues λ and the eigenvectors $\mathbf{u}$ depend on the coefficients a_{ij}, differentiate the right eigenvalue problem to get the FSE

$$\mathbf{A}\frac{\partial\mathbf{u}}{\partial a_{ij}} + \frac{\partial\mathbf{A}}{\partial a_{ij}}\mathbf{u} = \lambda\frac{\partial\mathbf{u}}{\partial a_{ij}} + \frac{\partial\lambda}{\partial a_{ij}}\mathbf{u}. \tag{13}$$

The difficulty that arises in this example is that there are two unknown derivatives of interest, the derivative of the eigenvalues $\partial\lambda/\partial a_{ij}$ and the derivative of the eigenvectors $\partial\mathbf{u}/\partial a_{ij}$. The purpose of the adjoint methodology is to produce one, and only one, additional auxiliary problem. That is, a single associated adjoint problem can only be used to find the derivative of the eigenvalues or the derivative of the eigenvectors, but not both simultaneously. As we will show, using the adjoint problem to find $\partial\lambda/\partial a_{ij}$ precludes the ability to find $\partial\mathbf{u}/\partial a_{ij}$, unless additional information is provided.

---

[1] As we will see shortly, the associated left eigenvalue problem is the adjoint problem for (12), namely $\mathbf{A}^T\mathbf{v} = \lambda\mathbf{v}$.

Let $\mathbf{v}$ be some nonzero, as yet unspecified, vector and take the inner product with the FSE (13) to get

$$\frac{\partial \lambda}{\partial a_{ij}} \langle \mathbf{u}, \mathbf{v} \rangle = \left\langle \frac{\partial \mathbf{A}}{\partial a_{ij}} \mathbf{u}, \mathbf{v} \right\rangle + \left\langle (\mathbf{A} - \lambda \mathbf{I}) \frac{\partial \mathbf{u}}{\partial a_{ij}}, \mathbf{v} \right\rangle. \tag{14}$$

Because $(\mathbf{A} - \lambda \mathbf{I})^T = \mathbf{A}^T - \lambda \mathbf{I}$, we can use the Lagrange identity for matrices, under the usual inner product, to get

$$\left\langle (\mathbf{A} - \lambda \mathbf{I}) \frac{\partial \mathbf{u}}{\partial a_{ij}}, \mathbf{v} \right\rangle = \left\langle \frac{\partial \mathbf{u}}{\partial a_{ij}}, (\mathbf{A}^T - \lambda \mathbf{I}) \mathbf{v} \right\rangle.$$

Now annihilate the second inner product by forcing the adjoint condition

$$\mathbf{A}^T \mathbf{v} = \lambda \mathbf{v}, \tag{15}$$

which is known as the left eigenvalue problem. For the original eigenvalue problem, the left eigenvalue problem is the associated adjoint problem. (For more details, see [18, 32].)

The properties of the left and right eigenvalue problems include:

- If the right eigenvalue problem has a solution, then the left eigenvalue also has a solution.
- The right and left eigenvectors $\mathbf{u}$ and $\mathbf{v}$ are distinct, for a specified eigenvalue λ.
- The right eigenvectors $\mathbf{u}^{(k)} = \left(u_1^{(k)} \ u_2^{(k)} \ \cdots \ u_N^{(k)} \right)^T$ and left eigenvectors $\mathbf{v}^{(l)} = \left(v_1^{(l)} \ v_2^{(l)} \ \cdots \ v_N^{(l)} \right)^T$ are orthogonal for $k \neq l$ and $\langle \mathbf{u}^{(k)}, \mathbf{v}^{(k)} \rangle \neq 0$ for $k = l$.
- Using the previous result, the right and left eigenvectors can be normalized, i.e., $\langle \mathbf{u}^{(k)}, \mathbf{v}^{(k)} \rangle = 1$.

Using the left eigenvalue problem (adjoint problem), Equation (14) reduces to

$$\frac{\partial \lambda}{\partial a_{ij}} \langle \mathbf{u}, \mathbf{v} \rangle = v_i \, u_j.$$

Since the right and left eigenvectors are normalized, the explicit expression for the derivative of the eigenvalue wrt. the coefficients a_{ij} is

$$\frac{\partial \lambda}{\partial a_{ij}} = v_i \, u_j. \tag{16}$$

To find an explicit expression for $\partial \mathbf{u}/\partial a_{ij}$, we must introduce additional information. The reason for this diversion is that no new information can be gleaned about $\partial \mathbf{u}/\partial a_{ij}$ from the adjoint problem. The key to making further progress is to recall that we have assumed that the $N \times N$ matrix $\mathbf{A}$ has N distinct eigenvalues, in which case there exists a complete set of N eigenvectors. We now make use of the fact that any vector in $\mathbb{C}^N$ can be expressed as a linear combination of the spanning eigenvectors. Since $\partial \mathbf{u}/\partial a_{ij}$ is an $N \times 1$ vector, we can write this derivative as a linear combination of the eigenvectors.

It will be helpful to introduce some additional notation describing the right and left eigenvector matrices $\mathbf{U}$ and $\mathbf{V}$, whose columns are the individual eigenvectors $\mathbf{u}^{(k)}$ and $\mathbf{v}^{(k)}$ respectively, and let Λ be the diagonal matrix of eigenvalues λ_k, that is

$$\mathbf{U} := \left(\mathbf{u}^{(1)} \ \mathbf{u}^{(2)} \ \cdots \ \mathbf{u}^{(N)} \right), \quad \mathbf{V} := \left(\mathbf{v}^{(1)} \ \mathbf{v}^{(2)} \ \cdots \ \mathbf{v}^{(N)} \right) \quad \text{and} \quad \Lambda := \begin{pmatrix} \lambda_1 & & & \mathbf{0} \\ & \lambda_2 & & \\ & & \ddots & \\ \mathbf{0} & & & \lambda_N \end{pmatrix}.$$

Using this notation, the right and left eigenvalue problems can be written as

$$\mathbf{AU} = \mathbf{U}\Lambda \qquad \text{and} \qquad \mathbf{A}^T\mathbf{V} = \mathbf{V}\Lambda. \tag{17}$$

Earlier we forced the right and left eigenvectors to be normalized, and therefore the matrix of eigenvectors satisfy the identity

$$\mathbf{V}^T\mathbf{U} = \mathbf{I}. \tag{18}$$

The derivative of the matrix of eigenvectors can written as a linear combination of the eigenspace;

$$\frac{\partial \mathbf{U}}{\partial a_{ij}} = \mathbf{UC}. \tag{19}$$

This equation defines the coefficient matrix

$$\mathbf{C} := \begin{pmatrix} c_1^{(1)} & c_1^{(2)} & c_1^{(3)} & \cdots & c_1^{(N)} \\ c_2^{(1)} & c_2^{(2)} & c_2^{(3)} & \cdots & c_2^{(N)} \\ \vdots & & \vdots & & \vdots \\ c_N^{(1)} & c_N^{(2)} & c_N^{(3)} & \cdots & c_N^{(N)} \end{pmatrix}, \tag{20}$$

where for a fixed eigenvector $\mathbf{u}^{(k)}$, the derivative can be expanded as the sum

$$\frac{\partial \mathbf{u}^{(k)}}{\partial a_{ij}} = c_1^{(k)}\mathbf{u}^{(1)} + \cdots + c_k^{(k)}\mathbf{u}^{(k)} + \cdots c_N^{(k)}\mathbf{u}^{(N)}. \tag{21}$$

We now describe how to define the coefficients $c_l^{(m)}$.

Differentiating the right eigenvector matrix Equation (17) gives

$$\mathbf{A}\frac{\partial \mathbf{U}}{\partial a_{ij}} + \frac{\partial \mathbf{A}}{\partial a_{ij}}\mathbf{U} = \mathbf{U}\frac{\partial \Lambda}{\partial a_{ij}} + \frac{\partial \mathbf{U}}{\partial a_{ij}}\Lambda. \tag{22}$$

Using Equation (17) and (19) and rearranging we get

$$\mathbf{U}[\Lambda, \mathbf{C}] = \mathbf{U}\frac{\partial \Lambda}{\partial a_{ij}} - \frac{\partial \mathbf{A}}{\partial a_{ij}}\mathbf{U}, \tag{23}$$

where $[\cdot,]$ denotes the commutator bracket $[\Lambda, \mathbf{C}] := \Lambda\mathbf{C} - \mathbf{C}\Lambda$.

Next, premultiply by the left eigenvector matrix and use the normalization condition, this equation reduces to

$$[\Lambda, \mathbf{C}] = \frac{\partial \Lambda}{\partial a_{ij}} - \mathbf{V}^T \frac{\partial \mathbf{A}}{\partial a_{ij}}\mathbf{U}. \tag{24}$$

Expanding the commutator bracket we find that

$$[\Lambda, \mathbf{C}] = \begin{pmatrix} 0 & c_1^{(2)}(\lambda_1 - \lambda_2) & c_1^{(3)}(\lambda_1 - \lambda_3) & \cdots & c_1^{(N)}(\lambda_1 - \lambda_N) \\ c_2^{(1)}(\lambda_2 - \lambda_1) & 0 & c_2^{(3)}(\lambda_2 - \lambda_3) & \cdots & c_2^{(N)}(\lambda_2 - \lambda_N) \\ c_3^{(1)}(\lambda_3 - \lambda_1) & c_3^{(2)}(\lambda_3 - \lambda_2) & 0 & \cdots & c_3^{(N)}(\lambda_3 - \lambda_N) \\ \vdots & & & \ddots & \vdots \\ c_N^{(1)}(\lambda_N - \lambda_1) & c_N^{(2)}(\lambda_N - \lambda_2) & c_N^{(3)}(\lambda_N - \lambda_3) & \cdots & 0 \end{pmatrix} \tag{25}$$

Since the right side of Equation (24) is known, and because we assumed that the eigenvalues are distinct, we can solve for the off-diagonal coefficients

$$c_l^{(m)} = -\frac{1}{\lambda_l - \lambda_m}\left[\mathbf{V}^T \frac{\partial \mathbf{A}}{\partial a_{ij}}\mathbf{U}\right]_{lm} \quad \text{for} \quad l \neq m. \tag{26}$$

The next task is to find the values of the diagonal coefficients. Once again, we make use of the fact that the eigenvectors form a basis for $\mathbb{C}^N$. To solve for the scalar diagonal coefficients $c_k^{(k)}$ in (21), we first transform this vector equation to a scalar equation by normalizing the right eigenvectors. That is, we force the condition $\langle \mathbf{u}^k, \mathbf{u}^k \rangle = 1$. Next, we fix the indexes i, j and differentiate this normalization condition to get

$$\mathbf{u}^{kT}\frac{\partial \mathbf{u}^k}{\partial a_{ij}} + \frac{\partial \mathbf{u}^{kT}}{\partial a_{ij}}\mathbf{u}^k = 0.$$

Because

$$\frac{\partial \mathbf{u}^{kT}}{\partial a_{ij}}\mathbf{u}^k = \mathbf{u}^{kT}\frac{\partial \mathbf{u}^k}{\partial a_{ij}},$$

it follows that $\mathbf{u}^k$ and $\partial \mathbf{u}^k / \partial a_{ij}$ are orthogonal, in which case we obtain the N equations

$$\left\langle \frac{\partial \mathbf{u}^k}{\partial a_{ij}}, \mathbf{u}^k \right\rangle = 0, \qquad \text{for} \quad k = 1, \dots N. \tag{27}$$

Next premultiply, the summed version of the derivative of the eigenvector (21), by $\mathbf{u}^{(k)}$ to get

$$c_1^{(k)} \langle \mathbf{u}^{(1)}, \mathbf{u}^{(k)} \rangle + \cdots + c_k^{(k)} \langle \mathbf{u}^{(k)}, \mathbf{u}^{(k)} \rangle + \cdots c_N^{(k)} \langle \mathbf{u}^{(N)}, \mathbf{u}^{(k)} \rangle = 0.$$

Since the individual eigenvectors have been normalized, we can solve for the diagonal coefficients in terms of the known off diagonal coefficients:

$$c_k^{(k)} = - \sum_{\substack{i=1 \\ i \neq k}}^{N} c_i^{(k)} \langle \mathbf{u}^{(i)}, \mathbf{u}^{(k)} \rangle. \tag{28}$$

4 Dimensionality Reduction

When considering a mathematical model where some of the variables may be redundant, one would like to be able to identify, with confidence, those variables that can be safely eliminated without affecting the validity of the model. To not inadvertently eliminate significant variables, one must identify *groups* of variables that are highly correlated. In essence, one is trying to identify those aspects of the model that are comprised of strongly interacting mechanisms. A problem arises when one uses data, which contain errors or noise, to estimate the correlation between these variables and use these estimates to determine which variables can be safely eliminated. Thus, uncertainty in the data can create uncertainty in the correlation estimates and ultimately in the reduced model.

For example, consider an imaginary disease for which a specific blood test can, with certainty, identify whether the patient has or does not have this disease. Now suppose that there exists a medication whose sole purpose is to treat this particular disease. When constructing a model of this scenario, the number of prescriptions for this medication and the positive blood test results are highly correlated. Assuming that the examining physician always prescribes this medication the correlation would in fact be 1.0. The information contained in these two data sets are redundant. Either the number of positive blood test results or the number of prescriptions provides sufficient information about the number of positively diagnosed infections. Taking a geometric perspective of this scenario, since the two data sets are so highly correlated, a projection from a 2-dimensional parameter space to a 1-dimensional space would be appropriate.

Now consider the more realistic scenario where public health officials are monitoring a seasonal outbreak of a disease. Syndromic surveillance or biosurveillance data of clinical symptoms such as fever, number of hospital admissions, over-the-counter medication consumption, respiratory complaints, school or work absences, etc., while readily available, does not directly provide accurate numerical quantification of the size of the outbreak. Furthermore, "noise" in the data causes inaccuracy of any specific numerical assessments or predictions. Additionally, symptoms such as fever and respiratory complaints have different levels of correlation for different diseases, and therefore difficulties arise in determining which factors are redundant and which factors are essential to the model. In other words, it would be desirable to identify the highly correlated variables, in which case we could reduce the dimension of the data, without significantly degrading the validity of the model, and minimize the effects of noise.

4.1 Principal Component Analysis

Principal component analysis (PCA) is a powerful method of modern data analysis that provides a systematic way to reduce the dimension of a complex data set to a lower dimension, and oftentimes reveals hidden simplified structures that would otherwise go unnoticed.

Consider an $M \times N$ matrix of data measurements $\mathbf{A}$ with M data types and N observations of each data type. Each $M \times 1$ column of $\mathbf{A}$ represents the measurement of the data types at some time t for which there are N time samples. Since any $M \times 1$ vector lies in an M-dimensional vector space, then there exists an M-dimensional orthonormal basis that spans the vector space. The goal of PCA is to transform the noisy, and possibly redundant data, set to a lower dimensional orthonormal basis. The desired result is that this new basis will effectively and successively filter out the noisy data and reveal hidden structures among the data types.

The way this is accomplished is based on the idea of noise, rotation, and covariance. When performing measurements, the problem of quantifying the effect of noise has on the data set is often defined by the signal-to-noise ratio (SNR) and is defined as the ratio of variances

$$SNR := \frac{\sigma^2{}_{\text{Signal}}}{\sigma^2{}_{\text{Noise}}}. \tag{29}$$

If the SNR is large, then the signal/measurements are accurate; whereas, if SNR is small, then the data is significantly contaminated by noise. Since one of the goals of PCA is transform the data to a basis that minimizes the effect of noise, PCA increases the SNR by maximizing the signal variance. Secondly, data identified having high covariance is used to guide in reducing the dimension of the data set.

4.2 Singular Value Decomposition (SVD)

Let $\mathbf{A}$ be a real $M \times N$ matrix and let r denote the rank of $\mathbf{A}$. Recall some essential geometric properties of matrices:

1. The matrix $\mathbf{A}$ maps the unit sphere in $\mathbb{R}^N$ and into a hyperellipsoid in $\mathbb{R}^M$.

2. The directions of the hyper-axes of the ellipsoid are denoted by the orthogonal basis $\{\mathbf{u}^{(k)}\}$, for $k = 1, \ldots M$ (singular vectors).
3. The stretching/compression factors, (singular values) are denoted by $\{\sigma_k\}$.
4. The vectors $\sigma_k \mathbf{u}^{(k)}$ define the principal semi-axes of the hyperellipsoid.

The SVD defines the particular factorization of $\mathbf{A}$, in terms of the above geometric properties, as

$$\mathbf{A} = \mathbf{U} \underset{\sim}{\Sigma} \mathbf{V}^T \tag{30}$$

where

- the $M \times M$ matrix $\mathbf{U}$ is unitary (i.e., $\mathbf{U}^T\mathbf{U} = \mathbf{I}$, where T denotes transpose and $\mathbf{I}$ is the $M \times M$ identity matrix) and the columns $\mathbf{u}^{(k)}$ form an orthogonal basis for $\mathbb{R}^M$,
- similarly, the $N \times N$ matrix $\mathbf{V}$ is also unitary and the column $\mathbf{v}^{(k)}$ form an orthogonal basis for $\mathbb{R}^N$, and
- the $M \times N$ diagonal matrix $\underset{\sim}{\Sigma}$ is

$$\underset{\sim}{\Sigma} = \begin{pmatrix} \sigma_1 & & & & & \mathbf{0} \\ & \ddots & & & & \\ & & \sigma_r & & & \\ & & & 0 & & \\ & & & & \ddots & \\ \mathbf{0} & & & & & 0 \end{pmatrix}, \tag{31}$$

where the singular values are ordered as $\sigma_1 > \sigma_2 > \cdots > \sigma_r > \sigma_{r+1} = \cdots = \sigma_p = 0$ and $p := \min(M, N)$.

The way to find the M columns $\mathbf{u}$ of $\mathbf{U}$, and the N columns $\mathbf{v}$ of $\mathbf{V}$, where

$$\mathbf{U} := \left(\mathbf{u}^{(1)} \, \mathbf{u}^{(2)} \, \cdots \, \mathbf{u}^{(M)}\right), \quad \mathbf{V} := \left(\mathbf{v}^{(1)} \, \mathbf{v}^{(2)} \, \cdots \, \mathbf{v}^{(N)}\right)$$

is to solve the left and right eigenvalue problems

$$\mathbf{A}\mathbf{v} = \sigma\mathbf{u}, \quad \text{and} \quad \mathbf{A}^T\mathbf{u} = \sigma\mathbf{v}. \tag{32}$$

Note that because the columns of U and V are the eigenvectors of AA^T, the norms of these matrix vector products are the same as the norms of the eigenvectors.

4.3 Sensitivity of SVD

Because the singular values σ and the singular vectors $\mathbf{u}$ and $\mathbf{v}$ depend on the coefficients a_{ij}, we can differentiate the left and right eigenvalue problems (32) to get the FSE

$$\mathbf{A}\frac{\partial \mathbf{v}}{\partial a_{ij}} + \frac{\partial \mathbf{A}}{\partial a_{ij}}\mathbf{v} = \sigma\frac{\partial \mathbf{u}}{\partial a_{ij}} + \frac{\partial \sigma}{\partial a_{ij}}\mathbf{u},\tag{33}$$

$$\mathbf{A}^T\frac{\partial \mathbf{u}}{\partial a_{ij}} + \frac{\partial \mathbf{A}^T}{\partial a_{ij}}\mathbf{u} = \sigma\frac{\partial \mathbf{v}}{\partial a_{ij}} + \frac{\partial \sigma}{\partial a_{ij}}\mathbf{v}.\tag{34}$$

Because the matrices $\mathbf{U}$ and $\mathbf{V}$ are unitary, the associated singular vectors $\mathbf{u}$ and $\mathbf{v}$ are normalized, i.e.,

$$\langle \mathbf{u}, \mathbf{u}\rangle = \langle \mathbf{v}, \mathbf{v}\rangle = 1.$$

Using this result we find the useful orthogonality condition

$$\mathbf{u}^T\frac{\partial \mathbf{u}}{\partial a_{ij}} = \mathbf{v}^T\frac{\partial \mathbf{v}}{\partial a_{ij}} = 0.\tag{35}$$

Premultiply the left FSE given in (33) by $\mathbf{u}^T$ and, using the orthogonality and normalizing conditions, the FSE reduces to

$$\mathbf{u}^T\mathbf{A}\frac{\partial \mathbf{v}}{\partial a_{ij}} + \mathbf{u}^T\frac{\partial \mathbf{A}}{\partial a_{ij}}\mathbf{v} = \frac{\partial \sigma}{\partial a_{ij}}.\tag{36}$$

The right eigenvalue problem, rewritten as $\mathbf{u}^T\mathbf{A} = \sigma\mathbf{v}^T$, is used with the orthogonality condition (35) to eliminate the first term in (36) to give:

$$\begin{aligned}\frac{\partial \sigma}{\partial a_{ij}} &= \mathbf{u}^T\frac{\partial \mathbf{A}}{\partial a_{ij}}\mathbf{v}\\ &= u_i v_j.\end{aligned}\tag{37}$$

for $i = 1,\ldots, M$ and $j = 1,\ldots, N$

Now using the matrix notation, the left and right eigenvalue problems can be written in matrix form

$$\mathbf{A}\,\mathbf{V} = \mathbf{U}\,\underset{\sim}{\Sigma} \quad \text{and} \quad \mathbf{A}^T\,\mathbf{U} = \mathbf{V}\,\underset{\sim}{\Sigma}^T.\tag{38}$$

Since the derivative of the singular vector is in $\mathbb{R}^M$, it can be written as a linear combination of the singular vectors, define the coefficient matrix as

$$\mathbf{C} := \begin{pmatrix} c_1^{(1)} & c_1^{(2)} & c_1^{(3)} & \cdots & c_1^{(M)} \\ c_2^{(1)} & c_2^{(2)} & c_2^{(3)} & \cdots & c_2^{(M)} \\ \vdots & & \vdots & & \vdots \\ c_M^{(1)} & c_M^{(2)} & c_M^{(3)} & \cdots & c_M^{(M)} \end{pmatrix},\tag{39}$$

so that the derivative of the eigenvector matrix can be written as

$$\frac{\partial \mathbf{U}}{\partial a_{ij}} = \mathbf{U}\mathbf{C}. \tag{40}$$

Differentiating the right eigenvector matrix equation gives

$$\mathbf{A}^T \frac{\partial \mathbf{U}}{\partial a_{ij}} + \frac{\partial \mathbf{A}^T}{\partial a_{ij}} \mathbf{U} = \mathbf{V} \frac{\partial \underset{\sim}{\Sigma}^T}{\partial a_{ij}} + \frac{\partial \mathbf{V}}{\partial a_{ij}} \underset{\sim}{\Sigma}^T. \tag{41}$$

Using (40), we get

$$\mathbf{A}^T \mathbf{U}\mathbf{C} - \frac{\partial \mathbf{V}}{\partial a_{ij}} \underset{\sim}{\Sigma}^T = \mathbf{V} \frac{\partial \underset{\sim}{\Sigma}^T}{\partial a_{ij}} - \frac{\partial \mathbf{A}^T}{\partial a_{ij}} \mathbf{U}. \tag{42}$$

To replace the derivative $\partial \mathbf{V}/\partial a_{ij}$ in terms of the product $\mathbf{U}\mathbf{C}$, differentiate the left eigenvalue problem to obtain

$$\mathbf{A} \frac{\partial \mathbf{V}}{\partial a_{ij}} = \mathbf{U} \frac{\partial \underset{\sim}{\Sigma}}{\partial a_{ij}} + \mathbf{U}\mathbf{C}\underset{\sim}{\Sigma} - \frac{\partial \mathbf{A}}{\partial a_{ij}} \mathbf{V}.$$

Next, premultiply Equation (42) by matrix $\mathbf{A}$, and using this result gives

$$\mathbf{A}\mathbf{A}^T \mathbf{U}\mathbf{C} - \mathbf{A} \frac{\partial \mathbf{V}}{\partial a_{ij}} \underset{\sim}{\Sigma}^T = \mathbf{A}\mathbf{V} \frac{\partial \underset{\sim}{\Sigma}^T}{\partial a_{ij}} - \mathbf{A} \frac{\partial \mathbf{A}^T}{\partial a_{ij}} \mathbf{U}$$

$$\mathbf{A}\mathbf{A}^T \mathbf{U}\mathbf{C} - \left(\mathbf{U} \frac{\partial \underset{\sim}{\Sigma}}{\partial a_{ij}} + \mathbf{U}\mathbf{C}\underset{\sim}{\Sigma} - \frac{\partial \mathbf{A}}{\partial a_{ij}} \mathbf{V} \right) \underset{\sim}{\Sigma}^T = \mathbf{A}\mathbf{V} \frac{\partial \underset{\sim}{\Sigma}^T}{\partial a_{ij}} - \mathbf{A} \frac{\partial \mathbf{A}^T}{\partial a_{ij}} \mathbf{U}.$$

Rearranging so as to isolate the expressions containing $\mathbf{U}\mathbf{C}$, on the left side of the equation, we get

$$\mathbf{A}\mathbf{A}^T \mathbf{U}\mathbf{C} - \mathbf{U}\mathbf{C}\underset{\sim}{\Sigma}\,\underset{\sim}{\Sigma}^T = \mathbf{A}\mathbf{V} \frac{\partial \underset{\sim}{\Sigma}^T}{\partial a_{ij}} - \mathbf{A} \frac{\partial \mathbf{A}^T}{\partial a_{ij}} \mathbf{U} + \mathbf{U} \frac{\partial \underset{\sim}{\Sigma}}{\partial a_{ij}} \underset{\sim}{\Sigma}^T - \frac{\partial \mathbf{A}}{\partial a_{ij}} \mathbf{V} \underset{\sim}{\Sigma}^T.$$

Consider the pair of expressions on the left side of this equation

$$\mathbf{A}\mathbf{A}^T \mathbf{U}\mathbf{C} - \mathbf{U}\mathbf{C}\underset{\sim}{\Sigma}\,\underset{\sim}{\Sigma}^T = \mathbf{A}\mathbf{V}\underset{\sim}{\Sigma}^T \mathbf{C} - \mathbf{U}\mathbf{C}\underset{\sim}{\Sigma}\,\underset{\sim}{\Sigma}^T$$

$$= \mathbf{U}\underset{\sim}{\Sigma}\,\underset{\sim}{\Sigma}^T \mathbf{C} - \mathbf{U}\mathbf{C}\underset{\sim}{\Sigma}\,\underset{\sim}{\Sigma}^T$$

$$= \mathbf{U}\left[\underset{\sim}{\Sigma}\,\underset{\sim}{\Sigma}^T, \mathbf{C} \right],$$

where $[\cdot,\cdot]$ denotes the commutator bracket $\left[\underset{\sim}{\Sigma}\underset{\sim}{\Sigma}^T, \mathbf{C}\right] := \underset{\sim}{\Sigma}\underset{\sim}{\Sigma}^T\mathbf{C} - \mathbf{C}\underset{\sim}{\Sigma}\underset{\sim}{\Sigma}^T$. Next, consider the two expressions

$$\mathbf{A}\mathbf{V}\frac{\partial \underset{\sim}{\Sigma}^T}{\partial a_{ij}} + \mathbf{U}\frac{\partial \underset{\sim}{\Sigma}}{\partial a_{ij}}\underset{\sim}{\Sigma}^T = \mathbf{U}\underset{\sim}{\Sigma}\frac{\partial \underset{\sim}{\Sigma}^T}{\partial a_{ij}} + \mathbf{U}\frac{\partial \underset{\sim}{\Sigma}}{\partial a_{ij}}\underset{\sim}{\Sigma}^T$$

$$= \mathbf{U}\frac{\partial}{\partial a_{ij}}\left[\underset{\sim}{\Sigma}\underset{\sim}{\Sigma}^T\right].$$

Now consider the remaining two expressions

$$\mathbf{A}\frac{\partial \mathbf{A}^T}{\partial a_{ij}}\mathbf{U} + \frac{\partial \mathbf{A}}{\partial a_{ij}}\mathbf{V}\underset{\sim}{\Sigma}^T = \mathbf{A}\frac{\partial \mathbf{A}^T}{\partial a_{ij}}\mathbf{U} + \frac{\partial \mathbf{A}}{\partial a_{ij}}\mathbf{A}^T\mathbf{U}$$

$$= \left(\frac{\partial}{\partial a_{ij}}\left[\mathbf{A}\mathbf{A}^T\right]\right)\mathbf{U}.$$

Using these simplifications in notation gives the system of equations in $c_k^{(l)}$

$$\mathbf{U}\left[\underset{\sim}{\Sigma}\underset{\sim}{\Sigma}^T, \mathbf{C}\right] = \mathbf{U}\frac{\partial}{\partial a_{ij}}\left[\underset{\sim}{\Sigma}\underset{\sim}{\Sigma}^T\right] - \left(\frac{\partial}{\partial a_{ij}}\left[\mathbf{A}\mathbf{A}^T\right]\right)\mathbf{U}.$$

Using the unitary condition $\mathbf{U}^T\mathbf{U} = \mathbf{I}$, where $\mathbf{I}$ is the $M \times M$ identity matrix, this equation simplifies to the final form

$$\left[\underset{\sim}{\Sigma}\underset{\sim}{\Sigma}^T, \mathbf{C}\right] = \frac{\partial}{\partial a_{ij}}\left[\underset{\sim}{\Sigma}\underset{\sim}{\Sigma}^T\right] - \mathbf{U}^T\left(\frac{\partial}{\partial a_{ij}}\left[\mathbf{A}\mathbf{A}^T\right]\right)\mathbf{U}. \tag{43}$$

Expanding the commutator bracket we find that

$$\left[\underset{\sim}{\Sigma}\underset{\sim}{\Sigma}^T, \mathbf{C}\right]_{kl} = \begin{cases} 0 & k = l \text{ or } k \text{ and } l > r, \\ c_k^{(l)}\left((\sigma_k)^2 - (\sigma_l)^2\right) & k, l \le r, \\ -c_k^{(l)}(\sigma_l)^2 & l \le r \text{ and } k \ge r + 1, \\ c_k^{(l)}(\sigma_k)^2 & k \le r \text{ and } l \ge r + 1. \end{cases} \tag{44}$$

Since the right side of Equation (43) is known, and since we have assumed that the singular values are distinct, we can solve for the off-diagonal coefficients.

The final task is to find the values of the diagonal coefficients. Once again, we make use of the fact that the singular vectors $\{\mathbf{u}^{(k)}\}$ form a basis for $\mathbb{R}^M$, that is, for a fixed eigenvector $\mathbf{u}^{(k)}$, the derivative is expanded as the sum

$$\frac{\partial \mathbf{u}^{(k)}}{\partial a_{ij}} = c_1^{(k)}\mathbf{u}^{(1)} + \cdots + c_k^{(k)}\mathbf{u}^{(k)} + \cdots c_M^{(k)}\mathbf{u}^{(M)}.$$

When we use the orthogonality of the derivative of the singular vector with the
singular vector we get

$$c_1^{(k)} \langle \mathbf{u}^{(1)}, \mathbf{u}^{(k)} \rangle + \cdots + c_k^{(k)} \langle \mathbf{u}^{(k)}, \mathbf{u}^{(k)} \rangle + \cdots c_M^{(k)} \langle \mathbf{u}^{(M)}, \mathbf{u}^{(k)} \rangle = 0.$$

Since the individual singular vectors are orthonormal, the diagonal coefficients are
all identically zero.

Using this same approach, we can find $\partial \mathbf{V} / \partial a_{ij}$. To accomplish this, write this
derivative as a linear combination of the singular vectors $\mathbf{v}^{(k)}$

$$\frac{\partial \mathbf{V}}{\partial a_{ij}} = \mathbf{VD},$$

where

$$\mathbf{D} := \begin{pmatrix} d_1^{(1)} & d_1^{(2)} & d_1^{(3)} & \cdots & d_1^{(N)} \\ d_2^{(1)} & d_2^{(2)} & d_2^{(3)} & \cdots & d_2^{(N)} \\ \vdots & & \vdots & & \vdots \\ d_N^{(1)} & d_N^{(2)} & d_N^{(3)} & \cdots & d_N^{(N)} \end{pmatrix},$$

and proceed as was done above.

5 Initial Value Problem

We now extend the initial value problem (IVP) (3) and (4) as the more general
system of equations

$$\frac{du_1}{dt} = f_1(u_1, u_2, p_1, p_2, p_3) \qquad u_1(0) = u_1^{(0)} \tag{45}$$

$$\frac{du_2}{dt} = f_2(u_1, u_2, p_1, p_2, p_3) \qquad u_2(0) = u_2^{(0)} \tag{46}$$

where the $u_1(t)$ and $u_2(t)$ denote the time dependent forward solutions, p_1, p_2, p_3
denote some fixed or steady state parameters, $u_1^{(0)}, u_2^{(0)}$ are the initial conditions
(IC's), and $t \in [0, b]$. To determine the sensitivity of an associated functional, or
response function, of the solution, we consider a generic form that encompasses
most functionals that one encounters [2, 13];

$$J[\mathbf{u}] := \int_{t=0}^{b} g(u_1, u_2, p_1, p_2, p_3)\, dt + h(u_1, u_2, p_1, p_2, p_3)\Big|_{t=b}. \tag{47}$$

Here the functions g and h are sufficiently differentiable in their arguments. We wish to determine how the functional J is affected by changes to the parameters or IC's. Specifically, we must calculate the derivatives

$$\frac{\partial J}{\partial p_1} = \int_{t=0}^{b} \left(\frac{\partial g}{\partial u_1} \frac{\partial u_1}{\partial p_1} + \frac{\partial g}{\partial u_2} \frac{\partial u_2}{\partial p_1} + \frac{\partial g}{\partial p_1} \right) dt$$

$$+ \left(\frac{\partial h}{\partial u_1} \frac{\partial u_1}{\partial p_1} + \frac{\partial h}{\partial u_2} \frac{\partial u_2}{\partial p_1} + \frac{\partial h}{\partial p_1} \right) \Big|_{t=b}$$

$$\frac{\partial J}{\partial p_2} = \int_{t=0}^{b} \left(\frac{\partial g}{\partial u_1} \frac{\partial u_1}{\partial p_2} + \frac{\partial g}{\partial u_2} \frac{\partial u_2}{\partial p_2} + \frac{\partial g}{\partial p_2} \right) dt$$

$$+ \left(\frac{\partial h}{\partial u_1} \frac{\partial u_1}{\partial p_2} + \frac{\partial h}{\partial u_2} \frac{\partial u_2}{\partial p_2} + \frac{\partial h}{\partial p_2} \right) \Big|_{t=b}$$

$$\frac{\partial J}{\partial p_3} = \int_{t=0}^{b} \left(\frac{\partial g}{\partial u_1} \frac{\partial u_1}{\partial p_3} + \frac{\partial g}{\partial u_2} \frac{\partial u_2}{\partial p_3} + \frac{\partial g}{\partial p_3} \right) dt$$

$$+ \left(\frac{\partial h}{\partial u_1} \frac{\partial u_1}{\partial p_3} + \frac{\partial h}{\partial u_2} \frac{\partial u_2}{\partial p_3} + \frac{\partial h}{\partial p_3} \right) \Big|_{t=b}$$

$$\frac{\partial J}{\partial u_1^{(0)}} = \int_{t=0}^{b} \left(\frac{\partial g}{\partial u_1} \frac{\partial u_1}{\partial u_1^{(0)}} + \frac{\partial g}{\partial u_2} \frac{\partial u_2}{\partial u_1^{(0)}} \right) dt$$

$$+ \left(\frac{\partial h}{\partial u_1} \frac{\partial u_1}{\partial u_1^{(0)}} + \frac{\partial h}{\partial u_2} \frac{\partial u_2}{\partial u_1^{(0)}} \right) \Big|_{t=b}$$

$$\frac{\partial J}{\partial u_2^{(0)}} = \int_{t=0}^{b} \left(\frac{\partial g}{\partial u_1} \frac{\partial u_1}{\partial u_2^{(0)}} + \frac{\partial g}{\partial u_2} \frac{\partial u_2}{\partial u_2^{(0)}} \right) dt$$

$$+ \left(\frac{\partial h}{\partial u_1} \frac{\partial u_1}{\partial u_2^{(0)}} + \frac{\partial h}{\partial u_2} \frac{\partial u_2}{\partial u_2^{(0)}} \right) \Big|_{t=b}.$$

5.1 Forward Sensitivity of the IVP

To evaluate the functional, all of the derivative terms $\partial u_1/\partial p_1$, $\partial u_1/\partial p_2$, etc., must be found. We start by differentiating the original IVP given in Equations (45), (46) wrt. all of the parameters and ICs. Assuming that the derivative operators d/dt and

$\partial/\partial p$ commute, the forward sensitivity equations (FSE) are given by

$$\frac{d}{dt}\left[\frac{\partial u_1}{\partial p_1}\right] = \frac{\partial f_1}{\partial u_1}\frac{\partial u_1}{\partial p_1} + \frac{\partial f_1}{\partial u_2}\frac{\partial u_2}{\partial p_1} + \frac{\partial f_1}{\partial p_1}$$

$$\frac{d}{dt}\left[\frac{\partial u_1}{\partial p_2}\right] = \frac{\partial f_1}{\partial u_1}\frac{\partial u_1}{\partial p_2} + \frac{\partial f_1}{\partial u_2}\frac{\partial u_2}{\partial p_2} + \frac{\partial f_1}{\partial p_2}$$

$$\frac{d}{dt}\left[\frac{\partial u_1}{\partial p_3}\right] = \frac{\partial f_1}{\partial u_1}\frac{\partial u_1}{\partial p_3} + \frac{\partial f_1}{\partial u_2}\frac{\partial u_2}{\partial p_3} + \frac{\partial f_1}{\partial p_3}$$

$$\frac{d}{dt}\left[\frac{\partial u_1}{\partial u_1^{(0)}}\right] = \frac{\partial f_1}{\partial u_1}\frac{\partial u_1}{\partial u_1^{(0)}} + \frac{\partial f_1}{\partial u_2}\frac{\partial u_2}{\partial u_1^{(0)}}$$

$$\frac{d}{dt}\left[\frac{\partial u_1}{\partial u_2^{(0)}}\right] = \frac{\partial f_1}{\partial u_1}\frac{\partial u_1}{\partial u_2^{(0)}} + \frac{\partial f_1}{\partial u_2}\frac{\partial u_2}{\partial u_2^{(0)}}$$

$$\frac{d}{dt}\left[\frac{\partial u_2}{\partial p_1}\right] = \frac{\partial f_2}{\partial u_1}\frac{\partial u_1}{\partial p_1} + \frac{\partial f_2}{\partial u_2}\frac{\partial u_2}{\partial p_1} + \frac{\partial f_2}{\partial p_1}$$

$$\frac{d}{dt}\left[\frac{\partial u_2}{\partial p_2}\right] = \frac{\partial f_2}{\partial u_1}\frac{\partial u_1}{\partial p_2} + \frac{\partial f_2}{\partial u_2}\frac{\partial u_2}{\partial p_2} + \frac{\partial f_2}{\partial p_2}$$

$$\frac{d}{dt}\left[\frac{\partial u_2}{\partial p_3}\right] = \frac{\partial f_2}{\partial u_1}\frac{\partial u_1}{\partial p_3} + \frac{\partial f_2}{\partial u_2}\frac{\partial u_2}{\partial p_3} + \frac{\partial f_2}{\partial p_3}$$

$$\frac{d}{dt}\left[\frac{\partial u_2}{\partial u_1^{(0)}}\right] = \frac{\partial f_2}{\partial u_1}\frac{\partial u_1}{\partial u_1^{(0)}} + \frac{\partial f_2}{\partial u_2}\frac{\partial u_2}{\partial u_1^{(0)}}$$

$$\frac{d}{dt}\left[\frac{\partial u_2}{\partial u_2^{(0)}}\right] = \frac{\partial f_2}{\partial u_1}\frac{\partial u_1}{\partial u_2^{(0)}} + \frac{\partial f_2}{\partial u_2}\frac{\partial u_2}{\partial u_2^{(0)}}.$$

In full FSA, the parameter FSE's entails a total of six separate numerical solutions perturbing each of the parameters, while the set of IC's FSE's requires a total of four additional numerical runs perturbing each of the ICs. A significant drawback of FSA is the proliferation of equations that occurs in the SA. In this example, we had to introduce ten additional equations, six for the parameters and four for the IC's. When working with large systems of IVPs, performing a FSA can be computationally prohibitive. Suppose that the original system of IVPs consists of j equations and, hence, j initial conditions. If there are k parameters, then the total number of IVPs that must be solved is $j(j + k + 1)$. For example, in constructing an age structured epidemiological model, it would not be unreasonable to have 10 equations with 20 parameters. In this simple case, to do a full FSA we would need to solve a total of 310 IVPs. A 31-fold increase in the number of equations needed to do a sensitivity analysis is a significant computational burden.

Sometimes this computational burden can be reduced if you are only interested in obtaining the numerical estimation of some of the FSEs. Suppose that you were interested in only $\partial u_2/\partial p_3$, then you could note that only other IVP that is involved with this equation is the equation for $(d/dt)[\partial u_1/\partial p_3]$ and these two equations together do not involve any of the other FSEs. Therefore, only these two FSE's along with the original forward problem need to be solved.

Before discussing the adjoint approach, we summarize the procedure for finding the FSE of the general first order IVP

$$\frac{d\mathbf{u}}{dt} = \mathbf{F}[\mathbf{u}(t;\mathbf{p})], \qquad \mathbf{u}(0) = \mathbf{u}_0, \tag{48}$$

where $\mathbf{u}$ is an $n \times 1$ forward solution vector and $\mathbf{p}$ is an $(k + n) \times 1$ vector which represents any of the k parameters or n initial conditions associated with the problem.

Differentiating the forward problem wrt. $\mathbf{p}$ produces the FSE

$$\frac{d}{dt}\left[\mathbf{D_p}[\mathbf{u}]\right] = \mathbf{D_u}[\mathbf{F}] \cdot \mathbf{D_p}[\mathbf{u}] + \mathbf{D_p}[\mathbf{F}], \tag{49}$$

where $\mathbf{D_p}[\mathbf{u}]$ is the $n \times (k + n)$ Jacobian of $\mathbf{u}$, wrt. the parameters $\mathbf{p}$ and IC's $\mathbf{u}^{(0)}$, $\mathbf{D_u}[\mathbf{F}]$ is the $n \times n$ Jacobian of $\mathbf{F}$, wrt. the forward solution $\mathbf{u}$, and $\mathbf{D_p}[\mathbf{F}]$ is the $n \times (k+n)$ Jacobian of $\mathbf{F}$, with respect to the parameters $\mathbf{p}$ and IC's $\mathbf{u}^{(0)}$. To calculate the derivatives which define $\mathbf{D_p}[\mathbf{u}]$, both the forward problem-IVP and the FSEs given in Equations (48) and (49) respectively must be solved simultaneously. The IC's for the FSE is determined by the choice of parameter of interest. Notice that in solving the FSE, the derivatives are obtained, in which case the Jacobian $\mathbf{D_p}[\mathbf{u}]$ is found.

If the sensitivity of an associated function(al) J is needed, then we must calculate the derivatives of J with respect to each component of the vector $\mathbf{p}$;

$$\frac{dJ}{d\mathbf{p}} = \int_{t=0}^{b} \left(\mathbf{D_p}^T[\mathbf{u}]\nabla_u g + \nabla_p g\right) dt + \left(\mathbf{D_p}^T[\mathbf{u}]\nabla_u h + \nabla_p h\right)\Big|_{t=b}. \tag{50}$$

As was noted above, the term $\mathbf{D_p}^T[\mathbf{u}]$ obtained from the FSE's is now used to find the desired derivative $\partial J/\partial\mathbf{p}$. As has been done in previous examples, we introduce an associated adjoint problem to circumvent calculating $\mathbf{D_p}^T[\mathbf{u}]$. Specifically, by cleverly choosing the adjoint problem and adjoint boundary conditions, eventually we will eliminate/replace the expressions $\mathbf{D_p}^T[\mathbf{u}]\nabla_u g$ and $\mathbf{D_p}^T[\mathbf{u}]\nabla_u h|_{t=b}$.

5.2 Adjoint Sensitivity Analysis of the IVP

As was noted in previous examples, the next step in our analysis is to construct the associated adjoint sensitivity equations (ASE). The key was to cleverly formulate the ASE so as to eliminate the direct evaluation of $\mathbf{D_p}[\mathbf{u}]$.

As in previous cases, the adjoint can be constructed only if an appropriate inner product space exists for the forward problem. In this case, the natural inner product is

$$\int_{t=0}^{b} \mathbf{v}^{T} \left(\frac{\mathrm{d}}{\mathrm{d}t} [\mathbf{D_p}[\mathbf{u}]] - \mathbf{D_u}[F] \cdot \mathbf{D_p}[\mathbf{u}] - \mathbf{D_p}[F] \right) dt = 0, \qquad (51)$$

where $\mathbf{v}$ is the associated adjoint variable. Expanding the $\mathbf{v}^{T}$ term and using integration by parts on the first integrand gives

$$\mathbf{v}^{T} \mathbf{D_p}[\mathbf{u}] \Big|_{t=0}^{b} + \int_{t=0}^{b} \left(-\frac{\mathrm{d}\mathbf{v}^{T}}{\mathrm{d}t} - \mathbf{v}^{T} \mathbf{D_u}[F] \right) \mathbf{D_p}[\mathbf{u}] \, dt - \int_{t=0}^{b} \mathbf{v}^{T} \mathbf{D_p}[F] \, dt = 0. \quad (52)$$

If we compare the terms in the first integrand of this equation with the first expression in the integrand of Equation (50) notice that two expressions are similar in form. This can be seen by using the transpose operation, namely

$$(\mathbf{D_p}^{T}[\mathbf{u}] \nabla_u g)^{T} = (\nabla_u g)^{T} \mathbf{D_p}[\mathbf{u}], \qquad (53)$$

in which case we force the adjoint condition

$$-\frac{\mathrm{d}\mathbf{v}^{T}}{\mathrm{d}t} - \mathbf{v}^{T} \mathbf{D_u}[F] = (\nabla_u g)^{T} \qquad (54)$$

Substituting and rearranging gives

$$\int_{t=0}^{b} (\nabla_u g)^{T} \mathbf{D_p}[\mathbf{u}] \, dt = \int_{t=0}^{b} \mathbf{v}^{T} \mathbf{D_p}[F] \, dt - \mathbf{v}^{T} \mathbf{D_p}[\mathbf{u}] \Big|_{t=b}. \qquad (55)$$

Take the transpose and substitute into the right hand side of dJ/dp

$$\frac{\mathrm{d}J}{\mathrm{d}\mathbf{p}} = \int_{t=0}^{b} (\mathbf{D_p}^{T}[F]\mathbf{v} + \nabla_p g) \, dt - \mathbf{D_p}^{T}[\mathbf{u}] \Big|_{t=0}^{b} + (\mathbf{D_p}^{T}[\mathbf{u}] \nabla_u h + \nabla_p h) \Big|_{t=b}. \qquad (56)$$

Notice that in this formulation, the definite integral does not contain the expression $\mathbf{D_p}^{T}[\mathbf{u}]$, only the boundary conditions contain this expression. Since $\mathbf{D_p}^{T}[\mathbf{u}]|_{t=0}$ is easily calculated while the expression $\mathbf{D_p}^{T}[\mathbf{u}]|_{t=b}$ can only be calculated by integrating the FSE's for $t \in [0, b]$, we can eliminate the upper BC by forcing

$$v(b) := \nabla_u h \Big|_{t=b}, \qquad (57)$$

which reduces the expression for the derivative of J to be

$$\frac{dJ}{d\mathbf{p}} = \int_{t=0}^{b} (\mathbf{D_p}^T[\mathbf{F}]\mathbf{v} + \nabla_p g) \, dt + \mathbf{D_p}^T[\mathbf{u}]\mathbf{v}\Big|_{t=0} + \nabla_p h\Big|_{t=b}. \tag{58}$$

Once again, by creating an associated adjoint problem, with appropriately chosen BC's, we are able to circumvent the problem of having to calculate $\mathbf{D_p}[\mathbf{u}]$.

6 Principal Component Analysis of the IVP

6.1 Multiparameter Variation

In the previous section we constructed the FSEs for the IVP and obtained local time dependent sensitivities for fixed parameter values. It was quite evident that as the number of IVPs and parameters increase, the calculation of the FSEs becomes burdensome. In this situation, the adjoint methodology becomes a more practical alternative. With these limitations in mind, we now consider the case where the FSEs are not too cumbersome to solve. With this caveat, suppose that the parameter vector $\mathbf{p} = (p_1 \ p_2 \ \dots \ p_K)^T$ has an uncertainty, that is, the parameters are not specified as precise values, but rather are given as some distribution, with expected value vector $\mathbb{E}[\mathbf{p}] = \mu_\mathbf{p}$. The distinction between this analysis and previous results is that here we wish to quantify the effects of uncertainty for multiparameter variations. In other words, we wish to estimate the variation of the output, due to the effective strength of coupling between parameters.

For "small" perturbations $\delta\mathbf{p} := \mathbf{p} - \mu_\mathbf{p}$ to the parameter vector, the variation of the output, to first order terms, is given by

$$\delta\mathbf{u} := \mathbf{u}(t; \mu_\mathbf{p} + \delta\mathbf{p}) - \mathbf{u}(t; \mu_\mathbf{p}) \approx \mathbf{D_p}[\mathbf{u}]\delta\mathbf{p},$$

where as above, $\mathbf{D_p}[\mathbf{u}]$ denotes the Jacobian of $\mathbf{u}$, wrt. the parameters $\mathbf{p}$. Now take the outer product $\delta\mathbf{u} \otimes \delta\mathbf{u} = \delta\mathbf{u} \cdot \delta\mathbf{u}^T$, to obtain an approximation of the variation matrix of the output

$$\delta\mathbf{u} \cdot \delta\mathbf{u}^T \approx \mathbf{D_p}[\mathbf{u}] \, \delta\mathbf{p} \cdot \delta\mathbf{p}^T \, \mathbf{D_p}[\mathbf{u}]^T. \tag{59}$$

Without giving all the details (see pp.120–126 [5], especially equation III.F.16 page 124), it can be shown that the temporal output covariance matrix, denoted as $\mathbf{C_u}$, can be written as

$$\mathbf{C_u} = \mathbf{D_p}[\mathbf{u}] \, \mathbb{E}\left[\delta\mathbf{p} \cdot \delta\mathbf{p}^T\right] \, \mathbf{D_p}[\mathbf{u}]^T. \tag{60}$$

This time dependent matrix provides an approximation to the evolution of how the coupling in the parameter variation affects the output.

Since covariance matrices are symmetric, we are guaranteed (see [15]) to have a decomposition of $\mathbf{C_u}$ given by

$$\mathbf{C_u} = \mathbf{Q} \underset{\sim}{\Lambda} \mathbf{Q}^T = \sum_{i=1}^{K} \lambda_i \mathbf{q}_i(t) \cdot \mathbf{q}_i^{\ T}(t), \qquad (61)$$

where $\mathbf{Q}$ is an orthonormal matrix whose columns consist of the eigenvectors $\mathbf{q}_i(t)$, for $i = 1, \ldots, K$, of $\mathbf{C_u}$, and $\underset{\sim}{\Lambda}$ is a diagonal matrix whose entries are the associated eigenvalues, λ_i, written in decreasing order. Using this result we can examine the effect of multiparameter variation in the principal component space. To accomplish this, consider the transformation from solution space to principal component space given by

$$\mathbf{v} := \mathbf{Q}^T \left(\mathbf{u}(t; \mu_\mathbf{p} + \delta\mathbf{p}) - \mathbf{u}(t; \mu_\mathbf{p}) \right) \approx \mathbf{Q}^T \mathbf{D_p}[\mathbf{u}]\delta\mathbf{p}.$$

Taking the outer product $\mathbf{v} \otimes \mathbf{v}$ allows us to define the covariance matrix $\mathbf{C_{PCS}}$ in pricipal component space as

$$\begin{aligned}
\mathbf{C_{PCS}} &= \mathbf{Q}^T \ \mathbf{D_p}[\mathbf{u}] \ \mathbb{E}\left[\delta\mathbf{p} \cdot \delta\mathbf{p}^T\right] \ \mathbf{D_p}[\mathbf{u}]^T \mathbf{Q} \\
&= \mathbf{Q}^T \mathbf{C_u} \mathbf{Q} \\
&= \mathbf{Q}^T \ \mathbf{Q}\underset{\sim}{\Lambda}\mathbf{Q}^T \mathbf{Q} \\
&= \underset{\sim}{\Lambda}.
\end{aligned}$$

Notice that the covariance matrix $\mathbf{C_{PCS}}$ is a diagonal matrix, which means that the transformed vectors in principal component space are independent. Furthermore, since the diagonal contains the eigenvalues, in decreasing order, the transformed vectors are projected along the principal component axes formed by the eigenvectors and in decreasing variance. This means that the greatest variation of $\mathbf{v}$ occurs along the first eigenvector $\mathbf{q}_1(t)$ with variance λ_1, the second largest variation occurs along $\mathbf{q}_2(t)$ with variance λ_2, etc.

7 Algorithmic Differentiation

When the problem of interest is to "find the derivative," we must be careful to distinguish which of the following two objectives we trying to accomplish:

1. explicitly finding a symbolic expression for the derivative, or
2. numerically estimating the derivative by a discrete approximation, such as finite difference or a finite element method.

The main focus of previous sections was to explicitly find the ubiquitous derivative in various settings. We discussed how to find the derivative of an output variable wrt. a particular parameter, or input variable. In this section, we provide a cursory introduction to the methodology of algorithmic differentiation (AD), that is, how a computer differentiates a algorithm. Since the researcher in epidemiology will eventually want to numerically calculate derivatives, without having to write computer code to accomplish this, standard packages such as ADIFOR, ADOL-C, ADOL-F, DAFOR, TAMC, etc., should be used [25]. This section provides the basic background needed in order to understand how AD works.

7.1 Sensitivity of the Reproductive Number R_0

We introduce the AD methodology in a familiar epidemiological setting by considering the SEIR model

$$\frac{dS}{dt} = bN - \mu S - \beta S \frac{I}{N}$$

$$\frac{dE}{dt} = \beta S \frac{I}{N} - (\mu + k) E$$

$$\frac{dI}{dt} = kE - (r + \mu) I$$

$$\frac{dR}{dt} = rI - \mu R,$$

where S, E, I, and R denote the susceptible, exposed, infectious, and recovered populations respectively, and $N = S + E + I + R$ is the total population. The parameter β quantifies the efficacy of the infection in the susceptible population, k is the per capita rate at which the exposed population becomes infectious, μ is the per capita death rate, r is the per capita recovery rate, and b is the intrinsic birth/migration rate.

A commonly used measure of the intensity of the infection is the basic reproductive number R_0 of the average number of susceptible individuals who have been infected by a particular infectious individual, over the lifetime of that infected individual. If $R_0 < 1$, then on average, each infectious individual infects less than one other individual, in which case we expect the infection to eventually subside. If $R_0 > 1$, then the infection is expected to spread throughout the susceptible population. This threshold condition provides a mathematical criteria for determining whether the infection will spread or subside. Additionally, since R_0 depends on the parameters of the model, SA provides a way to measure which parameters have the most effect on the spread or decrease in the infection.

A particular problem in obtaining R_0 is that there are numerous ways, which have specific strengths/weaknesses, of deriving R_0. Three of the most used approaches to derive R_0 are:

- Survival function method: This method is appropriate when explicit expressions are available for the survival probability, (probability that a newly infected individual remains infectious for time t) and the infectivity as a function of time.
- Next generation method: This method is appropriate when the population can naturally be divided into discrete and disjoint classes, such as age, social status (e.g., prostitute, day care worker, drug addict, etc..), demographic region, etc.
- Surrogate methods: The key concepts are the stability of the disease free equilibrium point, locating a transcritical bifurcation of the endemic equilibrium, etc.

The R_0 for the above SEIR model is given by

$$R_0 := \frac{k\beta}{(r + \mu)(k + \mu)}. \tag{62}$$

Because the parameter values depend on the particular strain of infection, R_0 will also depend on the specific infection. For example, consider the potentially life threatening flu, which we broadly categorize in two forms: (1) seasonal flu, with $R_0 \approx 1.5$, and (2) pandemic flu[2] with $R_0 \in [2, 3]$. For *illustrative purposes only*, the seasonal flu will be modeled using the parameter values, in dimensional units of days^{-1}, of $\beta = 0.375$, $k = 0.5$, $\mu = 3.7 \times 10^{-5}$), and $r = 0.25$, in which case $R_0 \approx 1.499$. Since the reproductive number is greater than 1, the infection is expected to spread. SA may now be used to determine how sensitive the spread is to each of the defining parameters.

For example suppose, through some intervention strategy, we are able to slightly alter the value of the parameter r, then the SI

$$SI_r = -\left(\frac{r}{r + \mu}\right) = -0.999852 < 0,$$

tells us that if we increase r by approximately 1%, then R_0 decreases by approximately 1%, and vice versa. This is easily verified by increasing $r : 0.25 \to 0.2525$, which decreases $R_0 : 1.49967 \to 1.48482$ and results in a -0.989954% decrease in R_0, as estimated from the normalized SI.

A significant advantage of having this type of local analysis available is that now the powerful tool of cost-benefit analysis is available. If the sensitivity of hypothetical intervention strategy **A** is $SI_1 = 0.75$ with associated cost of $\$1 \times 10^4$, while

---

[2] Recall the devastating 1918–1919 influenza pandemic: "An estimated one third of the world's population (or $\approx$ 500 million persons) were infected and had clinically apparent illnesses during the 1918–1919 influenza pandemic. The disease was exceptionally severe. Case-fatality rates were $> 2.5\%$, compared to $< 0.1\%$ in other influenza pandemics. Total deaths were estimated at $\approx$ 50 million and were arguably as high as 100 million." [14]

the sensitivity of intervention strategy **B** is $SI_2 = -0.25$ with associated cost of $\$4 \times 10^3$, then the cost-benefit ratios are

$$CB_1 = \frac{\$1 \times 10^4}{|0.75|} = \frac{\$13.3 \times 10^3}{\text{unit}}, \quad \text{and} \quad CB_2 = \frac{\$4 \times 10^3}{|-0.25|} = \frac{\$16 \times 10^4}{\text{unit}}.$$

All other things being equal, since the first cost-benefit ratio is the smaller, this suggests that intervention strategy **A** should be implemented. It should be noted that the signs of the SIs and input and output variables be examined carefully, as was noted in the beginning section discussing the definition of the SI.

7.2 Forward Sensitivity/Mode

We now describe the main idea behind AD, in the *forward mode*, without discussing any of the coding quality, rounding, memory allocation, computational overhead, etc., topics that are inherent to the actual implementation and execution of AD [25]. The basic idea in AD is quite simple, however the actual implementation is rather sophisticated. Essentially, AD is an automatic implementation of the standard chain rule from calculus. For example, consider the formal differential operations

$$d\left[\frac{u}{v^2}\right] = \frac{v^2\,du - u\,d\left[v^2\right]}{(v^2)^2}$$
$$= \frac{v^2\,du - u\,(2v\,dv)}{v^4}.$$

The basic algebraic and differential operations performed were applications of the

- derivative of a quotient,
- derivative of a function to a power, and
- algebraic simplification rule of a base to an exponent, to another exponent.

In the jargon of AD, the standard rules of calculus would be written as the "tangent operations," using the elemental differentials in Fig. 6, and pseudo code for

Fig. 6 Templates used in AD for the standard rules of calculus, where the symbols $\square$, $\triangle$, and $\heartsuit$ denote "elemental functions", and the symbols $d\triangle$ and $d\heartsuit$ denote the "elemental differentials"

$$\square = c$$
$$d\square = 0$$
$$\square = \triangle \pm \heartsuit$$
$$d\square = d\triangle \pm d\heartsuit$$
$$\square = \triangle * \heartsuit$$
$$d\square = d\triangle * \heartsuit + \triangle * d\heartsuit$$
$$\square = \triangle / \heartsuit$$
$$d\square = (\heartsuit * d\triangle - \triangle * d\heartsuit)/(\heartsuit^2)$$
etc.

calculating the SI of R_0 wrt. r, is first defined without any attempt at efficient coding.

The first step is the initialization of the parameters.

$$p\_1 = 0.375; \qquad\qquad // \quad p_1 = \beta$$

$$p\_2 = 0.5; \qquad\qquad // \quad p_2 = k$$

$$p\_3 = 3.7 * (10^{\wedge}(-5)); \qquad // \quad p_3 = \mu$$

$$p\_4 = 0.25; \qquad\qquad // \quad p_4 = r$$

Our intention is to calculate the normalized SI wrt. the parameter r, while the other parameters β, k, and μ are constant. Therefore, we initialize the derivatives as

$$dp\_1 = 0.0; \qquad\qquad // \quad \partial\beta/\partial r = 0$$

$$dp\_2 = 0.0; \qquad\qquad // \quad \partial k/\partial r = 0$$

$$dp\_3 = 0.0; \qquad\qquad // \quad \partial\mu/\partial r = 0$$

$$dp\_4 = 1.0; \qquad\qquad // \quad \partial r/\partial r = 1$$

In the jargon of AD, $p_1, \ldots, p_4, dp_1, \ldots, dp_4$ are referred to as the input variables.

Next, we perform the forward evaluation of the intermediate variables $u_1 = k\beta$, $u_2 = r + \mu$, $u_3 = k + \mu$, and $u_4 = (r + \mu)(k + \mu)$, along with the associated derivatives.

$$u\_1 = p\_2 * p\_1 = 0.1875; \qquad\qquad // \quad u_1 = k\beta$$

$$du\_1 = p\_2 * dp\_1 + dp\_2 * p\_1 = 0.0; \qquad // \quad \frac{\partial u_1}{\partial r} = k\frac{\partial \beta}{\partial r} + \frac{\partial k}{\partial r}\beta = 0$$

$$u\_2 = p\_4 + p\_3 = 0.250038; \qquad\qquad // \quad u_2 = r + \mu = 0.250038$$

$$du\_2 = dp\_4 + dp\_3 = 1.0; \qquad\qquad // \quad \frac{\partial u_2}{\partial r} = \frac{\partial r}{\partial r} + \frac{\partial \mu}{\partial r} = 1.0$$

$$u\_3 = p\_2 + p\_3 = 0.500038; \qquad\qquad // \quad u_3 = k + \mu = 0.500038$$

$$du\_3 = dp\_2 + dp\_3 = 0.0; \qquad\qquad // \quad \frac{\partial u_3}{\partial r} = \frac{\partial k}{\partial r} + \frac{\partial \mu}{\partial r} = 0.0.$$

$$u\_4 = u\_2 * u\_3 = 0.125028; \qquad\qquad // \quad \begin{aligned} u_4 &= (r + \mu)(k + \mu) \\ &= 0.125028 \end{aligned}$$

$$du\_4 = u\_2 * du\_3 + du\_2 * u\_3 = 0.500038; \quad // \quad \begin{aligned} \frac{\partial u_4}{\partial r} &= \frac{\partial}{\partial r}[(r + \mu)(k + \mu)] \\ &= 0.500038 \end{aligned}$$

Now form the reproductive number

$$R_0 = u_5 = \frac{u_1}{u_4} = \frac{u_1}{u_2 u_3} = \frac{\overbrace{k\beta}^{u_1}}{\underbrace{(r+\mu)}_{u_2}\underbrace{(k+\mu)}_{u_3}} \tag{63}$$

and the derivative $\partial R_0 / \partial r$.

$u\_5 = u\_1/u\_4 = 1.49967;$ // $u_5 = \dfrac{k\beta}{(r+\mu)(k+\mu)}$
$\qquad\qquad\qquad\qquad\qquad\qquad = 1.49967$

$du\_5 = (u\_4 * du\_1 - u\_1 * du\_4)/$

$(u\_4)^2 = -5.99778;$ // $\dfrac{\partial u_5}{\partial r} = \dfrac{\partial}{\partial r}\left[\dfrac{k\beta}{(r+\mu)(k+\mu)}\right]$
$\qquad\qquad\qquad\qquad\qquad\qquad = -5.99778$

Finally, the SI is calculated, as the output variable u_6

$u\_6 = (p\_4/u\_5) * du\_5 = -0.999852?;$ // $u_6 = \dfrac{r}{R_0}\dfrac{\partial R_0}{\partial r}$
$\qquad\qquad\qquad\qquad\qquad\qquad\qquad\qquad = -0.999852$

as was found by direct calculation.

The above pseudo code for calculating, in the forward mode, the SI $(r/R_0)\partial R_0/\partial r$ provides a glimpse into how AD is done. The execution of AD is that as one intermediate calculation is completed, that result, along with other intermediate results, become inputs for subsequent calculations. Furthermore, each forward evaluation is also differentiated as well. Evaluation of these functions can be thought of as the progression through a directed tree[3], with vertices $p_1, \ldots, p_4, u_1, \ldots, u_6$, and SI_{R_0} as shown in Fig. 7. The input/independent variables, denoted as $p_1, \ldots, p_4$ are referred to as the roots of the graph, and the leaves of the graph are the dependent variables $u_1, \ldots, u_6$, and SI_{R_0}. The standard convention is to place the roots to the left, and the leaves to the right in the graph.

As another unrelated however instructive example, consider the sequence of computations

$$u_1 := f_1[p_1, p_3]; \quad u_2 := f_2[p_2, u_1]; \quad u_3 := f_3[p_1, p_2, p_4, u_2];$$
$$u_4 := f_4[p_2, u_2, u_3]; \quad u := u_4;$$

---

[3] We are assuming that this particular algorithm does not have any loops, in which case the graph has no cycles, which means the graph will be a tree. In the more general case, this restriction is not necessary as sophisticated AD packages can handle these complications.

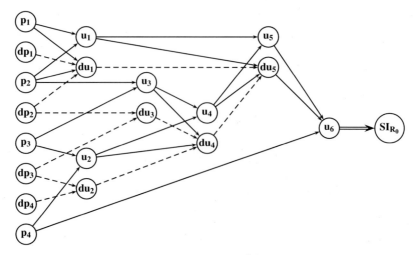

Fig. 7 Directed computational graph for R_0. *Solid arrows* denote forward evaluations and *dashed arrows* denote forward derivative evaluations. The parameters $p_1, \ldots, p_4$ and the derivative parameters $dp_1, \ldots, dp_4$ are first initialized. Next the intermediate forward variables $u_1, \ldots, u_6$ and the intermediate forward derivative variables $du_1, \ldots, du_6$ are calculated. The final step is the output variable SI_{R_0}

where $p_1, \ldots, p_4$ are the input variables, $u_1, \ldots, u_4$, are the intermediate outputs/variables, and u: final output/variable, with the associated computational graph as shown in Fig. 8

Suppose that we wish to calculate du/dp_3. In the forward mode, we start at the specified parameter p_3 and successively take derivatives of every intermediate variable by following the directed edges. Since there are two distinct directed paths from p_3 to u, namely $p_3 \rightarrow u_1 \rightarrow u_2 \rightarrow u_4 \rightarrow u$ and $p_3 \rightarrow u_1 \rightarrow u_2 \rightarrow u_3 \rightarrow u_4 \rightarrow u$, we expect that the final expression for du/dp_3 has two terms

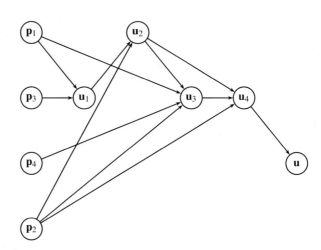

Fig. 8 Directed graph of an algorithm with input parameters $p_1, \ldots, p_4$, intermediate outputs/variables $u_1, \ldots, u_4$, and final output/variable u

reflecting this observation. If we had wanted to obtain du/dp_4, the progression would be $p_4 \rightarrow u_3 \rightarrow u_4 \rightarrow u$ and the associated derivative would contain only one expression.

Assuming that the input parameters are independent of each other, then to find du/dp_3 the following forward calculations, taken in order, are performed:

$$\frac{du_1}{dp_3} = \frac{\partial u_1}{\partial p_3}$$

$$\frac{du_2}{dp_3} = \frac{\partial u_2}{\partial u_1} \frac{du_1}{dp_3}$$

$$\frac{du_3}{dp_3} = \frac{\partial u_3}{\partial u_2} \frac{du_2}{dp_3}$$

$$\frac{du_4}{dp_3} = \frac{\partial u_4}{\partial u_2} \frac{du_2}{dp_3} + \frac{\partial u_4}{\partial u_3} \frac{du_3}{dp_3}$$

$$\frac{du}{dp_3} = \frac{\partial u}{\partial u_4} \frac{du_4}{dp_3}, \qquad \text{where} \quad \frac{\partial u}{\partial u_4} = 1$$

The actual progression needed to calculate the final output derivative is in the forward direction and the explicit output derivative is given by

$$\frac{du}{dp_3} = \underbrace{\frac{\partial u}{\partial u_4} \frac{\partial u_4}{\partial u_2} \frac{\partial u_2}{\partial u_1} \frac{\partial u_1}{\partial p_3}}_{p_3 \rightarrow u_1 \rightarrow u_2 \rightarrow u_4 \rightarrow u} + \underbrace{\frac{\partial u}{\partial u_4} \frac{\partial u_4}{\partial u_3} \frac{\partial u_3}{\partial u_2} \frac{\partial u_2}{\partial u_1} \frac{\partial u_1}{\partial p_3}}_{p_3 \rightarrow u_1 \rightarrow u_2 \rightarrow u_3 \rightarrow u_4 \rightarrow u}. \tag{64}$$

Using these examples as a template, suppose that we have K input parameters $p \in \{p_1, \ldots, p_K\}$ and N intermediate variables $u_1, \ldots, u_N$, defined as the differentiable functions $u_1 := f_1[p_1, \ldots, p_K]$, $u_i := f_i[p_1, \ldots, p_K, u_1, \ldots u_{i-1}]$, for $i = 2, \ldots N$, and the output variable only depends on u_N, i.e., $u = u_N$. The derivatives du_i/dp are given by

$$\frac{du_1}{dp} = \frac{\partial u_1}{\partial p} \tag{65}$$

$$\frac{du_i}{dp} = \sum_{j=1}^{i-1} \frac{\partial u_i}{\partial u_j} \frac{du_j}{dp} + \frac{\partial u_i}{\partial p} \tag{66}$$

$$\frac{du}{dp} = \frac{du_N}{dp} \tag{67}$$

for $i = 2, \ldots, N$.

7.3 Adjoint/Reverse Mode

In the forward mode, a particular parameter/input variable of interest was first chosen, then moving forward on the directed tree, derivatives of successive intermediate variables were taken. In the adjoint or reverse mode,[4] a final output variable is chosen and this output is differentiated wrt. each of the intermediate variables. The actual order of calculation however is reversed.

For the specific example given in Fig. 8 the differentiation proceeds as follows. The output variable u is directly affected by the intermediate variable u_4, in which case

$$\frac{du}{du_4} = \frac{\partial u_4}{\partial u_4} = 1.$$

Now u is affected by u_3 indirectly through u_4, in which case the chain rule gives

$$\frac{\partial u}{\partial u_3} = \frac{\partial u}{\partial u_4}\frac{\partial u_4}{\partial u_3} = \frac{\partial u_4}{\partial u_3}.$$

Similarly, since u_2 affects u indirectly through u_3 and u_4, then

$$\frac{\partial u}{\partial u_2} = \frac{\partial u}{\partial u_3}\frac{\partial u_3}{\partial u_2} + \frac{\partial u}{\partial u_4}\frac{\partial u_4}{\partial u_2}.$$

Lastly, u_1 affects u through u_2 and p_3 affects u through u_1, then

$$\frac{\partial u}{\partial u_1} = \frac{\partial u}{\partial u_2}\frac{\partial u_2}{\partial u_1} \quad \text{and} \quad \frac{du}{dp} = \frac{\partial u}{\partial u_1}\frac{\partial u_1}{\partial p_3}.$$

Notice that the order of evaluation is reversed, namely, the path now taken is $\partial u/\partial u_3 \to \cdots$, and the result du/dp_3, which is obtained by the composition of the derivatives, is the same as the result given in Equation (64).

For the reproduction number example given in Fig. 7, we will only calculate $\partial R_0/\partial r = \partial u_5/\partial p_4$. To follow standard conventions in AD, define the output variable $u := u_5$, in which case we wish to calculate $\partial u/\partial p_4$.

Examining Fig. 7, ignoring the paths containing du vertices, there is only one path from p_4 to u_5, namely $p_4 \to u_2 \to u_4 \to u_5$, and since p_4 does not affect u_1, pseudo code for the reverse/adjoint mode is given by

---

[4] The reader is cautioned about the usage of the terminology "backward mode." The standard methods in numerical analysis of the BDF (Backward Differentiation Formulas), which are used in the numerical solution of stiff IVP's, are not what is being discussed in the adjoint/reverse mode of AD. Hence to avoid any confusion, we will refer to the differentiation of the output variable, wrt. each of the intermediate variables as the adjoint or reverse mode.

$du\backslash du\_5 = 1.0;$ $//$ $\quad \dfrac{\partial u}{\partial u_5} = \dfrac{\partial u_5}{\partial u_5}$

$du\backslash du\_4 = du\backslash du\_5 * du\_5\backslash du\_4 = -11.9947;$ $//$ $\quad \dfrac{\partial u}{\partial u_4} = \dfrac{\partial u}{\partial u_5}\dfrac{\partial u_5}{\partial u_4}$

$du\backslash du\_3 = du\backslash du\_4 * du\_4\backslash du\_3 = -2.9991;$ $//$ $\quad \dfrac{\partial u}{\partial u_3} = \dfrac{\partial u}{\partial u_4}\dfrac{\partial u_4}{\partial u_3}$

$du\backslash du\_2 = du\backslash du\_4 * du\_4\backslash du\_2 = -5.9998;$ $//$ $\quad \dfrac{\partial u}{\partial u_2} = \dfrac{\partial u}{\partial u_4}\dfrac{\partial u_4}{\partial u_2}$

$du\backslash du\_1 = du\backslash du\_5 * du\_5\backslash du\_1 = 7.9982;$ $//$ $\quad \dfrac{\partial u}{\partial u_1} = \dfrac{\partial u}{\partial u_5}\dfrac{\partial u_5}{\partial u_1}$

$du\backslash dr = du\backslash du\_2 * du\_2\backslash dr = -5.9979;$ $//$ $\quad \dfrac{\partial u}{\partial p_4} = \dfrac{\partial u}{\partial u_2}\dfrac{\partial u_2}{\partial p_4}$

in which case $SI_{R_0} = (r/R_0)\partial R_0/\partial r = (0.25/1.49967)(-5.9979) = -0.99987$ as agrees with the previous results.

For the general problem, in the actual order they are evaluated, the ASE are given by

$$\frac{\partial u}{\partial u_N} = \frac{\partial u_N}{\partial u_N} = 1$$

$$\frac{\partial u}{\partial u_{N-1}} = \frac{\partial u}{\partial u_N}\frac{\partial u_N}{\partial u_{N-1}}$$

$$\frac{\partial u}{\partial u_{N-2}} = \frac{\partial u}{\partial u_{N-1}}\frac{\partial u_{N-1}}{\partial u_{N-2}} + \frac{\partial u}{\partial u_N}\frac{\partial u_N}{\partial u_{N-2}}$$

$$\frac{\partial u}{\partial u_{N-3}} = \frac{\partial u}{\partial u_{N-2}}\frac{\partial u_{N-2}}{\partial u_{N-3}} + \frac{\partial u}{\partial u_{N-1}}\frac{\partial u_{N-1}}{\partial u_{N-3}} + \frac{\partial u}{\partial u_N}\frac{\partial u_N}{\partial u_{N-3}}$$

$$\vdots$$

$$\frac{\partial u}{\partial u_1} = \frac{\partial u}{\partial u_2}\frac{\partial u_2}{\partial u_1} + \frac{\partial u}{\partial u_3}\frac{\partial u_3}{\partial u_1} + \cdots + \frac{\partial u}{\partial u_N}\frac{\partial u_N}{\partial u_1} \tag{68}$$

and finally

$$\frac{du}{dp} = \sum_{i=1}^{N} \frac{\partial u}{\partial u_i}\frac{\partial u_i}{\partial p}. \tag{69}$$

The astute reader is probably wondering why the insistence on using the phrase "adjoint mode," rather than the more transparent "reverse mode," since it is quite clear that the derivative terms are being evaluated in reverse order, as compared to the forward mode. To justify this terminology, reverse the order of the above ASE, given in (68). Without giving all the details, this system can be concisely written in matrix form involving the transpose of the Jacobian[5] $\mathbf{D}[\mathbf{u}]$

$$
\mathbf{D}[\mathbf{u}] = \begin{pmatrix}
1 & 0 & \cdots & & & 0 \\
\dfrac{\partial u_2}{\partial u_1} & 1 & 0 & \cdots & & 0 \\
\dfrac{\partial u_3}{\partial u_1} & \dfrac{\partial u_3}{\partial u_2} & 1 & 0 & \cdots & 0 \\
\vdots & \vdots & & & \ddots & \vdots \\
\dfrac{\partial u_N}{\partial u_1} & \dfrac{\partial u_N}{\partial u_2} & \cdots & & \dfrac{\partial u_N}{\partial u_{N-1}} & 1
\end{pmatrix}.
\tag{70}
$$

To summarize, the essence of the calculations of the forward and the adjoint/reverse modes is shown in the following diagram:

Forward Mode   Adjoint/Reverse Mode

vs.

$$\frac{du_1}{dp} \to \frac{du_2}{dp} \to \cdots \to \frac{du_N}{dp} \to \frac{du}{dp} \qquad \frac{\partial u}{\partial u_N} \to \frac{\partial u}{\partial u_{N-1}} \to \cdots \to \frac{\partial u}{\partial u_1} \to \frac{du}{dp}$$

For those readers who need more detail on the theory, implementation, software, and generalizations see [25]. One cautionary note is in order: the input and output variables *must* be independent variables; only the intermediate variables can be dependent.

Input Variables	Intermediate Variables	Output Variables
$u_{-K}, \ldots, u_{-2}, u_1$	$u_1, u_2, \ldots, u_M$	$u_{M+1}, u_{M+2}, \ldots, u_{M+L}$
Independent	Dependent	Independent

8 Optimization Problems

A major objective of epidemiology is to identify and quantify the relevant mechanisms that determine how a disease propagates through a susceptible population. This information can be used to develop intervention strategies that will effectively and efficiently minimize the outbreak and the subsequent deleterious effects. Inherent in the decision-making process is the fact that resources used to intervene, such as money, vaccines, antibiotics, trained medical personnel, isolation, diagnosis using syndromic surveillance, etc., are limited. Determining what the optimal strategy should be, and how to implement such a strategy, is not a trivial matter. In

---

[5] For those readers who want more details on the theory and implementation of AD see [25].

this section we discuss two commonly occurring optimization problems from the decision-making sciences, namely the linear and quadratic programming problems. Additionally, we introduce an optimization/control problem in the context of an influenza pandemic.

8.1 Linear Programming Problem: BVD Disease

In the realm of veterinary epidemiology, bovine viral diarrhoea (BVD) [20] has, and will continue to have, a significant economic impact on the farming industry. Since this is such a competitive market, any losses caused by the disease must be balanced with the associated costs of eradication, prevention and treatment strategies. For example, replacement of the breeding stock will change the age structure of the herd. This strategy affects the productivity of the herd and disease outbreak.

In light of these and many other practical aspects, it may be more realistic to examine the economic options available to the farmer, which will have direct consequences on the epidemiology of the spread of BVD, rather than modeling the disease as an outbreak in isolation. In other words the economically motivated actions taken by the farmer has significant implications for the epidemiology of the disease and the bottom line. This viewpoint provides farm management with quantitative information about the potential variability in income and hence a measure of potential economic risk.

For this application, the constraints take on a wide range of aspects such as total land area, silage area, silage consumption by cows and heifers, calving rates, subsidies, labor rates, available capital, etc.. Decisions that affect the size and quality of the herd, and the spread of disease include how many female or male calfs are sold, how much graze land is used, number of replacement heifers, double fencing of pastures, vermin control, etc.. Since the primary motivation for any business is profit, financial aspects are of primary concern to management. However, it is well known that there is an associated risk in trying to maximize profit, as is easily demonstrated by the stock market. A whole-farm business model [11] in this context would quantify the cost of disease intervention strategies verses the variability of income. Furthermore, a SA of the optimal solution, wrt. the constraints and limited resources, would give quantitative information about which aspects have the most/least effect on the risk and a cost-benefit analysis.

A commonly used methodology in the decision-making sciences is to formulate this problem as a linear programming problem (LPP) [31]. The essential components of a LPP are (1) an objective function which is to be minimized (e.g. cost, risk, etc.,) or maximized (e.g. profit, productivity, etc.,) and (2) constraints (limited resources such as money, silage land, etc.).

Definition 1 (Standard/Forward/Primal LPP). *Let $u_1, u_2, \ldots, u_n$ denote the individual production levels of n commodities with associated unit profits $c_1, c_2, \ldots, c_n$. Let a_{ij} denote the unit amount of resource b_i consumed in the production of commodity j. The* **Standard/Forward/Primal LPP** *is defined as*

Maximize the profit function

$$J(u_1, u_2, \ldots, u_n) := c_1 u_1 + c_2 u_2 + \cdots + c_n u_n = \mathbf{c}^T \mathbf{u},$$

subject to the linear inequality constraints

$$a_{11} u_1 + a_{12} u_2 + \cdots + a_{1n} u_n \leq b_1$$
$$a_{21} u_1 + a_{22} u_2 + \cdots + a_{2n} u_n \leq b_2$$
$$\vdots$$
$$a_{m1} u_1 + a_{m2} u_2 + \cdots + a_{mn} u_n \leq b_m$$
$$u_1, u_2, \cdots, u_m \geq 0,$$

or in matrix form, the constraints are written as $A\mathbf{u} \leq \mathbf{b}$.

It is standard practice to assume that the parameters a_{ij}, b_i and c_j are nonnegative. When this is not the case, then usually a simple change of variables can map the original parameters to a situation where it is true.

Sensitivity analysis allows the analyst a way to determine which of the parameters a_{ij}, b_i, or c_j, defining the problem, has the most effect on the profit function. Since we are interested in how the profit function is affected by perturbations to the defining parameters, we must explicitly find the derivative of the profit function, wrt. changes in the defining parameters. Let p denote any of the parameters a_{ij}, b_i, or c_j, in which case we wish to find

$$\frac{\partial J}{\partial p} = \mathbf{c}^T \frac{\partial \mathbf{u}}{\partial p} + \frac{\partial \mathbf{c}^T}{\partial p} \mathbf{u}. \tag{71}$$

Although rarely discussed, the associated adjoint or dual problem is crucial in finding the sensitivity of the profit function. The main difficulty is in evaluating the derivative expression $\mathbf{c}^T \partial \mathbf{u}/\partial p$ term. To eliminate this problem, the associated adjoint/dual problem will naturally occur, in which case a derivative does not need to be explicitly calculated. Instead, we only need to obtain the solutions to the forward and adjoint/dual problems. Since the simplex method produces both solutions simultaneously, no extra calculations are needed. For completeness, recall the associated adjoint/dual LPP:

Definition 2 (Adjoint/Dual LPP). *The **Adjoint/Dual LPP** is defined as*

Minimize the cost function

$$J(v_1, v_2, \ldots, v_m) := b_1 v_1 + b_2 v_2 + \cdots + b_m v_m = \mathbf{b}^T \mathbf{v},$$

subject to the inequality constraints

$$a_{11}v_1 + a_{21}v_2 + \cdots + a_{m1}v_m \geq c_1$$
$$a_{12}v_1 + a_{22}v_2 + \cdots + a_{m2}v_m \geq c_2$$
$$\vdots$$
$$a_{1n}v_1 + a_{2n}v_2 + \cdots + a_{mn}v_m \geq c_n$$
$$v_1, v_2, \cdots, v_m \geq 0,$$

or in matrix form $A^T v \geq c$.

Sensitivity of the Parameter Space

Many of the commonly occurring optimization problems can be written in the form

Maximize/Minimize a given objective function

$$J(\mathbf{u}) = F(u_1, \ldots, u_n)$$

subject to the K equality and L inequality constraints

$$f_k(\mathbf{u}) = 0 \qquad \text{where} \quad k = 1, \ldots, K$$
$$g_l(\mathbf{u}) \leq 0 \qquad \text{where} \quad l = 1, \ldots, L.$$

To determine the sensitivity of the profit function to perturbations in the parameters, we form a modified Lagrange function based on the Karush-Kuhn-Tucker (KKT) theorem [17]. Recall from multivariable calculus that the technique of the method of Lagrange multipliers was used to find the maximum/minimum of a given function, subject to specified *equality* constraints. In the field of optimization, there exists an analogous method when a mixture of equality and inequality constraints are present.

The procedure is based on a modified Lagrangian function, which is a result of the KKT theorem. In applying this theorem, an adjoint problem naturally arises. This modified Lagrangian function is constructed by forming a linear combination of the objective functional and the constraints as

$$\mathcal{L}(\mathbf{u}; \mu, \lambda) := F(\mathbf{u}) + \sum_{k=1}^{K} \mu_k f_k(\mathbf{u}) + \sum_{l=1}^{L} \lambda_l g_l(\mathbf{u}), \tag{72}$$

where μ_k and λ_l are called the Lagrange multipliers. as we shall see, the Lagrange multipliers are in fact adjoint variables.

Theorem 1 (Karush/Kuhn/Tucker Theorem). *An optimal solution is found by solving the associated equations*

$$\frac{\partial F(\boldsymbol{u}^*)}{\partial u_j} + \sum_{k=1}^{K} \mu_k \frac{\partial f_k(\boldsymbol{u}^*)}{\partial u_j} + \sum_{l=1}^{L} \lambda_l \frac{\partial g_l(\boldsymbol{u}^*)}{\partial u_j} = 0 \qquad for \quad j = 1, \ldots n$$

$$\mu_k f_k(\boldsymbol{u}^*) = 0, \qquad for \quad k = 1, \ldots L$$

$$\lambda_l g_l(\boldsymbol{u}^*) = 0, \qquad for \quad l = 1, \ldots L$$

where $\boldsymbol{u}^*$ is optimal in the sense that $F(\boldsymbol{u}^*) \leq F(\boldsymbol{u})$, where $\boldsymbol{u}$ is any admissible solution.

We begin by changing the linear inequality constraints in the forward problem into equality constraints by introducing slack variables $s_1, s_2, \ldots, s_m$ as follows:

$$\begin{aligned}
a_{11}u_1 + a_{12}u_2 + \cdots + a_{1n}u_n + (s_1)^2 &= b_1 \\
a_{21}u_1 + a_{22}u_2 + \cdots + a_{2n}u_n \qquad + (s_2)^2 &= b_2 \\
&\vdots \\
a_{m1}u_1 + a_{m2}u_2 + \cdots + a_{mn}u_n \qquad + (s_m)^2 &= b_m \\
u_1, u_2, \cdots, u_m &\geq 0.
\end{aligned}$$

Notice that we have deviated from the usual procedure of introducing nonnegative slack variables as $(s_i)^2$ rather than just s_i.

To apply the KKT theorem, we next construct the associated Lagrange function

$$\begin{aligned}
\mathcal{L} := {}& c_1u_1 + c_2u_2 + \cdots c_nu_n \\
&+ v_1 \left(b_1 - a_{11}u_1 - a_{12}u_2 - \cdots - a_{1n}u_n - (s_1)^2 \right) \\
&+ v_2 \left(b_2 - a_{21}u_1 - a_{22}u_2 - \cdots - a_{2n}u_n - (s_2)^2 \right) \\
&\vdots \\
&+ v_m \left(b_m - a_{m1}u_1 - a_{m2}u_2 - \cdots - a_{mn}u_n - (s_m)^2 \right),
\end{aligned}$$

where the v_i are called the Lagrange multipliers. Using the usual inner product notation, the Lagrange function can be written in the more concise form

$$\mathcal{L} := \mathbf{c}^T \mathbf{u} + \mathbf{v}^T \left(\mathbf{b} - \mathbf{A}\mathbf{u} - \begin{pmatrix} (s_1)^2 \\ (s_2)^2 \\ \vdots \\ (s_m)^2 \end{pmatrix} \right).$$

The optimal solution occurs at a critical point of the Lagrange function, that is, when the system of equations

$$\frac{\partial \mathcal{L}}{\partial u_j} = 0, \qquad \frac{\partial \mathcal{L}}{\partial s_i} = 0, \qquad \text{and} \qquad \frac{\partial \mathcal{L}}{\partial v_i} = 0$$

are satisfied. These equations respectively reduce to the adjoint problem:

$$\mathbf{A}^T \mathbf{v} = \mathbf{c}, \tag{73}$$

the orthogonality conditions:

$$v_i s_i = 0, \qquad \text{for} \quad i = 1, \ldots m, \tag{74}$$

and lastly to the forward problem:

$$\mathbf{A}\mathbf{u} + \begin{pmatrix} (s_1)^2 \\ (s_2)^2 \\ \vdots \\ (s_m)^2 \end{pmatrix} = \mathbf{b}. \tag{75}$$

Taking the transpose of the adjoint problem given in Equation (73) and substituting into the derivative of the profit function given in Equation (71) gives

$$\frac{\partial J}{\partial p} = \mathbf{v}^T \mathbf{A} \frac{\partial \mathbf{u}}{\partial p} + \frac{\partial \mathbf{c}^T}{\partial p} \mathbf{u}. \tag{76}$$

To evaluate this expression, we must somehow evaluate the derivative $\partial \mathbf{u}/\partial p$. We will circumvent this problem by relating this derivative with the adjoint solution $\mathbf{v}$. To obtain this relationship, differentiate the forward problem given in Equation (75) wrt. the parameter p to get

$$\mathbf{A}\frac{\partial \mathbf{u}}{\partial p} + \frac{\partial \mathbf{A}}{\partial p}\mathbf{u} + 2 \begin{pmatrix} s_1 \frac{\partial s_1}{\partial p} \\ s_2 \frac{\partial s_2}{\partial p} \\ \vdots \\ s_m \frac{\partial s_m}{\partial p} \end{pmatrix} = \frac{\partial \mathbf{b}}{\partial p}.$$

Now premultiply by $\mathbf{v}^T$ and use the orthogonality conditions given in Equation (74) to obtain

$$\mathbf{v}^T \mathbf{A} \frac{\partial \mathbf{u}}{\partial p} = \mathbf{v}^T \left(\frac{\partial \mathbf{b}}{\partial p} - \frac{\partial \mathbf{A}}{\partial p} \mathbf{u} \right),$$

in which case

$$\frac{\partial J}{\partial p} = \mathbf{v}^T \mathbf{A} \frac{\partial \mathbf{u}}{\partial p} + \frac{\partial \mathbf{c}^T}{\partial p} \mathbf{u}$$

$$= \mathbf{v}^T \left(\frac{\partial \mathbf{b}}{\partial p} - \frac{\partial \mathbf{A}}{\partial p} \mathbf{u} \right) + \frac{\partial \mathbf{c}^T}{\partial p} \mathbf{u}.$$

The utility of this formula is that to calculate $\partial J/\partial p$, only static/fixed quantities need to be known, specifically the solutions to the forward and adjoint problems, namely $\mathbf{u}$ and $\mathbf{v}$. Since the simplex method calculates both solutions simultaneously, there is no need to make perturbations to the simplex tableau, and reapply the simplex method for each change.

For the cases where $p = b_i$, $p = a_{ij}$, or $p = c_j$ the respective derivatives reduce to

$$\frac{\partial J}{\partial b_i} = v_i \qquad \text{for} \quad i = 1, \ldots, m,$$

$$\frac{\partial J}{\partial a_{ij}} = -v_i u_j \qquad \text{for} \quad i = 1, \ldots, m, \quad \text{and} \quad j = 1, \ldots, n, \qquad \text{and}$$

$$\frac{\partial J}{\partial c_j} = u_j \qquad \text{for} \quad j = 1, \ldots, n.$$

Notice that $\partial J/\partial b_i$ and $\partial J/\partial c_j \geq 0$, while $\partial J/\partial a_{ij} \leq 0$. This means that as the limited resources b_i, or unit profits c_j are increased, the profit is increased, whereas if the unit consumption quantities a_{ij} are increased, the profit is decreased, as is expected.

8.2 Quadratic Programming Problem: Wheat Selection

In 1952, Harry Markowitz [24] published a seminal paper titled "Portfolio Selection" which laid the foundation for what is now called modern portfolio theory. Markowitz constructed the mathematical framework for the well known and accepted observation that investors, although seeking a maximum return on their investments, also simultaneously want to minimize the associated risk. What his work espoused was that the proper mixture of various investments can significantly reduce the overall volatility of the portfolio, while maintaining a "high" rate of return. More precisely, Markowitz was able to quantitatively provide two solutions: a maximum amount of return for a given level of risk, or a minimum level of risk for a given amount of return.

Since cereal grains, such as wheat, provide a substantial portion of the caloric needs of humans worldwide, issues such as disease management and prevention are of the utmost importance. In the United States, Kansas is the leading wheat grower in the nation, and is acutely aware of the effects of soil type, average rainfall, disease tolerance, etc., on the yield, and hence the bottom line. To further complicate the problem, agricultural researchers are attempting to produce perennial grain crops that will displace the annual crops that are currently planted. The commonly used practices, that reduce disease inoculum in annual crops, such as tillage, delayed planting, or crop rotation, are not applicable to perennial crops. In this situation, farmers would need to plant blends of seeds from a mixture of cultivars (varieties). This strategy of using mixtures of cultivars has been shown to be effective in the management/prevention of disease.

In the jargon of modern portfolio theory, investment in securities, stocks or bonds is replaced with the planting of multiple wheat cultivars. The objective of maximizing the expected rate of return on the investments is replaced with maximizing the wheat yield. Finally, minimize the financial risks is replaced by minimizing the variation in wheat yield due to "genotype-environment interaction," that is, how each cultivar responds to the inevitable unpredictable environmental conditions. Once quantitative values can be established for the average yield, and the variance and covariance of yields of each cultivar, an optimal portfolio is found by solving a Quadratic Programming Problem (QPP) [6].

In the case of modern portfolio theory, risk is defined in terms of the standard deviation/variance of the return on the assets, and is in fact a quadratic functional. Since the risk in the wheat portfolio is also a function of the variance, this problem will also be a QPP. Lastly, a SA of the optimal solution(s) provides quantitative information on which aspects have the most effect on the optimal solution(s).

Definition 3 (Quadratic Programming Problem QPP). *The Quadratic Programming Problem (QPP) is defined as*

Maximize the profit function

$$J(u_1, u_2, \ldots, u_n) := c^T u - \frac{1}{2} u^T Q u,$$

subject to the linear inequality constraints

$$a_{11}u_1 + a_{12}u_2 + \cdots + a_{1n}u_n \leq b_1$$
$$a_{21}u_1 + a_{22}u_2 + \cdots + a_{2n}u_n \leq b_2$$
$$\vdots$$
$$a_{m1}u_1 + a_{m2}u_2 + \cdots + a_{mn}u_n \leq b_m$$
$$u_1, u_2, \cdots, u_m \geq 0,$$

or in matrix form, the constraints are written as $Au \leq b$.

---

[6] For the general LPP discussed earlier, it is assumed that the profit function is strictly linear in terms of the production level of the associated products. Intuitively this assumption cannot hold true for arbitrary levels of production. One would expect that if the level of production was sufficiently high, the profit would decrease. A common way of incorporating this behavior into the model is to subtract a quadratic term from the objective function. In essence, the quadratic expression can be thought of as a penalty function for excessive production [3, 4].

The matrix $\mathbf{Q}$ is assumed to be a symmetric, positive semi-definite matrix; it is sometimes referred to as the Hessian matrix. The expression $(1/2)\mathbf{u}^T \mathbf{Q}\mathbf{u}$ is a quadratic form and represents the penalty of excess production.

8.2.1 Sensitivity of the Parameter Space

As was done in the LPP, the inequality constraints are transformed into equality constraints by the introduction of slack variables, as given in Equation (75). To apply the Karush-Kuhn-Tucker theorem, construct the extended Lagrange function

$$
\mathcal{L} := \mathbf{c}^T \mathbf{u} - \frac{1}{2}\mathbf{u}^T \mathbf{Q}\mathbf{u} + \mathbf{v}^T \left(\mathbf{b} - \mathbf{A}\mathbf{u} - \begin{pmatrix} (s_1)^2 \\ (s_2)^2 \\ \vdots \\ (s_m)^2 \end{pmatrix} \right).
$$

Once again, the optimal solution occurs at a critical point of the Lagrange function, that is, when the system of equations

$$
\frac{\partial \mathcal{L}}{\partial u_j} = 0, \qquad \frac{\partial \mathcal{L}}{\partial s_i} = 0, \qquad \text{and} \qquad \frac{\partial \mathcal{L}}{\partial v_i} = 0
$$

are satisfied. These equations respectively reduce to the nonhomogeneous adjoint problem:

$$
\mathbf{A}^T \mathbf{v} = \mathbf{c} - \mathbf{Q}\mathbf{u}, \tag{77}
$$

the orthogonality conditions given in Equation (74), and lastly to the forward problem given in Equation (75). Notice that if the matrix $\mathbf{Q}$ is the zero matrix, then the nonhomogeneous adjoint problem for the QPP reduces to the homogeneous adjoint problem for the LPP, as is to be expected.

Let p denote any of the parameters a_{ij}, b_i, c_j, or q_{ij}, where q_{ij} denotes the i, j entry of the matrix $\mathbf{Q}$. Next, differentiate the cost function, wrt. parameter p:

$$
\frac{\partial J}{\partial p} = \frac{\partial \mathbf{c}^T}{\partial p}\mathbf{u} - \frac{1}{2}\mathbf{u}^T \frac{\partial \mathbf{Q}}{\partial p}\mathbf{u} + \frac{1}{2}\left(2\mathbf{c}^T \frac{\partial \mathbf{u}}{\partial p} - \mathbf{u}^T \mathbf{Q}\frac{\partial \mathbf{u}}{\partial p} - \frac{\partial \mathbf{u}^T}{\partial p}\mathbf{Q}\mathbf{u} \right). \tag{78}
$$

Since the matrix $\mathbf{Q}$ is symmetric, then

$$
\left(\mathbf{Q}\frac{\partial \mathbf{u}}{\partial p} \right)^T = \frac{\partial \mathbf{u}^T}{\partial p}\mathbf{Q},
$$

in which case Equation (78) reduces to

$$
\frac{\partial J}{\partial p} = \frac{\partial \mathbf{c}^T}{\partial p}\mathbf{u} - \frac{1}{2}\mathbf{u}^T \frac{\partial \mathbf{Q}}{\partial p}\mathbf{u} + \left(\mathbf{c}^T - \mathbf{u}^T \mathbf{Q} \right)\frac{\partial \mathbf{u}}{\partial p}.
$$

The last expression in this equation contains the derivative term $\partial \mathbf{u}/\partial p$ and will be replaced by an expression containing the forward and adjoint solutions. This expression is found by differentiating the forward problem given in Equation (75).

Next, premultiply this result by the modified adjoint solution $\mathbf{v}^T$, and lastly use the orthogonality conditions given in Equation (74). Specifically,

$$\mathbf{v}^T \mathbf{A} \frac{\partial \mathbf{u}}{\partial p} = \left(\mathbf{c}^T - \mathbf{u}^T \mathbf{Q} \right) \frac{\partial \mathbf{u}}{\partial p}$$

$$= \mathbf{v}^T \left(\frac{\partial \mathbf{b}}{\partial p} - \frac{\partial \mathbf{A}}{\partial p} \mathbf{u} \right),$$

in which case

$$\frac{\partial J}{\partial p} = \mathbf{v}^T \left(\frac{\partial \mathbf{b}}{\partial p} - \frac{\partial \mathbf{A}}{\partial p} \mathbf{u} \right) + \frac{\partial \mathbf{c}^T}{\partial p} \mathbf{u} - \underbrace{\frac{1}{2} \mathbf{u}^T \frac{\partial \mathbf{Q}}{\partial p} \mathbf{u}}_{\text{Additional Term}} . \tag{79}$$

Notice that only the solutions to the forward and adjoint problems are needed to find the derivative of the objective function.

Comparing this result with the LPP, if the matrix $\mathbf{Q}$ is the zero matrix then the QPP reduces to the LPP as expected. For the parameters a_{ij}, b_i, and c_j, the derivatives $\partial J/\partial a_{ij}$, $\partial J/\partial b_i$, and $\partial J/\partial c_j$ are the same form as given for the LPP. However, it should be noted that the adjoint solution $\mathbf{v}$ of Equation (77) is not the same as in the LPP.

8.3 Adjoint Operator, Problem, and Sensitivity

This section provides the generalization for constructing the adjoint problem in its most powerful form. The crucial requirements to take note of are:

- there must be a natural way to define an inner product on the FSE
- the associated adjoint problem must provide a way to allow a natural evaluation of the derivative $\partial \mathbf{u}/\partial p$, or some functional $J(\mathbf{u})$.

The following sketch [19, 20] provides an overview of how the generalized adjoint problem is constructed. The types of problems which are amenable to the adjoint methodology are those that can be expressed in the form

$$F(u) = f,$$

where F is a linear/nonlinear operator $F : X \rightarrow Y$, and f is the forward forcing function. The domain and range X and Y are assumed to have sufficiently nice topological properties. For example, both X and Y could be Hilbert or Sobolov spaces. Also, associated with the forward problem is the task of determining the sensitivity of some desired response function(al) $J(u)$.

The adjoint problem arises naturally by the introduction of an adjoint variable $v \in X$, through the calculation of the Gâteaux derivative:

$$F'(u)v := \lim_{\epsilon \to 0} \frac{F(u + \epsilon v) - F(u)}{\epsilon}.$$

This definition can be thought of as a directional derivative of the operator F at the point u, and in the direction of the adjoint variable v. The somewhat awkward notation $F'(u)v$ is intended to suggest that the operator F takes the forward variable u, and maps it to an operator F', which now depends on both u and the adjoint variable v.

The next piece of necessary machinery is to formulate an extended representation of the operator F. This is accomplished by assuming that F is sufficiently Gâteaux differentiable. Application of the intermediate-value theorem of operators, about the point u_0, permits us to rewrite the forward operator F in extended form:

$$\Phi(u)u = F(u),$$

where the operator Φ is defined in integral form

$$\Phi(u)v := F(u_0) + \int_{\tau=0}^{1} F'(u_0 + \tau(u - u_0)) \, d\tau (v - u_0),$$

Given that an appropriate inner product has been defined, consider the adjoint operation

$$\langle \Phi(u)v, w \rangle = \text{SC1} + \langle v, \Phi^{\dagger}(u)w \rangle,$$

where SC1 denotes the 1st solvability condition, and $\Phi^{\dagger}$ denotes the adjoint operator associated with the forward operator Φ. When SC1 = 0, the result is referred to as the Lagrange identity. The associated generalized adjoint problem is defined as

$$\Phi^{\dagger}(u)v = g,$$

where the adjoint forcing function g has not yet been specified. As was illustrated in the linear system problem, not specifying g at this time is advantageous, since it may be cleverly related to the response functional J.

A second solvability condition SC2 occurs when the forward and adjoint problems are related. Assuming that the Lagrange identity is satisfied, i.e. SC1 = 0, then taking the dot product of the forward problem with the adjoint solution gives

$$\langle \Phi(u)u, v \rangle = \langle f, v \rangle,$$

while taking the dot product of the adjoint problem with the forward solution gives

$$
\begin{aligned}
\langle \Phi^{\dagger}(u)v, u\rangle &= \langle g, u\rangle \\
\langle v, \Phi(u)u\rangle &= \langle g, u\rangle \\
\langle v, f\rangle &= \langle g, u\rangle .
\end{aligned}
$$

This invariance condition, or second solvability condition SC2, relates the forward and adjoint solutions and forcing functions by

$$\langle g, u\rangle = \langle f, v\rangle .$$

Finally, the adjoint forcing function g is cleverly chosen so that

$$\langle g, u\rangle = J(u).$$

We summarize the construction of the adjoint problem in the following diagram (see Fig. 9 below):

For the linear system, the adjoint methodology produces the result that the adjoint problem is $\mathbf{A}^T\mathbf{v} = \mathbf{c}$, provided the operator equation $F(\mathbf{u}) = f$ is constructed from the forward sensitivity equation. Specifically, the results follow when

$$
F(\mathbf{u}) := \mathbf{A}\frac{\partial \mathbf{u}}{\partial q} + \frac{\partial \mathbf{A}}{\partial q}\mathbf{u}, \qquad f := \frac{\partial \mathbf{b}}{\partial q},
$$
$$
\text{and} \qquad J(\mathbf{u}) := \left\langle \frac{\partial \mathbf{u}}{\partial q}, \mathbf{c} \right\rangle .
$$

$$
\begin{array}{ccc}
\overbrace{\Phi(u)u = f}^{\text{Forward Problem}} & \leftrightarrow & \overbrace{\Phi^{\dagger}(u)v = g}^{\text{Adjoint Problem}} \\
\downarrow & & \downarrow \\
\overbrace{\langle \Phi(u)v, v\rangle = \langle f, v\rangle}^{\text{Adjoint Product}} & \leftrightarrow & \overbrace{\langle \Phi^{\dagger}(u)v, u\rangle = \langle g, u\rangle}^{\text{Forward Product}} \\
\downarrow & & \downarrow \\
\underbrace{J(u) = \langle f, v\rangle}_{\text{Adjoint Response}} & \leftrightarrow & \underbrace{J(u) = \langle g, u\rangle}_{\text{Forward Response}}
\end{array}
$$

Fig. 9 Construction of the Adjoint Problem

9 Examples

In this section we highlight a warning: "Let the buyer beware!" The warnings are a discussion of some of the pitfalls/shortcomings that can occur in FSA and ASA. Here we list situations where the reader should proceed with caution:

- In order for an adjoint problem to be defined, an associated inner product structure must exist. **No inner product $\implies$ No adjoint**.
- To determine the sensitivity of the associated functional $J = J(u)$, using the adjoint methodology, the functional must be cleverly written in terms of the inner product.
- Once an adjoint problem has been defined, if more than one sensitivity is required, (e.g., recall the case of the sensitivity of the eigenvalues and eigenvectors), additional information must be introduced to make further progress.
- SA as discussed here is local in nature. The estimates of derivatives are valid only in some "small" neighborhood of the specified nominal values of the parameters. For a more global approach, uncertainty quantification methodology should be used.

In the following examples we provide some insight into how one might attain explicit formula for derivatives of aspects of solutions, which cannot be defined in terms of an inner product. The basic tool is not exotic, rather ubiquitous: the chain rule. As another disclaimer, the following examples are provided in the hopes that they might be useful in your program of SA, and stimulate ideas that would allow you to build additional tools of SA in your own specific realm of research.

9.1 Sensitivity of the Doubling Time

Suppose we have an IVP and we are interested in the time it takes for the solution $u = u(t)$ to double its initial value, i.e., $u(t_D) = 2u_0$. For example, we might wish to know the doubling time for the number of people infected in an epidemic and how it it affected by changes to specific parameters. The typical difficulty is that, in general, we do not have the explicit forward solution, in which case explicit expressions for the desired derivatives are not available. However, numerical values for these derivatives can be calculated using the numerical solution of the forward sensitivity equation(s). The derivatives of interest are found by application of the following lemma.

Lemma 1 (Sensitivity of time to attain a multiple of the initial condition). *Let $u = u(t; p, u_0)$ be the solution to the first order IVP*

$$\frac{du}{dt} = f(u, t; p) \qquad with \qquad u(0) = u_0, \tag{80}$$

where f is differentiable in u, t, and p. Let t_k denote the time t for which u attains the value $u(t_k) = ku_0$, where $k > 0$. The derivative dt_k/dp is given by

$$\frac{dt_k}{dp} = -\frac{\left.\frac{\partial u}{\partial p}\right|_{t=t_k}}{f(ku_0, t_k; p)}, \tag{81}$$

and dt_k/du_0 is given by

$$\frac{dt_k}{du_0} = -\frac{k - \left.\frac{\partial u}{\partial u_0}\right|_{t=t_k}}{f(ku_0, t_k; p)} = 0. \tag{82}$$

Proof. When $t = t_k$ the solution u satisfies the condition $u(t_k) = ku_0$ and upon differentiation wrt. the parameter p, we obtain

$$\left.\frac{d}{dp}[u(t; p, u_0)]\right|_{t=t_k} = \frac{d}{dp}[ku_0].$$

Assuming that k and u_0 are independent of the parameter p, this equation reduces to

$$\left.\frac{du}{dt}\right|_{t=t_k}\frac{dt_k}{dp} + \left.\frac{\partial u}{\partial p}\right|_{t=t_k} = 0,$$

and upon solving for $\partial t_k/\partial p$, we obtain the result given in Equation (81). Similarly, differentiate $u_k = ku_0$ wrt. u_0 to get

$$\left.\frac{d}{du_0}[u(t; p, u_0)]\right|_{t=t_k} = \frac{d}{du_0}[ku_0].$$

Assuming that k and p are independent of u_0, this equation reduces to

$$\left.\frac{du}{dt}\right|_{t=t_k}\frac{dt_k}{du_0} + \left.\frac{\partial u}{\partial u_0}\right|_{t=t_k} = k.$$

But when $t = t_k$ then $u(t_k) = ku_0$, which means $\partial u/\partial u_0|_{t=t_k} = k$, in which case $dt_k/du_0 = 0$.

9.2 Sensitivity of a Critical Point

An important application of SA is to determine which parameter(s), of an IVP modeling the spread of an epidemic, has the most effect on the peak of the infection. In other words, we want to determine the sensitivity of a critical point, to parameters or initial conditions. Specifically we must calculate the derivatives $\partial u/\partial p|_{t=t_{cp}}$ and $\partial t/\partial p|_{t=t_{cp}}$ where t_{cp} denotes the time when the solution is at a critical point u_{cp}.

Lemma 2 (Sensitivity of Critical Points). *The derivative* dt_{cp}/dp *is given by*

$$\frac{dt_{cp}}{dp} = -\frac{\left(\dfrac{\partial f}{\partial p} + \dfrac{\partial f}{\partial u}\dfrac{\partial u}{\partial p}\right)\bigg|_{t=t_{cp}}}{\dfrac{\partial f}{\partial u}\bigg|_{t=t_{cp}}}, \tag{83}$$

and $\partial u/\partial p|_{t=t_{cp}}$ *is found numerically by solving the FSE*

$$\frac{d}{dt}\left[\frac{\partial u}{\partial p}\right] = \frac{\partial f}{\partial u}\frac{\partial u}{\partial p} + \frac{\partial f}{\partial p}. \tag{84}$$

Similarly, the derivative dt_{cp}/dp *is given by*

$$\frac{dt_{cp}}{du_0} = -\frac{\dfrac{\partial f}{\partial u}\dfrac{\partial u}{\partial u_0}\bigg|_{t=t_{cp}}}{\dfrac{\partial f}{\partial u}\bigg|_{t=t_{cp}}}, \tag{85}$$

and $\partial u/\partial u_0|_{t=t_{cp}}$ *is found numerically by solving the FSE*

$$\frac{d}{dt}\left[\frac{\partial u}{\partial u_0}\right] = \frac{\partial f}{\partial u}\frac{\partial u}{\partial u_0}. \tag{86}$$

Proof. Now a critical point u_{cp} at time t_{cp} satisfies the property that

$$f(u_c, t_c; p) = 0. \tag{87}$$

Differentiating this equation wrt. the parameter p gives the single equation

$$\frac{\partial f}{\partial u}\frac{\partial u}{\partial p}\bigg|_{t=t_{cp}} + \frac{\partial f}{\partial t}\frac{\partial t}{\partial p}\bigg|_{t=t_{cp}} + \frac{\partial f}{\partial p}\bigg|_{t=t_{cp}} = 0. \tag{88}$$

in the two unknowns $\partial u/\partial p|_{t=t_{cp}}$, $\partial t/\partial p|_{t=t_{cp}}$. Solving this equation for $\partial t/\partial p|_{t=t_{cp}}$ and numerically solving the above mentioned FSE for $\partial u/\partial p|_{t=t_{cp}}$ gives the desired result. The other result is obtained in a similar fashion.

9.3 Sensitivity of Periodic Solutions to Parameters

Consider the IVP where the forward solution u approaches a limit cycle of period T as $t \to \infty$. As is almost aways the case, a closed form of the forward solution is not available, in which case the derivative $\partial T / \partial p$ can not be explicitly obtained.

As seen from the previous examples, the key to obtaining the desired derivative is to state, mathematically, the desired property, apply the chain rule, and possibly utilize the solution to the FSEs. In this example, the key observation is that if u is periodic with period T, where $t \in [0, \infty)$, u_0 and u_0' are given initial conditions, and p is a parameter, then

$$u(t + T; u_0, u_0', p) = u(t; u_0, u_0', p), \qquad \forall t \in [0, \infty).$$

We will differentiate this expression wrt. the parameter p and find a numerical expression for dT/dp, in terms of the forward sensitivity derivatives. The following lemma gives the desired expressions.

Lemma 3 (Sensitivity of a periodic function). *Let $u = u(t; u_0, u_0', p)$ be a family of periodic functions with period T, that is,*

$$u(t + T; u_0, u_0', p) = u(t; u_0, u_0', p), \tag{89}$$

$\forall t \in [0, \infty)$ and where u is differentiable in t, u_0, u_0', and p. The derivative of the period T with respect to the parameter p is given by

$$\frac{dT}{dp} = \frac{\dfrac{\partial u(t; u_0, u_0', p)}{\partial p} - \dfrac{\partial u(s; u_0, u_0', p)}{\partial p}\bigg|_{s=t+T}}{\dfrac{du(t; u_0, u_0', p)}{dt}}. \tag{90}$$

The astute reader is no doubt immediately suspicious of this result, since the left hand side seems to be independent of time, while the right hand side is apparently time dependent. However, this "contradiction" will be addressed shortly.

Proof. Differentiate Equation (89) wrt. the parameter p to get

$$\frac{d}{dp}\left[u(s; u_0, u_0', p)\right]\bigg|_{s=t+T} = \frac{d}{dp}\left[u(t; u_0, u_0', p)\right],$$

or in expanded form

$$\frac{du(s;u_0,u_0',p)}{ds}\bigg|_{s=t+\mathcal{T}}\frac{d[t+\mathcal{T}]}{dp}+\frac{\partial u(s;u_0,u_0',p)}{\partial u_0}\bigg|_{s=t+\mathcal{T}}$$

$$\frac{du_0}{dp}+\frac{\partial u(s;u_0,u_0',p)}{\partial u_0'}\bigg|_{s=t+\mathcal{T}}\frac{du_0'}{dp}+\frac{\partial u(s;u_0,u_0',p)}{\partial p}\bigg|_{s=t+\mathcal{T}}$$

$$=\frac{du(t;u_0,u_0',p)}{dt}\frac{dt}{dp}+\frac{\partial u(t;u_0,u_0',p)}{\partial u_0}\frac{du_0}{dp}$$

$$+\frac{\partial u(t;u_0,u_0',p)}{\partial u_0'}\frac{du_0'}{dp}+\frac{\partial u(t;u_0,u_0'p)}{\partial p}. \tag{91}$$

Since t, u_0, and u_0' are independent of p, then $dt/dp = du_0/dp = du_0'/dp = 0$, in which case this equation reduces to

$$\frac{du(s;u_0,u_0',p)}{ds}\bigg|_{s=t+\mathcal{T}}\frac{d\mathcal{T}}{dp}+\frac{\partial u(s;u_0,u_0',p)}{\partial p}\bigg|_{s=t+\mathcal{T}}=\frac{\partial u(t;u_0,u_0',p)}{\partial p}.$$

Now solve for $d\mathcal{T}/dp$ and use the fact that since u is periodic in t, then

$$\frac{du(s;u_0,u_0',p)}{ds}\bigg|_{s=t+\mathcal{T}}=\frac{du(t;u_0,u_0',p)}{dt},$$

to obtain the result stated as Equation (89).

A cautionary note is needed to prevent misapplication of this result. The formula given in Equation (89) is for an arbitrary time t as compared to previous examples, where the formula for the derivative of a particular aspect of a problem was valid only at a particular specified point in time. In other words, for a fixed value of the parameter p and initial conditions u_0, and u_0' the expression $d\mathcal{T}/dp$ should remain constant if the period $\mathcal{T}$ is independent of time. That is, we must assume that the periodicity of the solution is not changing, or, at worst, is approaching a fixed value.

Acknowledgments This research was supported by the Department of Energy under contract DE-AC52-06NA25396 and DOE ASCR Applied Mathematical Sciences Program.

References

1. Bailey N, Duppenthaler J (1980) Sensitivity Analysis in the Modelling of Infectious Disease Dynamics. J Math Biology 10:113–131.
2. Bartlett R (2008) A Derivation of Forward and Adjoint Sensitivities for ODEs and DAEs. Tech. Rep. SAND2007-6699, Sandia National Laboratories.

3. Barkley A, Bowden R, Shroyer J (2006) Kansas Wheat Variety Selection: Combining Economics and Agronomy to Maximize Profits and Minimize Risk. Risk and Profit Conference.
4. Barkley A, Peterson H (2008) Wheat Variety Selection: An to Application of Portfolio Theory to Improve Returns. NCCC-134 Confererce on Applied Commodity Price Analysis, Forecasting, and Market Risk.
5. Cacuci D (1981a) Sensitivity Theory for Nonlinear Systems. I. Nonlinear Functional Analysis Approach. J Math Phys 22:2794–2802.
6. Cacuci D (1981b) Sensitivity Theory for Nonlinear Systems. II. Extensions to Additional Classes of Responses. J Math Phys 22:2803–2812.
7. Cacuci D (2003) Sensitivity and Uncertainty Analysis: Theory, vol. I. Chapman & Hall/CRC.
8. Cacuci D (2005) Sensitivity and Uncertainty Analysis: Applications to Large–Scale Systems, vol. II. Chapman & Hall/CRC.
9. Cacuci D, Ionescu-Bujor M, Navon I (2005) Sensitivity and Uncertainty Analysis: Applications to Large–Scale Systems, vol. II. Chapman & Hall/CRC.
10. Cacuci D, Weber C, Oblow E, Marable J (1980) Sensitivity Theory for General Systems of Nonlinear Equations. Nucl Sci Eng 75:88–110.
11. Endrud G (1986) Optimize your farm. ii. lp for whole-farm modeling . . . linear programming as a management decision tool. AgriComp 4:39–44.
12. Errico R (1997) What is an Adjoint model?. Bull Am Meteorol Soc 78:2577–2591.
13. Frank P (1978) Introduction to System Sensitivity Theory. Academic Press.
14. Garrett L (1995) The Coming Plague: Newly Emerging Diseases in a World Out of Balance. Penguin.
15. Golub GH, Loan CFV (1996) Matrix Computations. Johns Hopkins University Press.
16. Hora S (1997) Sensitivity, Uncertainty, and Decision Analyses in the Prioritization of Research. J Statist Comput Simul 57:175–196.
17. Nocedal SJWJ (2006) Numerical Optimization. Springer Publishing.
18. Lancaster P, Tismenetsky M (1985) The Theory of Matrices. Academic Press.
19. Levy A (2001) Solution Sensitivity From General Principles. SIAM J Control Optim 40:1–38.
20. Lindberg ALE (2003) Bovine viral diarrhoea virus infections and its control – a review. Vet Q 25:1–16.
21. Marchuk G (1995) Adjoint Equations and Analysis of Complex Systems. Kluwer Academic Pulishers.
22. Marchuk G, Agoshkov V (1988) Conjugate Operators and Algorithms of Perturbation in Nonlinear Problems I. Principles of Construction of Conjugate Operators. Sov J Numer Anal Math Modell 3:21–46.
23. Marchuk G, Agoshkov V, Shutyaev V (1996) Adjoint Equations and Perturbation Algorithms in Nonlinear Problems. CRC Press.
24. Markowitz H (1952) Portfolio Selection. J Finance 7:77–91.
25. Martins JRRA, Sturdza P, Alonso JJ (2003) The complex-step derivative approximation. ACM Transactions on Mathematical Software (TOMS) 29:245 – 262.
26. Murray J (1986) Mathematical Biology I: An Introduction. Springer-Verlag.
27. Saltelli A (1999) Sensitivity Analysis: Could Better Methods by Used?. J Geophys Res 104:3789–3793.
28. Saltelli A, Chan K, Scott E (eds) (2000) Sensitivity Analysis, Wiley Series in Probability and Statistics. John Wiley & Sons.
29. Saltelli A, Ratto M, Andres T, Campolongo F, Cariboni J, Gatelli D, Saisan M, Tarantola S (2008) Global Sensitivity Analysis: The Primer. John Wiley & Sons, Ltd.
30. Saltelli A, Tarantola S, Campolongo F, Ratto M (2004) Sensitivity Analysis in Practice: A Guide to Assessing Scientific Models. John Wiley & Sons, Ltd.
31. Vanderbei RJ (2007) Linear Programming: Foundations and Extensions. Springer.
32. Wallace S (2000) Decision Making Under Uncertainty: Is Sensitivity Analysis of Any Use?. Operat Res 48:20–25.
33. Wilkinson JH (1988) The Algebraic Eigenvalue Problem. Oxford University Press.

An Inverse Problem Statistical Methodology Summary

**H. Thomas Banks, Marie Davidian,
John R. Samuels, Jr., and Karyn L. Sutton**

Abstract We discuss statistical and computational aspects of inverse or parameter estimation problems for deterministic dynamical systems based on Ordinary Least Squares and Generalized Least Squares with appropriate corresponding data noise assumptions of constant variance and nonconstant variance (relative error), respectively. Among the topics included here are mathematical model, statistical model and data assumptions, and some techniques (residual plots, sensitivity analysis, model comparison tests) for verifying these. The ideas are illustrated throughout with the popular logistic growth model of Verhulst and Pearl as well as with a recently developed population level model of pneumococcal disease spread.

Keywords Inference · Least squares inverse problems · Parameter estimation · Sensitivity and generalized sensitivity functions

1 Introduction

In this Chapter we discuss mathematical and statistical aspects of *inverse* or *parameter estimation* problems for deterministic differential equation models. While we briefly discuss *maximum likelihood estimators* (MLE), our focus here will be on *ordinary least squares* (OLS) and *generalized least squares* (GLS) estimation formulations and issues related to use of these techniques in practice. Although we choose a general nonlinear ordinary differential equation *mathematical model* to discuss concepts and ideas, the discussions are also applicable to partial differential equation models and other deterministic dynamical systems. As we shall explain, the choice of an appropriate *statistical model* is of critical importance, and we discuss at length the difference between constant variance and nonconstant variance noise in the observation process, the consequences for incorrect choices in this regard, and computational techniques for investigating whether a good decision has

H. Thomas Banks (✉)
Center for Research in Scientific Computation and Center for Quantitative Sciences in Biomedicine, North Carolina State University, Raleigh, NC 27695-8212, USA

G. Chowell et al. (eds.), *Mathematical and Statistical Estimation Approaches in Epidemiology*, DOI 10.1007/978-90-481-2313-1_11,
© Springer Science+Business Media B.V. 2009

been made. In particular, we illustrate the use of residual plots to suggest whether or not a correct statistical model has been specified in an inverse problem formulation. We illustrate these and other techniques with examples including the well known Verhulst-Pearl logistic population model and a specific epidemiological model (a pneumococcal disease dynamics model). We discuss the use of sensitivity equations coupled with the asymptotic theory for sampling distributions and the computation of associated covariances, standard errors and confidence intervals for the estimators of model parameters. We also discuss *sensitivity functions* (*traditional* and *generalized*) and their emerging use in design of experiments for data specific to models and mechanism investigation. Traditional sensitivity involves sensitivity of outputs to parameters while the recent concept of generalized sensitivity in inverse problems pertains to sensitivity of parameters (to be estimated) to data or observations. That is, generalized sensitivity quantifies the relevance of data measurements for identification of parameters in a typical parameter estimation problem. In a final section we present and illustrate some methods for model comparison. Specifically, we discuss statistical tests that can be used with inverse problems when one wishes to compare the "goodness of fit" to data of two deterministic models, one of which includes the other by a simplification through a reduction of mechanisms/ interactions.

Our presentation is intended for scientists who have an interest in fitting models to data (inverse or parameter estimation problems) and who possess a modest background in mathematics and elementary statistics. However, we do not assume a specific detailed factual knowledge in either but do provide a number of references for further reading as well as for background material. We note that our presentation illustrates how inverse problems for completely deterministic systems result in the need for statistical analysis in the usual situation where one has noisy data for use in the inverse problems.

2 Parameter Estimation: MLE, OLS, and GLS

2.1 The Underlying Mathematical and Statistical Models

2.1.1 The Mathematical Model

We consider inverse or parameter estimation problems in the context of a parameterized (with vector parameter $\vec{\theta}$) dynamical system or *mathematical model*

$$\frac{d\vec{x}}{dt}(t) = \vec{g}(t, \vec{x}(t), \vec{\theta}) \tag{1}$$

with *observation process*

$$\vec{y}(t) = \mathcal{C}\vec{x}(t; \vec{\theta}). \tag{2}$$

The mathematical model is a deterministic system (here we treat ordinary differential equations, but as noted above, our discussions are relevant to problems involving parameter dependent partial differential equations, delay differential equations, etc., as long as the system is assumed to be well-posed, i.e., to possess unique solutions that depend smoothly on the parameters and initial data). Following usual convention (which corresponds to the form of data usually available from experiments), we assume a discrete form of the observations in which one has n longitudinal observations corresponding to

$$\vec{y}(t_j) = C\vec{x}(t_j; \vec{\theta}), \quad j = 1, \ldots, n, \tag{3}$$

where C is an observation operator as described below. In general the corresponding observations or data $\{\vec{y}_j\}$ will not be exactly $\vec{y}(t_j)$. Because of the nature of the phenomena leading to this discrepancy, we treat this uncertainty pertaining to the observations with a statistical model for the observation process.

2.1.2 The Statistical Model

In our discussions here we consider a *statistical model* of the form

$$\vec{Y}_j = \vec{f}(t_j, \vec{\theta}_0) + \vec{\epsilon}_j, \quad j = 1, \ldots, n, \tag{4}$$

where $\vec{f}(t_j, \vec{\theta}) = C\vec{x}(t_j; \vec{\theta})$, $j = 1, \ldots, n$, corresponds to the solution of the mathematical model (1) at the jth covariate or observation time for a particular vector of parameters $\vec{\theta} \in R^p, \vec{x} \in R^N, \vec{f} \in R^m$, and C is an $m \times N$ matrix. The term $\vec{\theta}_0$ represents the "truth" or the parameters that generate the observations $\{\vec{Y}_j\}_{j=1}^n$. (The assumption of existence of a truth parameter $\vec{\theta}_0$ is standard in statistical formulations and this along with the assumption that the means $E[\vec{\epsilon}_j]$ are zero yields implicitly that the (1) is a correct description of the process being modeled.) The terms $\vec{\epsilon}_j$ are random variables which can represent observation or measurement error, "system fluctuations" or other phenomena that cause observations to not fall exactly on the points $\vec{f}(t_j, \vec{\theta})$ from the smooth path $\vec{f}(t, \vec{\theta})$. Since these fluctuations are unknown to the modeler, we will assume $\vec{\epsilon}_j$ is generated from a probability distribution (with mean zero throughout our discussions) that reflects the assumptions regarding these phenomena. For instance, in a statistical model for pharmacokinetics of drug in human blood samples, a natural distribution for $\vec{\epsilon} = (\epsilon_1, \ldots, \epsilon_n)^T$ might be a multivariate normal distribution. In other applications the distribution for $\vec{\epsilon}$ might be much more complicated [22].

The purpose of our presentation here is to discuss methodology related to the estimation of the true value of the parameters $\vec{\theta}_0$ from a set Θ of admissible parameters, and its dependence on what is assumed about the variance $\text{var}(\vec{\epsilon}_j)$ of the error $\vec{\epsilon}_j$. We discuss two inverse problem methodologies that can be used to calculate estimates $\hat{\theta}$ for $\vec{\theta}_0$: the ordinary least-squares (OLS) and generalized least-squares (GLS) formulations as well as the popular maximum likelihood estimate (MLE) formulation in the case one assumes the distributions of the error process $\{\vec{\epsilon}_j\}$ are known.

2.2 Known Error Processes: Normally Distributed Error

In the introduction of the statistical model we initially made no mention of the probability distribution that generates the error $\vec{\epsilon}_j$. In many situations one readily assumes that the errors $\vec{\epsilon}_j = 1, \ldots, n$, are independent and identically distributed (we make the *standing assumptions of independence across j* throughout our discussions in this Chapter). We discuss a case where one is able to make further assumptions on the error, namely that the distribution is known. In this case, maximum likelihood techniques may be used. We discuss first one such case for a scalar observation system, i.e., $m = 1$. If, in addition, there is sufficient evidence to suspect the error is generated by a normal distribution then we may be willing to assume $\epsilon_j \sim \mathcal{N}(0, \sigma_0^2)$, and hence $Y_j \sim \mathcal{N}(f(t_j, \vec{\theta}_0), \sigma_0^2)$. We can then obtain an expression for determining $\vec{\theta}_0$ and σ_0 by seeking the maximum over $(\vec{\theta}, \sigma^2) \in \Theta \times (0, \infty)$ of the likelihood function for $\epsilon_j = Y_j - f(t_j, \vec{\theta})$ which is defined by

$$L(\vec{\theta}, \sigma^2 | \vec{Y}) = \prod_{j=1}^{n} \frac{1}{\sqrt{2\pi\sigma^2}} \exp\left\{ -\frac{1}{2\sigma^2} [Y_j - f(t_j, \vec{\theta})]^2 \right\}. \tag{5}$$

The resulting solutions θ_{MLE} and σ_{MLE}^2 are the maximum likelihood *estimators* (MLEs) for $\vec{\theta}_0$ and σ_0^2, respectively. We point out that these solutions $\theta_{\text{MLE}} = \theta_{\text{MLE}}^n(\vec{Y})$ and $\sigma_{\text{MLE}}^2 = \sigma_{\text{MLE}}^{2\,n}(\vec{Y})$ are *random variables* by virtue of the fact that $\vec{Y}$ is a random variable. The corresponding maximum likelihood *estimates* are obtained by maximizing (5) with $\vec{Y} = (Y_1, \ldots, Y_n)^T$ replaced by a given realization $\vec{y} = (y_1, \ldots, y_n)^T$ and will be denoted by $\hat{\theta}_{\text{MLE}} = \hat{\theta}_{\text{MLE}}^n$ and $\hat{\sigma}_{\text{MLE}} = \hat{\sigma}_{\text{MLE}}^n$ respectively. In our discussions here and below, almost every quantity of interest is dependent on n, the *size of the set of observations* or the *sampling size*. On occasion we will express this dependence explicitly by use of superscripts or subscripts, especially when we wish to remind the reader of this dependence. However, for notational convenience we will often suppress the notation of explicit dependence on n.

Maximizing (5) is equivalent to maximizing the log likelihood

$$\log L(\vec{\theta}, \sigma^2 | \vec{Y}) = -\frac{n}{2} \log(2\pi) - \frac{n}{2} \log \sigma^2 - \frac{1}{2\sigma^2} \sum_{j=1}^{n} [Y_j - f(t_j, \vec{\theta})]^2. \tag{6}$$

We determine the maximum of (6) by differentiating with respect to $\vec{\theta}$ (with σ^2 fixed) and with respect to σ^2 (with $\vec{\theta}$ fixed), setting the resulting equations equal to zero and solving for $\vec{\theta}$ and σ^2. With σ^2 fixed we solve $\frac{\partial}{\partial \vec{\theta}} \log L(\vec{\theta}, \sigma^2 | \vec{Y}) = 0$ which is equivalent to

$$\sum_{j=1}^{n} [Y_j - f(t_j, \vec{\theta})] \nabla f(t_j, \vec{\theta}) = 0, \tag{7}$$

where as usual $\nabla f = \frac{\partial}{\partial \vec{\theta}} f = f_{\vec{\theta}}$. We see that solving (7) is the same as the least squares optimization

$$\theta_{\text{MLE}}(\vec{Y}) = \arg \min_{\vec{\theta} \in \Theta} J(\vec{Y}, \vec{\theta}) = \arg \min_{\vec{\theta} \in \Theta} \sum_{j=1}^{n} [Y_j - f(t_j, \vec{\theta})]^2. \qquad (8)$$

We next fix $\vec{\theta}$ to be θ_{MLE} and solve $\frac{\partial}{\partial \sigma^2} \log L(\theta_{\text{MLE}}, \sigma^2 | \vec{Y}) = 0$, which yields

$$\sigma_{\text{MLE}}^2(\vec{Y}) = \frac{1}{n} J(\vec{Y}, \theta_{\text{MLE}}). \qquad (9)$$

Note that we can solve for θ_{MLE} and σ_{MLE}^2 separately – a desirable feature, but one that does not arise in more complicated formulations discussed below. The 2nd derivative test (which is omitted here) verifies that the expressions above for θ_{MLE} and σ_{MLE}^2 do indeed maximize (6).

If, however, we have a vector of observations for the jth covariate t_j then the statistical model is reformulated as

$$\vec{Y}_j = \vec{f}(t_j, \vec{\theta}_0) + \vec{\epsilon}_j \qquad (10)$$

where $\vec{f} \in R^m$ and

$$V_0 = \text{var}(\vec{\epsilon}_j) = \text{diag}(\sigma_{0,1}^2, \ldots, \sigma_{0,m}^2) \qquad (11)$$

for $j = 1, \ldots, n$. In this setting we have allowed for the possibility that the observation coordinates Y_j^i may have different *constant* variances $\sigma_{0,i}^2$, i.e., $\sigma_{0,i}^2$ does not necessarily have to equal $\sigma_{0,k}^2$. If (again) there is sufficient evidence to claim the errors are independent and identically distributed and generated by a normal distribution then $\vec{\epsilon}_j \sim \mathcal{N}_m(0, V_0)$. We thus can obtain the maximum likelihood estimators $\theta_{\text{MLE}}(\{\vec{Y}_j\})$ and $V_{\text{MLE}}(\{\vec{Y}_j\})$ for θ_0 and V_0 by determining the maximum of the log of the likelihood function for $\vec{\epsilon}_j = \vec{Y}_j - \vec{f}(t_j, \vec{\theta})$ defined by

$$\log L(\vec{\theta}, V | \{Y_j^1, \ldots, Y_j^m\}) = -\frac{n}{2} \sum_{i=1}^{m} \log \sigma_{0,i}^2 - \frac{1}{2} \sum_{i=1}^{m} \frac{1}{\sigma_{0,i}^2} \sum_{j=1}^{n} [Y_j^i - f^i(t_j, \vec{\theta})]^2$$

$$= -\frac{n}{2} \sum_{i=1}^{m} \log \sigma_{0,i}^2 - \sum_{j=1}^{n} [\vec{Y}_j - \vec{f}(t_j, \vec{\theta})]^T V^{-1} [\vec{Y}_j - \vec{f}(t_j, \vec{\theta})].$$

Using arguments similar to those given for the scalar case, we determine the maximum likelihood estimators for $\vec{\theta}_0$ and V_0 to be

$$\theta_{\mathrm{MLE}} = \arg\min_{\vec{\theta} \in \Theta} \sum_{j=1}^{n} [\vec{Y}_j - \vec{f}(t_j, \vec{\theta})]^T V_{\mathrm{MLE}}^{-1} [\vec{Y}_j - \vec{f}(t_j, \vec{\theta})] \tag{12}$$

$$V_{\mathrm{MLE}} = \mathrm{diag}\left(\frac{1}{n} \sum_{j=1}^{n} [\vec{Y}_j - \vec{f}(t_j, \theta_{\mathrm{MLE}})][\vec{Y}_j - \vec{f}(t_j, \theta_{\mathrm{MLE}})]^T \right). \tag{13}$$

Unfortunately, this is a coupled system, which requires some care when solving numerically. We will discuss this issue further in Sections 2.3.2 and 2.3.5 below.

2.3 Unspecified Error Distributions and Asymptotic Theory

In Section 2.2 we examined the estimates of $\vec{\theta}_0$ and V_0 under the assumption *that the error is normally distributed, independent and has constant variance longitudinally.* But what if it is suspected that the error is not normally distributed, or the error distribution is unknown to the modeler beyond the assumptions on $E[\vec{Y}_j]$ embodied in the model and the assumptions made on $\mathrm{var}(\vec{\epsilon}_j)$ (as in most applications)? How should we proceed in estimating $\vec{\theta}_0$ and σ_0 (or V_0) in these circumstances? In this section we will review two estimation procedures for such situations: ordinary least squares (OLS) and generalized least squares (GLS).

2.3.1 Ordinary Least Squares (OLS)

The statistical model in the scalar case takes the form

$$Y_j = f(t_j, \vec{\theta}_0) + \epsilon_j \tag{14}$$

where the variance $\mathrm{var}(\epsilon_j) = \sigma_0^2$ is assumed constant in longitudinal data (note that the error's distribution is not specified). We also note that the assumption that the observation errors are uncorrelated across j (i.e., time) may be a reasonable one when the observations are taken with sufficient intermittency or when the primary source of error is measurement error. If we define

$$\theta_{\mathrm{OLS}}(\vec{Y}) = \theta_{\mathrm{OLS}}^n(\vec{Y}) = \arg\min_{\vec{\theta} \in \Theta} \sum_{j=1}^{n} [Y_j - f(t_j, \vec{\theta})]^2 \tag{15}$$

then θ_{OLS} can be viewed as minimizing the distance between the data and model where all observations are treated as of equal importance. We note that minimizing in (15) corresponds to solving for $\vec{\theta}$ in

$$\sum_{j=1}^{n} [Y_j - f(t_j, \vec{\theta})] \nabla f(t_j, \vec{\theta}) = 0. \tag{16}$$

We point out that θ_{OLS} is a *random variable* ($\epsilon_j = Y_j - f(t_j, \vec{\theta})$ is a random variable); hence if $\{y_j\}_{j=1}^n$ is a realization of the *random process* $\{Y_j\}_{j=1}^n$ then solving

$$\hat{\theta}_{OLS} = \hat{\theta}_{OLS}^n = \arg\min_{\vec{\theta} \in \Theta} \sum_{j=1}^n [y_j - f(t_j, \vec{\theta})]^2 \qquad (17)$$

provides a realization for θ_{OLS}. (A remark on notation: for a random variable or estimator θ we will always denote a corresponding realization or estimate with an over hat, e.g., $\hat{\theta}$ is an estimate for θ.)

Noting that

$$\sigma_0^2 = \frac{1}{n} E \left[\sum_{j=1}^n [Y_j - f(t_j, \vec{\theta}_0)]^2 \right] \qquad (18)$$

suggests that once we have solved for θ_{OLS} in (15), we may obtain an estimate $\hat{\sigma}_{OLS}^2 = \hat{\sigma}_{MLE}^2{}^n$ for σ_0^2.

Even though the error's distribution is not specified we can use asymptotic theory to approximate the mean and variance of the random variable θ_{OLS} [31]. As will be explained in more detail below, as $n \to \infty$, we have that

$$\theta_{OLS} = \theta_{OLS}^n \sim \mathcal{N}_p(\vec{\theta}_0, \Sigma_0^n) \approx \mathcal{N}_p(\vec{\theta}_0, \sigma_0^2 [\chi^{nT}(\vec{\theta}_0)\chi^n(\vec{\theta}_0)]^{-1}) \qquad (19)$$

where the sensitivity matrix $\chi(\vec{\theta}) = \chi^n(\vec{\theta}) = \{\chi_{jk}^n\}$ is defined as

$$\chi_{jk}^n(\vec{\theta}) = \frac{\partial f(t_j, \vec{\theta})}{\partial \theta_k}, \quad j = 1, \ldots, n, \quad k = 1, \ldots, p,$$

and

$$\Sigma_0^n \equiv \sigma_0^2 [n\Omega_0]^{-1} \qquad (20)$$

with

$$\Omega_0 \equiv \lim_{n \to \infty} \frac{1}{n} \chi^{nT}(\vec{\theta}_0)\chi^n(\vec{\theta}_0), \qquad (21)$$

where the limit is assumed to exist-see [31]. However, $\vec{\theta}_0$ and σ_0^2 are generally unknown, so one usually will instead use the *realization* $\vec{y} = (y_1, \ldots, y_n)^T$ of the random process $\vec{Y}$ to obtain the estimate

$$\hat{\theta}_{OLS} = \arg\min_{\vec{\theta} \in \Theta} \sum_{j=1}^n [y_j - f(t_j, \vec{\theta})]^2 \qquad (22)$$

and the *bias adjusted* estimate

$$\hat{\sigma}_{\text{OLS}}^2 = \frac{1}{n-p} \sum_{j=1}^{n} [y_j - f(t_j, \hat{\theta})]^2 \tag{23}$$

to use as an approximation in (19).

We note that (23) represents the estimate for σ_0^2 of (18) with the factor $\frac{1}{n}$ replaced by the factor $\frac{1}{n-p}$ (in the linear case the estimate with $\frac{1}{n}$ can be shown to be biased downward and the same behavior can be observed in the general nonlinear case–see Chapter 12 of [31] and p. 28 of [22]). We remark that (18) is true even in the general nonlinear case (it does not rely on any asymptotic theories although it does depend on the assumption of constant variance being correct).

Both $\hat{\theta} = \hat{\theta}_{\text{OLS}}$ and $\hat{\sigma}^2 = \hat{\sigma}_{\text{OLS}}^2$ will then be used to approximate the covariance matrix

$$\Sigma_0^n \approx \hat{\Sigma}^n \equiv \hat{\sigma}^2 [\chi^{nT}(\hat{\theta}) \chi^n(\hat{\theta})]^{-1}. \tag{24}$$

We can obtain the standard errors $SE(\hat{\theta}_{\text{OLS},k})$ (discussed in more detail in the next section) for the kth element of $\hat{\theta}_{\text{OLS}}$ by calculating $SE(\hat{\theta}_{\text{OLS},k}) \approx \sqrt{\hat{\Sigma}_{kk}^n}$. Also note the similarity between the MLE Equations (8) and (9), and the scalar OLS Equations (22) and (23). That is, under a normality assumption for the error, the MLE and OLS formulations are equivalent.

If, however, we have a vector of observations for the jth covariate t_j and we assume the variance is still constant in longitudinal data, then the statistical model is reformulated as

$$\vec{Y}_j = \vec{f}(t_j, \vec{\theta}_0) + \vec{\epsilon}_j \tag{25}$$

where $\vec{f} \in R^m$ and

$$V_0 = \text{var}(\vec{\epsilon}_j) = \text{diag}(\sigma_{0,1}^2, \ldots, \sigma_{0,m}^2) \tag{26}$$

for $j = 1, \ldots, n$. Just as in the MLE case we have allowed for the possibility that the observation coordinates Y_j^i may have different *constant* variances $\sigma_{0,i}^2$, i.e., $\sigma_{0,i}^2$ does not necessarily have to equal $\sigma_{0,k}^2$. We note that this formulation also can be used to treat the case where V_0 is used to simply scale the observations, i.e., $V_0 = \text{diag}(v_1, \ldots, v_m)$ is known. In this case the formulation is simply a *vector OLS* (sometimes also called a weighted least squares (WLS)). The problem will consist of finding the minimizer

$$\theta_{\text{OLS}} = \arg \min_{\vec{\theta} \in \Theta} \sum_{j=1}^{n} [\vec{Y}_j - \vec{f}(t_j, \vec{\theta})]^T V_0^{-1} [\vec{Y}_j - \vec{f}(t_j, \vec{\theta})], \tag{27}$$

where the procedure weights elements of the vector $\vec{Y}_j - \vec{f}(t_j, \vec{\theta})$ according to their variability. (Some authors refer to (27) as a generalized least squares (GLS) procedure, but we will make use of this terminology in a different formulation in subsequent discussions). Just as in the scalar OLS case, θ_{OLS} is a *random variable* (again because $\vec{\epsilon}_j = \vec{Y}_j - \vec{f}(t_j, \vec{\theta})$ is); hence if $\{\vec{y}_j\}_{j=1}^n$ is a realization of the *random process* $\{\vec{Y}_j\}_{j=1}^n$ then solving

$$\hat{\theta}_{\mathrm{OLS}} = \arg\min_{\theta \in \Theta} \sum_{j=1}^n [\vec{y}_j - \vec{f}(t_j, \vec{\theta})]^T V_0^{-1} [\vec{y}_j - \vec{f}(t_j, \vec{\theta})] \tag{28}$$

provides an estimate (realization) $\hat{\theta} = \hat{\theta}_{\mathrm{OLS}}$ for θ_{OLS}. By the definition of variance

$$V_0 = \mathrm{diag}\, E\left(\frac{1}{n} \sum_{j=1}^n [\vec{Y}_j - \vec{f}(t_j, \vec{\theta}_0)][\vec{Y}_j - \vec{f}(t_j, \vec{\theta}_0)]^T \right),$$

so an unbiased estimate of V_0 for the realization $\{\vec{y}_j\}_{j=1}^n$ is

$$\hat{V} = \mathrm{diag}\left(\frac{1}{n-p} \sum_{j=1}^n [\vec{y}_j - \vec{f}(t_j, \hat{\theta})][\vec{y}_j - \vec{f}(t_j, \hat{\theta})]^T \right). \tag{29}$$

However, the estimate $\hat{\theta}$ requires the (generally unknown) matrix V_0 and V_0 requires the unknown vector $\vec{\theta}_0$ so we will instead use the following expressions to calculate $\hat{\theta}$ and $\hat{V}$:

$$\vec{\theta}_0 \approx \hat{\theta} = \arg\min_{\theta \in \Theta} \sum_{j=1}^n [\vec{y}_j - \vec{f}(t_j, \vec{\theta})]^T \hat{V}^{-1} [\vec{y}_j - \vec{f}(t_j, \vec{\theta})] \tag{30}$$

$$V_0 \approx \hat{V} = \mathrm{diag}\left(\frac{1}{n-p} \sum_{j=1}^n [\vec{y}_j - \vec{f}(t_j, \hat{\theta})][\vec{y}_j - \vec{f}(t_j, \hat{\theta})]^T \right). \tag{31}$$

Note that the expressions for $\hat{\theta}$ and $\hat{V}$ constitute a coupled system of equations, which will require greater effort in implementing a numerical scheme.

Just as in the scalar case we can determine the asymptotic properties of the OLS estimator (27). As $n \to \infty$, θ_{OLS} has the following asymptotic properties [22, 31]:

$$\theta_{\mathrm{OLS}} \sim \mathcal{N}(\vec{\theta}_0, \Sigma_0^n), \tag{32}$$

where

$$\Sigma_0^n \approx \left(\sum_{j=1}^{n} D_j^T(\vec{\theta}_0) V_0^{-1} D_j(\vec{\theta}_0) \right)^{-1}, \tag{33}$$

and the $m \times p$ matrix $D_j(\vec{\theta}) = D_j^n(\vec{\theta})$ is given by

$$\begin{pmatrix} \dfrac{\partial f_1(t_j, \vec{\theta})}{\partial \theta_1} & \dfrac{\partial f_1(t_j, \vec{\theta})}{\partial \theta_2} & \cdots & \dfrac{\partial f_1(t_j, \vec{\theta})}{\partial \theta_p} \\ \vdots & \vdots & & \vdots \\ \dfrac{\partial f_m(t_j, \vec{\theta})}{\partial \theta_1} & \dfrac{\partial f_m(t_j, \vec{\theta})}{\partial \theta_2} & \cdots & \dfrac{\partial f_m(t_j, \vec{\theta})}{\partial \theta_p} \end{pmatrix}.$$

Since the true value of the parameters $\vec{\theta}_0$ and V_0 are unknown their estimates $\hat{\theta}$ and $\hat{V}$ will be used to approximate the asymptotic properties of the least squares estimator θ_{OLS}:

$$\theta_{\text{OLS}} \sim \mathcal{N}_p(\vec{\theta}_0, \Sigma_0^n) \approx \mathcal{N}_p(\hat{\theta}, \hat{\Sigma}^n) \tag{34}$$

where

$$\Sigma_0^n \approx \hat{\Sigma}^n = \left(\sum_{j=1}^{n} D_j^T(\hat{\theta}) \hat{V}^{-1} D_j(\hat{\theta}) \right)^{-1}. \tag{35}$$

The standard errors can then be calculated for the kth element of $\hat{\theta}_{\text{OLS}}$ ($SE(\hat{\theta}_{\text{OLS},k})$) by $SE(\hat{\theta}_{\text{OLS},k}) \approx \sqrt{\hat{\Sigma}_{kk}}$. Again, we point out the similarity between the MLE Equations (12) and (13), and the OLS Equations (30) and (31) for the vector statistical model (25).

2.3.2 Numerical Implementation of the OLS Procedure

In the scalar statistical model (14), the estimates $\hat{\theta}$ and $\hat{\sigma}$ can be solved for separately (this is also true of the vector OLS in the case $V_0 = \sigma_0^2 I_m$, where I_m is the $m \times m$ identity) and thus the numerical implementation is straightforward – first determine $\hat{\theta}_{\text{OLS}}$ according to (22) and then calculate $\hat{\sigma}_{\text{OLS}}^2$ according to (23). The estimates $\hat{\theta}$ and $\hat{V}$ in the case of the vector statistical model (25), however, require more effort since they are coupled:

$$\hat{\theta} = \arg\min_{\vec{\theta} \in \Theta} \sum_{j=1}^{n} [\vec{y}_j - \vec{f}(t_j, \vec{\theta})]^T \hat{V}^{-1} [\vec{y}_j - \vec{f}(t_j, \vec{\theta})] \tag{36}$$

$$\hat{V} = \text{diag} \left(\frac{1}{n-p} \sum_{j=1}^{n} [\vec{y}_j - \vec{f}(t_j, \hat{\theta})][\vec{y}_j - \vec{f}(t_j, \hat{\theta})]^T \right). \tag{37}$$

To solve this coupled system the following iterative process will be followed:

1. Set $\hat{V}^{(0)} = \mathbf{I}$ and solve for the initial estimate $\hat{\theta}^{(0)}$ using (36). Set $k = 0$.
2. Use $\hat{\theta}^{(k)}$ to calculate $\hat{V}^{(k+1)}$ using (37).
3. Re-estimate $\vec{\theta}$ by solving (36) with $\hat{V} = \hat{V}^{(k+1)}$ to obtain $\hat{\theta}^{(k+1)}$.
4. Set $k = k + 1$ and return to 2. Terminate the process and set $\hat{\theta}_{\text{OLS}} = \hat{\theta}^{(k+1)}$ when two successive estimates for $\hat{\theta}$ are sufficiently close to one another.

2.3.3 Generalized Least Squares (GLS)

Although in Section 2.3.1 the error's distribution remained unspecified, we did however require that the error remain constant in variance in longitudinal data. That assumption may not be appropriate for data sets whose error is not constant in a longitudinal sense. A common *relative error* model (e.g., one in which the size of the observation error is assumed proportional to the size of the observed quantity, an assumption which might be reasonable when counting individuals in a population) that experimenters use in this instance for the scalar observation case [22] is

$$Y_j = f(t_j, \vec{\theta}_0)\left(1 + \epsilon_j\right) \tag{38}$$

where $E(Y_j) = f(t_j, \vec{\theta}_0)$ and $\text{var}(Y_j) = \sigma_0^2 f^2(t_j, \vec{\theta}_0)$ which derives from the assumptions that $E[\epsilon_j] = 0$ and $\text{var}(\epsilon_j) = \sigma_0^2$. We see that the variance generated in this fashion is model dependent and hence generally is longitudinally non-constant variance. The method we will use to estimate $\vec{\theta}_0$ and σ_0^2 can be viewed as a particular form of the Generalized Least Squares (GLS) method.

To define the *random variable* θ_{GLS} the following equation must be solved for the estimator θ_{GLS}:

$$\sum_{j=1}^{n} w_j[Y_j - f(t_j, \theta_{\text{GLS}})]\nabla f(t_j, \theta_{\text{GLS}}) = 0, \tag{39}$$

where Y_j obeys (38) and $w_j = f^{-2}(t_j, \theta_{\text{GLS}})$. We note these are the normal equations (obtained by equating to zero the gradient of the weighted least squares criterion in the case the weights w_j are not dependent on θ). The quantity θ_{GLS} is a random variable, hence if $\{y_j\}_{j=1}^{n}$ is a *realization* of the random process Y_j then solving

$$\sum_{j=1}^{n} f^{-2}(t_j, \hat{\theta})[y_j - f(t_j, \hat{\theta})]\nabla f(t_j, \hat{\theta}) = 0, \tag{40}$$

for $\hat{\theta}$ we obtain an estimate $\hat{\theta}_{\text{GLS}}$ for θ_{GLS}.

The GLS estimator $\theta_{\text{GLS}} = \theta_{\text{GLS}}^n$ has the following asymptotic properties [22]:

$$\theta_{\text{GLS}} \sim \mathcal{N}_p(\vec{\theta}_0, \Sigma_0^n) \tag{41}$$

where

$$\Sigma_0^n \approx \sigma_0^2 \left(F_{\vec{\theta}}^T(\vec{\theta}_0) W(\vec{\theta}_0) F_{\vec{\theta}}(\vec{\theta}_0) \right)^{-1}, \tag{42}$$

$$F_{\vec{\theta}}(\vec{\theta}) = F_{\vec{\theta}}^n(\vec{\theta}) = \begin{pmatrix} \dfrac{\partial f(t_1, \vec{\theta})}{\partial \theta_1} & \dfrac{\partial f(t_1, \vec{\theta})}{\partial \theta_2} & \cdots & \dfrac{\partial f(t_1, \vec{\theta})}{\partial \theta_p} \\ \vdots & & & \vdots \\ \dfrac{\partial f(t_n, \vec{\theta})}{\partial \theta_1} & \dfrac{\partial f(t_n, \vec{\theta})}{\partial \theta_2} & \cdots & \dfrac{\partial f(t_n, \vec{\theta})}{\partial \theta_p} \end{pmatrix} = \begin{pmatrix} \nabla f(t_1, \vec{\theta})^T \\ \vdots \\ \nabla f(t_n, \vec{\theta})^T \end{pmatrix}$$

and $W^{-1}(\vec{\theta}) = \text{diag}\left(f^2(t_1, \vec{\theta}), \ldots, f^2(t_n, \vec{\theta}) \right)$. Note that because $\vec{\theta}_0$ and σ_0^2 are unknown, the estimates $\hat{\theta} = \hat{\theta}_{\text{GLS}}$ and $\hat{\sigma}^2 = \hat{\sigma}_{\text{GLS}}^2$ will be used in (42) to calculate

$$\Sigma_0^n \approx \hat{\Sigma}^n = \hat{\sigma}^2 \left(F_{\vec{\theta}}^T(\hat{\theta}) W(\hat{\theta}) F_{\vec{\theta}}(\hat{\theta}) \right)^{-1},$$

where [22] we take the approximation

$$\sigma_0^2 \approx \hat{\sigma}_{\text{GLS}}^2 = \frac{1}{n - p} \sum_{j=1}^{n} \frac{1}{f^2(t_j, \hat{\theta})} [y_j - f(t_j, \hat{\theta})]^2.$$

We can then approximate the standard errors of $\hat{\theta}_{\text{GLS}}$ by taking the square roots of the diagonal elements of $\hat{\Sigma}$. We will also mention that the solutions to (30) and (40) depend upon the numerical method used to find the minimum or root, and since Σ_0 depends upon the estimate for $\vec{\theta}_0$, the standard errors are therefore affected by the numerical method chosen.

2.3.4 GLS Motivation

We note the similarity between (16) and (40). The GLS Equation (40) can be motivated by examining the weighted least squares (WLS) estimator

$$\theta_{\text{WLS}} = \arg\min_{\vec{\theta} \in \Theta} \sum_{j=1}^{n} w_j [Y_j - f(t_j, \vec{\theta})]^2. \tag{43}$$

In many situations where the observation process is well understood, the weights $\{w_j\}$ may be known. The WLS estimate can be thought of minimizing the distance between the data and model while taking into account unequal quality of the observations [22]. If we differentiate the sum of squares in (43) with respect to $\vec{\theta}$, and *then* choose $w_j = f^{-2}(t_j, \vec{\theta})$, an estimate $\hat{\theta}_{\text{GLS}}$ is obtained by solving

$$\sum_{j=1}^{n} w_j [y_j - f(t_j, \vec{\theta})] \nabla f(t_j, \vec{\theta}) = 0$$

for $\vec{\theta}$. However, we note the GLS relationship (40) does *not* follow from minimizing the weighted least squares with weights chosen as $w_j = f^{-2}(t_j, \vec{\theta})$.

Another motivation for the GLS estimating Equation (40) can be found in [18]. In the text the authors claim that if the data are distributed according to the gamma distribution, then the maximum-likelihood estimator for $\vec{\theta}$ is the solution to

$$\sum_{j=1}^{n} f^{-2}(t_j, \vec{\theta})[Y_j - f(t_j, \vec{\theta})]\nabla f(t_j, \vec{\theta}) = 0,$$

which is equivalent to (40). The connection between the MLE and our GLS method is reassuring, but it also poses another interesting question: What if the variance of the data is assumed to not depend on the model output $f(t_j, \vec{\theta})$, but rather on some function $g(t_j, \vec{\theta})$ (i.e., $\text{var}(Y_j) = \sigma_0^2 g^2(t_j, \vec{\theta}) = \sigma_0^2/w_j$)? Is there a corresponding maximum likelihood estimator of $\vec{\theta}$ whose form is equivalent to the appropriate GLS estimating equation ($w_j = g^{-2}(t_j, \vec{\theta})$)

$$\sum_{j=1}^{n} g^{-2}(t_j, \vec{\theta})[Y_j - f(t_j, \vec{\theta})]\nabla f(t_j, \vec{\theta}) = 0 \ ? \tag{44}$$

In their text, Carroll and Rupert [18] briefly describe how distributions belonging to the exponential family of distributions generate maximum-likelihood estimating equations equivalent to (44).

2.3.5 Numerical Implementation of the GLS Procedure

Recall that an estimate $\hat{\theta}_{\text{GLS}}$ can either be solved for directly according to (40) or iteratively using the equations outlined in Section 2.3.3. The iterative procedure as described in [22] is summarized below:

1. Estimate $\hat{\theta}_{\text{GLS}}$ by $\hat{\theta}^{(0)}$ using the OLS Equation (15). Set $k = 0$.
2. Form the weights $\hat{w}_j = f^{-2}(t_j, \hat{\theta}^{(k)})$.
3. Re-estimate $\hat{\theta}$ by solving

$$\hat{\theta}^{(k+1)} = \arg\min_{\theta \in \Theta} \sum_{j=1}^{n} \hat{w}_j \left(y_j - f(t_j, \vec{\theta})\right)^2$$

   to obtain the $k + 1$ estimate $\hat{\theta}^{(k+1)}$ for $\hat{\theta}_{\text{GLS}}$.
4. Set $k = k + 1$ and return to 2. Terminate the process when two of the successive estimates for $\hat{\theta}_{\text{GLS}}$ are sufficiently close.

We note that the above iterative procedure was formulated by minimizing (over $\vec{\theta} \in \Theta$)

$$\sum_{j=1}^{n} f^{-2}(t_j, \tilde{\theta})[y_j - f(t_j, \vec{\theta})]^2$$

and then updating the weights $w_j = f^{-2}(t_j, \tilde{\theta})$ after each iteration. One would hope that after a sufficient number of iterations $\hat{w}_j$ would converge to $f^{-2}(t_j, \hat{\theta}_{\mathrm{GLS}})$. Fortunately, under reasonable conditions, if the process enumerated above is continued a sufficient number of times [22], then $\hat{w}_j \rightarrow f^{-2}(t_j, \hat{\theta}_{\mathrm{GLS}})$.

3 Computation of $\hat{\Sigma}^n$, Standard Errors and Confidence Intervals

We return to the case of n scalar longitudinal observations and consider the OLS case of Section 2.3.1 (the extension of these ideas to vectors is completely straightforward). These n scalar observations are represented by the statistical model

$$Y_j \equiv f(t_j, \vec{\theta}_0) + \epsilon_j, \quad j = 1, 2, \ldots, n, \tag{45}$$

where $f(t_j, \vec{\theta}_0)$ is the model for the observations in terms of the state variables and $\vec{\theta}_0 \in \mathbb{R}^p$ is a set of theoretical "true" parameter values (assumed to exist in a standard statistical approach). We further assume that the errors ϵ_j, $j = 1, 2, \ldots, n$, are independent identically distributed (*i.i.d.*) random variables with mean $E[\epsilon_j] = 0$ and constant variance $\mathrm{var}(\epsilon_j) = \sigma_0^2$, where σ_0^2 is unknown. The observations Y_j are then *i.i.d.* with mean $E[Y_j] = f(t_j, \vec{\theta}_0)$ and variance $\mathrm{var}(Y_j) = \sigma_0^2$.

Recall that in the ordinary least squares (OLS) approach, we seek to use a realization $\{y_j\}$ of the observation process $\{Y_j\}$ along with the model to determine a vector $\hat{\theta}_{\mathrm{OLS}}^n$ where

$$\hat{\theta}_{\mathrm{OLS}}^n = \arg \min J_n(\vec{\theta}) = \sum_{j=1}^n [y_j - f(t_j, \vec{\theta})]^2. \tag{46}$$

Since Y_j is a random variable, the corresponding estimator $\theta^n = \theta_{\mathrm{OLS}}^n$ (here we wish to emphasize the dependence on the sample size n) is also a random variable with a distribution called the *sampling distribution*. Knowledge of this sampling distribution provides uncertainty information (e.g., standard errors) for the numerical values of $\hat{\theta}^n$ obtained using a specific data set $\{y_j\}$. In particular, loosely speaking the sampling distribution characterizes the distribution of possible values the estimator could take on across all possible realizations with data of size n that could be collected. The standard errors thus approximate the extent of variability in possible values across all possible realizations, and hence provide a measure of the extent of uncertainty involved in estimating θ using the specific estimator and sample size n in actual data collection.

Under reasonable assumptions on smoothness and regularity (the smoothness requirements for model solutions are readily verified using continuous dependence results for differential equations in most examples; the regularity requirements include, among others, conditions on *how the observations are taken* as sample size increases, i.e., as $n \to \infty$), the standard nonlinear regression approximation theory ([22, 26, 29], and Chapter 12 of [31]) for *asymptotic* (as $n \to \infty$) *distributions* can be invoked. As stated above, this theory yields that the sampling distribution for the estimator $\theta^n(\vec{Y})$, where $\vec{Y} = (Y_1, \ldots, Y_n)^T$, is approximately a p-multivariate Gaussian with mean $E[\theta^n(\vec{Y})] \approx \vec{\theta}_0$ and covariance matrix $\mathrm{var}(\theta^n(\vec{Y})) \approx \Sigma_0^n = \sigma_0^2[n\Omega_0]^{-1} \approx \sigma_0^2[\chi^{nT}(\vec{\theta}_0)\chi^n(\vec{\theta}_0)]^{-1}$. Here $\chi^n(\vec{\theta}) = F_{\vec{\theta}}(\vec{\theta})$ is the $n \times p$ sensitivity matrix with elements

$$\chi_{jk}(\vec{\theta}) = \frac{\partial f(t_j, \vec{\theta})}{\partial \theta_k} \quad \text{and} \quad F_{\vec{\theta}}(\vec{\theta}) \equiv (f_{1\vec{\theta}}(\vec{\theta}), \ldots, f_{n\vec{\theta}}(\vec{\theta}))^T,$$

where $f_{j\vec{\theta}}(\vec{\theta}) = \frac{\partial f}{\partial \vec{\theta}}(t_j, \vec{\theta})$. That is, for n large, the sampling distribution approximately satisfies

$$\theta_{\mathrm{OLS}}^n(\vec{Y}) \sim \mathcal{N}_p(\vec{\theta}_0, \Sigma_0^n) \approx \mathcal{N}_p(\vec{\theta}_0, \sigma_0^2[\chi^{nT}(\vec{\theta}_0)\chi^n(\vec{\theta}_0)]^{-1}). \tag{47}$$

There are typically several ways to compute the matrix $F_{\vec{\theta}}$ (which are actually the well known sensitivity functions widely used in applied mathematics and engineering–see the discussions in Section 6 below). First, the elements of the matrix $\chi = (\chi_{jk})$ can always be estimated using the forward difference

$$\chi_{jk}(\vec{\theta}) = \frac{\partial f(t_j, \vec{\theta})}{\partial \theta_k} \approx \frac{f(t_j, \vec{\theta} + h_k) - f(t_j, \vec{\theta})}{|h_k|},$$

where h_k is a p-vector with a nonzero entry in only the kth component. But, of course, the choice of h_k can be problematic in practice.

Alternatively, if the $f(t_j, \vec{\theta})$ correspond to longitudinal observations $\vec{y}(t_j) = C\vec{x}(t_j; \vec{\theta})$ of solutions $\vec{x} \in \mathbb{R}^N$ to a parameterized N-vector differential equation system $\dot{\vec{x}} = \vec{g}(t, \vec{x}(t), \vec{\theta})$ as in (1), then one can use the $N \times p$ matrix *sensitivity equations* (see [4, 9] and the references therein)

$$\frac{d}{dt}\left(\frac{\partial \vec{x}}{\partial \vec{\theta}}\right) = \frac{\partial \vec{g}}{\partial \vec{x}}\frac{\partial \vec{x}}{\partial \vec{\theta}} + \frac{\partial \vec{g}}{\partial \vec{\theta}} \tag{48}$$

to obtain

$$\frac{\partial f(t_j, \vec{\theta})}{\partial \theta_k} = C\frac{\partial \vec{x}(t_j, \vec{\theta})}{\partial \theta_k}.$$

Finally, in some cases the function $f(t_j, \vec{\theta})$ may be sufficiently simple so as to allow one to derive analytical expressions for the components of $F_{\vec{\theta}}$.

Since $\vec{\theta}_0, \sigma_0$ are unknown, we will use their estimates to make the approximation

$$\Sigma_0^n \approx \sigma_0^2[\chi^{nT}(\vec{\theta}_0)\chi^n(\vec{\theta}_0)]^{-1} \approx \hat{\Sigma}^n(\hat{\theta}_{\mathrm{OLS}}^n) = \hat{\sigma}^2[\chi^{nT}(\hat{\theta}_{\mathrm{OLS}}^n)\chi^n(\hat{\theta}_{\mathrm{OLS}}^n)]^{-1}, \tag{49}$$

where the approximation $\hat{\sigma}^2$ to σ_0^2, as discussed earlier, is given by

$$\sigma_0^2 \approx \hat{\sigma}^2 = \frac{1}{n-p} \sum_{j=1}^{n} [y_j - f(t_j, \hat{\theta}_{\text{OLS}}^n)]^2. \tag{50}$$

Standard errors to be used in the confidence interval calculations are thus given by $SE_k(\hat{\theta}^n) = \sqrt{\Sigma_{kk}(\hat{\theta}^n)}$, $k = 1, 2, \ldots, p$ (see [19]).

In order to compute the confidence intervals (at the $100(1 - \alpha)\%$ level) for the estimated parameters in our example, we define the confidence level parameters associated with the estimated parameters so that

$$P\{\theta_k^n - t_{1-\alpha/2} SE_k(\theta^n) < \theta_{0k} < \theta_k^n + t_{1-\alpha/2} SE_k(\theta^n)\} = 1 - \alpha, \tag{51}$$

where $\alpha \in [0, 1]$ and $t_{1-\alpha/2} \in \mathbb{R}_+$. Given a small α value (e.g., $\alpha = .05$ for 95% confidence intervals), the critical value $t_{1-\alpha/2}$ is computed from the Student's t distribution t^{n-p} with $n - p$ degrees of freedom. The value of $t_{1-\alpha/2}$ is determined by $P\{T \geq t_{1-\alpha/2}\} = \alpha/2$ where $T \sim t^{n-p}$. In general, a confidence interval is constructed so that, if the confidence interval could be constructed for each possible realization of data of size n that could have been collected, $100(1 - \alpha)\%$ of the intervals so constructed would contain the true value θ_{0k}. Thus, a confidence interval provides further information on the extent of uncertainty involved in estimating θ_0 using the given estimator and sample size n.

When one is taking longitudinal samples corresponding to solutions of a dynamical system, the $n \times p$ sensitivity matrix depends explicitly on where in time the observations are taken when $f(t_j, \vec{\theta}) = Cx(t_j, \vec{\theta})$ as mentioned above. That is, the sensitivity matrix

$$\chi(\vec{\theta}) = F_{\vec{\theta}}(\vec{\theta}) = \left(\frac{\partial f(t_j, \vec{\theta})}{\partial \theta_k} \right)$$

depends on the number n and the nature (for example, how taken) of the sampling times $\{t_j\}$. Moreover, it is the matrix $[\chi^T \chi]^{-1}$ in (49) and the parameter $\hat{\sigma}^2$ in (50) that ultimately determine the standard errors and confidence intervals. At first investigation of (50), it appears that an increased number n of samples might drive $\hat{\sigma}^2$ (and hence the SE) to zero as long as this is done in a way to maintain a bound on the residual sum of squares in (50). However, we observe that the *condition number* of the matrix $\chi^T \chi$ is also very important in these considerations and increasing the sampling could potentially adversely affect the inversion of $\chi^T \chi$. In this regard, we note that among the important hypotheses in the asymptotic statistical theory (see p. 571 of [31]) is the existence of a matrix function $\Omega(\vec{\theta})$ such that

$$\frac{1}{n} \chi^{nT}(\vec{\theta}) \chi^n(\vec{\theta}) \to \Omega(\vec{\theta}) \quad \text{uniformly in } \vec{\theta} \text{ as } n \to \infty,$$

with $\Omega_0 = \Omega(\vec{\theta}_0)$ a **nonsingular** matrix. It is this condition that is rather easily violated in practice when one is dealing with data from differential equation systems, especially near an equilibrium or steady state (see the examples of [4]).

All of the above theory readily generalizes to vector systems with partial, non-scalar observations. Suppose now we have the vector system (1) with partial vector observations given by Equation (3), that is, we have m coordinate observations where $m \leq N$. In this case, we have

$$\frac{d\vec{x}}{dt}(t) = \vec{g}(t, \vec{x}(t), \vec{\theta}) \tag{52}$$

and

$$\vec{y}_j = \vec{f}(t_j, \vec{\theta}_0) + \vec{\epsilon}_j = C\vec{x}(t_j, \vec{\theta}_0) + \vec{\epsilon}_j, \tag{53}$$

where C is an $m \times N$ matrix and $\vec{f} \in R^m$, $\vec{x} \in R^N$. As already explained in Section 2.3.1, if we assume that different observation coordinates f_i may have different variances σ_i^2 associated with different coordinates of the errors ϵ_j, then we have that $\vec{\epsilon}_j$ is an m-dimensional random vector with

$$E[\vec{\epsilon}_j] = 0, \quad \mathrm{var}(\vec{\epsilon}_j) = V_0,$$

where $V_0 = \mathrm{diag}(\sigma_{0,1}^2, ..., \sigma_{0,m}^2)$, and we may follow a similar asymptotic theory to calculate approximate covariances, standard errors and confidence intervals for parameter estimates.

Since the computations for standard errors and confidence intervals (and also *model comparison tests*) depend on *an asymptotic limit distribution theory*, one should interpret the findings as sometimes crude indicators of uncertainty inherent in the inverse problem findings. Nonetheless, it is useful to consider the formal mathematical requirements underpinning these techniques.

Among the more readily checked hypotheses are those of the statistical model requiring that the errors ϵ_j, $j = 1, 2, \ldots, n$, are independent and identically distributed (*i.i.d.*) random variables with mean $E[\epsilon_j] = 0$ and constant variance $\mathrm{var}(\epsilon_j) = \sigma_0^2$.

- After carrying out the estimation procedures, one can readily plot the *residuals* $r_j = y_j - f(t_j, \hat{\theta}_{\mathrm{OLS}}^n)$ vs. time t_j and the *residuals vs. the resulting estimated model/observation* $f(t_j, \hat{\theta}_{\mathrm{OLS}}^n)$ *values*. A random pattern for the first is strong support for validity of independence assumption; a non increasing, random pattern for latter suggests assumption of constant variance may be reasonable.
- The underlying assumption that sampling size n must be large (recall the theory is asymptotic in that it holds as $n \to \infty$) is not so readily "verified"–often ignored (albeit at the user's peril in regard to the quality of the uncertainty findings).

Often asymptotic results provide remarkably good approximations to the true sampling distributions for finite n. However, in practice there is no way to ascertain whether theory holds for a specific example.

4 Investigation of Statistical Assumptions

The form of error in the data (which of course is rarely known) dictates which method from those discussed above one should choose. The OLS method is most appropriate for constant variance observations of the form $Y_j = f(t_j, \vec{\theta}_0) + \epsilon_j$ whereas the GLS should be used for problems in which we have nonconstant variance observations $Y_j = f(t_j, \vec{\theta}_0)(1 + \epsilon_j)$.

We emphasize that in order to obtain *the correct standard errors* in an inverse problem calculation, the OLS method (and *corresponding asymptotic formulas*) must be used with constant variance generated data, while the GLS method (and *corresponding asymptotic formulas*) should be applied to nonconstant variance generated data.

Not doing so can lead to incorrect conclusions. In either case, the standard error calculations are not valid unless the correct formulas (which depends on the error structure) are employed. Unfortunately, it is very difficult to ascertain the structure of the error, and hence the correct method to use, without a priori information. Although the error structure cannot definitively be determined, the two residuals tests can be performed *after* the estimation procedure has been completed to assist in concluding whether or not the correct asymptotic statistics were used.

4.1 Residual Plots

One can carry out simulation studies with a proposed mathematical model to assist in understanding the behavior of the model in inverse problems with different types of data with respect to mis-specification of the statistical model. For example, we consider a statistical model with constant variance noise

$$Y_j = f(t_j, \vec{\theta}_0) + \frac{k}{100}\epsilon_j, \qquad \mathrm{Var}(Y_j) = \frac{k^2}{10000}\sigma^2,$$

and nonconstant variance noise

$$Y_j = f(t_j, \vec{\theta}_0)\left(1 + \frac{k}{100}\epsilon_j\right), \qquad \mathrm{Var}(Y_j) = \frac{k^2}{10000}\sigma^2 f^2(t_j, \vec{\theta}_0).$$

We can obtain a data set by considering a *realization* $\{y_j\}_{j=1}^n$ of the random process $\{Y_j\}_{j=1}^n$ through a realization of $\{\epsilon_j\}_{j=1}^n$ and then calculate an estimate $\hat{\theta}$ of $\vec{\theta}_0$ using the OLS or GLS procedure.

We will then use the *residuals* $r_j = y_j - f(t_j, \hat{\theta})$ to test whether the data set is *i.i.d.* and possesses the assumed variance structure. If a data set has constant variance error then

$$Y_j = f(t_j, \vec{\theta}_0) + \epsilon_j \quad \text{or} \quad \epsilon_j = Y_j - f(t_j, \vec{\theta}_0).$$

Since it is assumed that the error ϵ_j is *i.i.d.* a plot of the residuals $r_j = y_j - f(t_j, \hat{\theta})$ vs. t_j should be random. Also, the error in the constant variance case does not depend on $f(t_j, \theta_0)$, and so a plot of the residuals $r_j = y_j - f(t_j, \hat{\theta})$ vs. $f(t_j, \hat{\theta})$ should also be random. Therefore, *if* the error has constant variance then a plot of the residuals $r_j = y_j - f(t_j, \hat{\theta})$ against t_j and against $f(t_j, \hat{\theta})$) should both be random. If not, then the constant variance assumption is suspect.

We turn next to questions of what to expect if this residual test is applied to a data set that has nonconstant variance generated error. That is, we wish to investigate what happens if the data are incorrectly assumed to have constant variance error when in fact they have nonconstant variance error. Since in the nonconstant variance example, $R_j = Y_j - f(t_j, \vec{\theta}_0) = f(t_j, \vec{\theta}_0)\epsilon_j$ depends upon the deterministic model $f(t_j, \vec{\theta}_0)$, we should expect that a plot of the residuals $r_j = y_j - f(t_j, \hat{\theta})$ vs. t_j should exhibit some type of pattern. Also, the residuals actually depend on $f(t_j, \hat{\theta})$ in the nonconstant variance case, and so as $f(t_j, \hat{\theta})$ increases the variation of the residuals $r_j = y_j - f(t_j, \hat{\theta})$ should increase as well. Thus $r_j = y_j - f(t_j, \hat{\theta})$ vs. $f(t_j, \hat{\theta})$ should have a fan shape in the nonconstant variance case.

In summary, if a data set has nonconstant variance generated data, then

$$Y_j = f(t_j, \vec{\theta}_0) + f(t_j, \vec{\theta}_0)\epsilon_j \quad \text{or} \quad \epsilon_j = \frac{Y_j - f(t_j, \vec{\theta}_0)}{f(t_j, \vec{\theta}_0)}.$$

If the distribution ϵ_j is *i.i.d.*, then a plot of the *modified residuals* $r_j^m = (y_j - f(t_j, \hat{\theta}))/f(t_j, \hat{\theta})$ vs. t_j should be random in nonconstant variance generated data. A plot of $r_j^m = (y_j - f(t_j, \hat{\theta}))/f(t_j, \hat{\theta})$ vs. $f(t_j, \hat{\theta})$ should also be random.

Another question of interest concerns the case in which the data are incorrectly assumed to have nonconstant variance error when in fact they have constant variance error. Since $Y_j - f(t_j, \vec{\theta}_0) = \epsilon_j$ in the constant variance case, we should expect that a plot of $r_j^m = (y_j - f(t_j, \hat{\theta}))/f(t_j, \hat{\theta})$ vs. t_j as well as that for $r_j^m = (y_j - f(t_j, \hat{\theta}))/f(t_j, \hat{\theta})$ vs. $f(t_j, \hat{\theta})$ will possess some distinct pattern.

Two further issues regarding residual plots: As we shall see by examples, some data sets might have values that are repeated or nearly repeated a large number of times (for example when sampling near an equilibrium for the mathematical model or when sampling a periodic system over many periods). If a certain value is repeated numerous times (e.g., f_{repeat}) then any plot with $f(t_j, \hat{\theta})$ along the horizontal axis should have a cluster of values along the vertical line $x = f_{\text{repeat}}$. This feature can easily be removed by excluding the data points corresponding to these high frequency values (or simply excluding the corresponding points in the residual plots). Another common technique when plotting against model predictions is to plot against $\log f(t_j, \hat{\theta})$ instead of $f(t_j, \hat{\theta})$ itself which has the effect of "stretching out" plots at the ends. Also, note that the model value $f(t_j, \hat{\theta})$ could possibly be zero or very near zero, in which case the modified residuals $R_j^m = \frac{Y_j - f(t_j, \hat{\theta})}{f(t_j, \hat{\theta})}$ would be undefined or extremely large. To remedy this situation one might exclude values very close to zero (in either the plots or in the data themselves). We chose here to reduce the data sets (although this sometimes could lead to a deterioration in the estimation results obtained). In our examples below, estimates obtained using a truncated data set will be denoted by $\hat{\theta}_{OLS}^{tcv}$ for constant variance data and $\hat{\theta}_{OLS}^{tncv}$ for nonconstant variance data.

4.2 Example Using Residual Plots

We illustrate residual plot techniques by exploring a widely studied model – the logistic population growth model of Verhulst/Pearl

$$\dot{x} = rx(1 - \frac{x}{K}), \quad x(0) = x_0. \tag{54}$$

Here K is the population's carrying capacity, r is the intrinsic growth rate and x_0 is the initial population size. This well-known logistic model describes how populations grow when constrained by resources or competition. The closed form solution of this simple model is given by

$$x(t) = \frac{K x_0 e^{rt}}{K + x_0 (e^{rt} - 1)}. \tag{55}$$

The left plot in Fig. 1 depicts the solution of the logistic model for $K = 17.5, r = .7$ and $x_0 = 1$ for $0 \le t \le 25$. If high frequency repeated or nearly repeated values (i.e., near the initial value x_0 or near the asymptote $x = K$) are removed from the original plot, the resulting truncated plot is given in the right panel of Fig. 1 (there are no near zero values for this function).

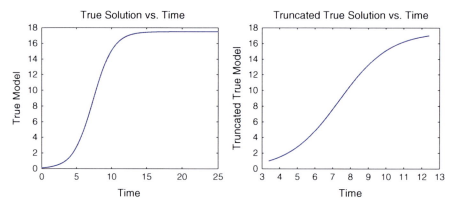

Fig. 1 Original and truncated logistic curve with $K = 17.5, r = .7$ and $x_0 = .1$

Table 1 Estimation using the OLS procedure with constant variance data for $k = 5$

k	$\vec{\theta}_{init}$	$\vec{\theta}_0$	$\hat{\theta}_{OLS}^{cv}$	$SE(\hat{\theta}_{OLS}^{cv})$	$\hat{\theta}_{OLS}^{tcv}$	$SE(\hat{\theta}_{OLS}^{tcv})$
5	17	17.5	1.7500e+001	1.5800e−003	1.7494e+001	6.4215e−003
5	.8	.7	7.0018e−001	4.2841e−004	7.0062e−001	6.5796e−004
5	1.2	.1	9.9958e−002	3.1483e−004	9.9702e−002	4.3898e−004

Table 2 Estimation using the GLS procedure with constant variance data for $k = 5$

k	$\vec{\theta}_{init}$	$\vec{\theta}_0$	$\hat{\theta}_{GLS}^{cv}$	$SE(\hat{\theta}_{GLS}^{cv})$	$\hat{\theta}_{GLS}^{tcv}$	$SE(\hat{\theta}_{GLS}^{tcv})$
5	17	17.5	1.7500e+001	1.3824e−004	1.7494e+001	9.1213e−005
5	.8	.7	7.0021e−001	7.8139e−005	7.0060e−001	1.6009e−005
5	1.2	.1	9.9938e−002	6.6068e−005	9.9718e−002	1.2130e−005

For this example we generated both constant variance and nonconstant variance noisy data (we sampled from $\mathcal{N}(0, 1)$ random variables to obtain realizations of ϵ_j) and obtained estimates $\hat{\theta}$ of $\vec{\theta}_0 = (K, r, x_0)$ by applying either the OLS or GLS method to a realization $\{y_j\}_{j=1}^n$ of the random process $\{Y_j\}_{j=1}^n$. The initial guesses $\vec{\theta}_{init} = \hat{\theta}^{(0)}$ along with estimates for each method and error structure are given in Tables 1-4 (the superscript tcv and tncv denote the estimate obtained using the truncated data set). As expected, both methods do a good job of estimating $\vec{\theta}_0$, however the error structure was not always correctly specified since incorrect asymptotic formulas were used in some cases.

When the OLS method was applied to nonconstant variance data and the GLS method was applied to constant variance data, the residual plots given below do reveal that the error structure was misspecified. For instance, the plot of the residuals for $\hat{\theta}_{OLS}^{ncv}$ given in Figs. 4 and 5 reveal a fan shaped pattern, which indicates the constant variance assumption is suspect. In addition, the plot of the residuals for $\hat{\theta}_{GLS}^{cv}$ given in Figs. 6 and 7 reveal an inverted fan shaped pattern, which indicates the nonconstant variance assumption is suspect. As expected, when the correct error

Table 3 Estimation using the OLS procedure with nonconstant variance data for $k = 5$

k	$\vec{\theta}_{init}$	$\vec{\theta}_0$	$\hat{\theta}_{OLS}^{ncv}$	$SE(\hat{\theta}_{OLS}^{ncv})$	$\hat{\theta}_{OLS}^{tncv}$	$SE(\hat{\theta}_{OLS}^{tncv})$
5	17	17.5	1.7499e+001	2.2678e−002	1.7411e+001	7.1584e−002
5	.8	.7	7.0192e−001	6.1770e−003	7.0955e−001	7.6039e−003
5	1.2	.1	9.9496e−002	4.5115e−003	9.4967e−002	4.8295e−003

Table 4 Estimation using the GLS procedure with nonconstant variance data for $k = 5$

k	$\vec{\theta}_{init}$	$\vec{\theta}_0$	$\hat{\theta}_{GLS}^{ncv}$	$SE(\hat{\theta}_{GLS}^{ncv})$	$\hat{\theta}_{GLS}^{tncv}$	$SE(\hat{\theta}_{GLS}^{tncv})$
5	17	17.5	1.7498e+001	9.4366e−005	1.7411e+001	3.1271e−004
5	.8	.7	7.0217e−001	5.3616e−005	7.0959e−001	5.7181e−005
5	1.2	.1	9.9314e−002	4.4976e−005	9.4944e−002	4.1205e−005

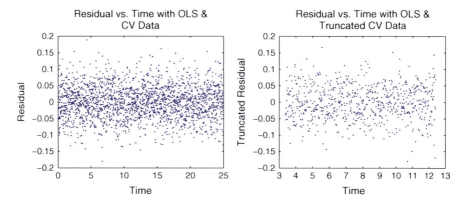

Fig. 2 Residual vs. time plots: Original and truncated logistic curve for $\hat{\theta}_{OLS}^{cv}$ with $k = 5$

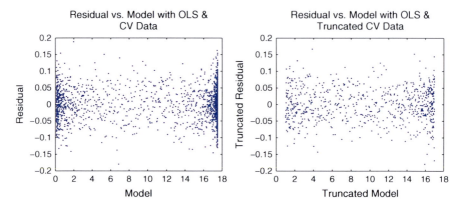

Fig. 3 Residual vs. model plots: Original and truncated logistic curve for $\hat{\theta}_{OLS}^{cv}$ with $k = 5$

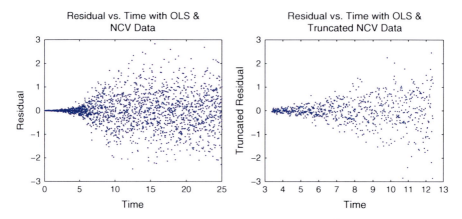

Fig. 4 Residual vs. time plots: Original and truncated logistic curve for $\hat{\theta}_{OLS}^{ncv}$ with $k = 5$

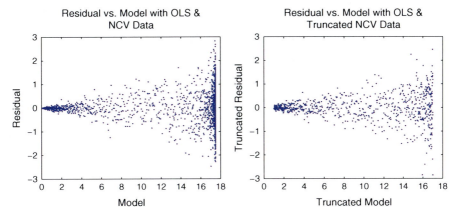

Fig. 5 Residual vs. model plots: Original and truncated logistic curve for $\hat{\theta}_{\mathrm{OLS}}^{ncv}$ with $k = 5$

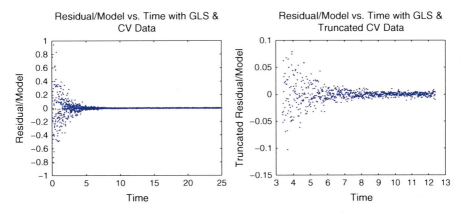

Fig. 6 Residual vs. time plots: Original and truncated logistic curve for $\hat{\theta}_{\mathrm{GLS}}^{cv}$ with $k = 5$

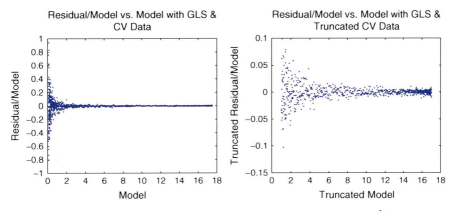

Fig. 7 Modified residual vs. model plots: Original and truncated logistic curve for $\hat{\theta}_{\mathrm{GLS}}^{cv}$ with $k = 5$

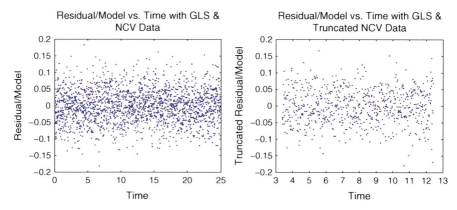

Fig. 8 Modified residual vs. time plots: Original and truncated logistic curve for $\hat{\theta}_{GLS}^{ncv}$ with $k = 5$

structure is specified, the *i.i.d.* test and the model dependence test each display a random pattern (Figs. 2, 3, 8, and 9).

Also, included in the right panel of Figs. 2–9 are the residual plots with the truncated data sets. In those plots only model values between one and seventeen were considered (i.e. $1 \leq y_j \leq 17$). Doing so removed the dense vertical lines in the plots with $f(t_j, \hat{\theta})$ along the x-axis. Nonetheless, the conclusions regarding the error structure remain the same.

In addition to the residual plots, we can also compare the standard errors obtained for each simulation. At a quick glance of Tables 1–4, the standard error of the parameter K in the truncated data set is larger than the standard error of K in the original data set. This behavior is expected. If we remove the "flat" region in the logistic curve, we actually discard measurements with high information content about the carrying capacity K [4]. Doing so reduces the quality of the estimator K. Another interesting observation is that the standard errors of the GLS estimate are

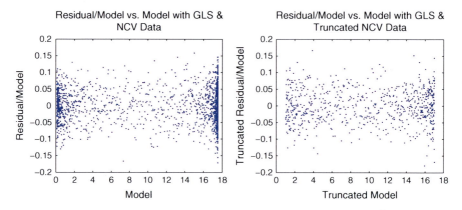

Fig. 9 Modified residual vs. model plots: Original and truncated logistic curve for $\hat{\theta}_{GLS}^{ncv}$ with $k = 5$

more optimistic than that of the OLS estimate, even when the non-constant variance assumption is wrong. This example further solidifies the conclusion we will make with the epidemiological model described below – before one reports an estimate and corresponding standard errors, there needs to be some assurance that the proper error structure has been specified.

5 Pneumococcal Disease Dynamics Model

To explore these ideas in the context of epidemiology, we discuss a population level model of pneumococcal disease dynamics as an example. This model has previously been applied to surveillance data available via the Australian National Notifiable Diseases Surveillance System in [32]. Monthly case notifications of invasive pneumococcal disease (IPD) and annual vaccination information were used to estimate unknown model parameters and to assess the impact of a newly implemented vaccination policy. Here we illustrate, with this example, the effects of incorrect versus correct statistical models assumed to represent observed data in reporting parameter values and their corresponding standard errors. Most importantly, we discuss relevant residual plots and how to use these to determine if reasonable assumptions on observed error have been made.

In this model, shown in Fig. 10, individuals are classified according to their epidemiological status with respect to invasive pneumococcal diseases, which include pneumonia, bacteremia, meningitis and are defined as the presence of *Streptococcus pneumoniae* in any normal sterile fluid in the body. Individuals are considered susceptible, or in the S class, in the absence of this bacteria. The E class represents individuals whose nasopharyngeal regions are asymptomatically colonized by S.

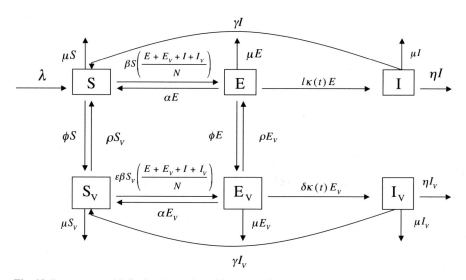

Fig. 10 Pneumococcal infection dynamics with vaccination

pneumoniae, a stage that is typically transient, but always precedes infection. Should a colony of *S. pneumoniae* be successful in establishing an infection, the individual then exhibits a clinical condition described above, and is then considered infected or in the I class. We consider vaccines which prevent progression to infection, or possibly, asymptomatic colonization. This protection is not complete, and the efficacy with which this is accomplished is $1 - \delta$ and $1 - \epsilon$, respectively. Once vaccinated, individuals may enter any of the epidemiological states, S_V, E_V, and I_V, although they do so with altered rates. The model equations (for detailed derivations, see [32]) are given by

$$\frac{dS}{dt} = \lambda - \beta S \frac{E + E_V + I + I_V}{N} + \alpha E + \gamma I - \phi S + \rho S_V - \mu S \tag{56}$$

$$\frac{dE}{dt} = \beta S \frac{E + E_V + I + I_V}{N} - \alpha E - l\kappa(t)E - \phi E + \rho E_V - \mu E \tag{57}$$

$$\frac{dS_V}{dt} = \phi S - \epsilon \beta S_V \frac{E + E_V + I + I_V}{N} + \alpha E_V + \gamma I_V - \rho S_V - \mu S_V \tag{58}$$

$$\frac{dE_V}{dt} = \epsilon \beta S_V \frac{E + E_V + I + I_V}{N} - \alpha E_V + \phi E - \rho E_V - \delta \kappa(t)E_V - \mu E_V \tag{59}$$

$$\frac{dI}{dt} = l\kappa(t)E - (\gamma + \eta + \mu)I \tag{60}$$

$$\frac{dI_V}{dt} = \delta \kappa(t)E_V - (\gamma + \eta + \mu)I_V. \tag{61}$$

Seasonality of invasive pneumococcal diseases has been observed and studies support a seasonal infection rate, κ, rather than a seasonal effective contact rate, β. Thus, we assume the form

$$\kappa(t) = \kappa_0 \left(1 + \kappa_1 \cos[\omega(t - \tau)]\right),$$

for $\kappa(t)$ to reflect seasonal changes in host susceptibility to pneumococcal infection.

5.1 Statistical Models of Case Notification Data

Monthly case notifications $f(t_j, \vec{\theta})$ are best represented as integrals of the new infection rates,

$$f(t_j, \vec{\theta}) = \int_{t_j}^{t_{j+1}} [l\kappa(s)E(s) + \delta\kappa(s)E_V(s)]\,ds,$$

(including those in the vaccinated class) over each month, since they represent the number of cases reported during the month and do not provide any information on how long individuals remain in an infected state. We use these data to estimate

$\vec{\theta} = (\beta, \kappa_0, \kappa_1)^T$. Before using the model with surveillance data, we test the model and methodology capabilities with simulated "data". Following the procedures in the logistic example discussions in Section 4, we generate data according to two statistical models:

$$Y_j = f(t_j, \theta_0) + \epsilon_j, \tag{62}$$

$$Y_j = f(t_j, \theta_0)(1 + \epsilon_j), \tag{63}$$

for $j = 1, \ldots, n$, where $\vec{\theta}_0$ are the "true" values of the parameters used to generate the data. In both (62) and (63), the ϵ_j are independent and identically distributed (*i.i.d.*) random variables with $E[\epsilon_j] = 0$ and $\mathrm{var}(\epsilon_j) = \sigma_0^2$. In model (62), however, the residual is then $R_j = Y_j - f(t_j, \vec{\theta}_0) = \epsilon_j$ and thus R_j satisfies $E[R_j] = 0$ and $\mathrm{var}(R_j) = \sigma_0^2$. As before, we will refer to this error with *constant variance*, or CV. The second case, (63), has residuals of the form $R_j = Y_j - f(t_j, \vec{\theta}_0) = \epsilon_j f(t_j, \vec{\theta}_0)$, so the residual is actually proportional to the model, $f(t_j, \vec{\theta}_0)$, at each time point t_j, and thus this is an example of error with *nonconstant variance*, or NCV. We note that in this case $E[R_j] = 0$ and $\mathrm{var}(R_j) = \sigma_0^2 f^2(t_j, \vec{\theta}_0)$ or $\dfrac{R_j}{f(t_j, \vec{\theta}_0)}$ has mean zero and variance σ_0^2.

For illustration, we consider the same four cases as with the logistic example in Section 4:

1. OLS estimation of $\hat{\theta}$ using data generated by model (62) with constant variance observational error: $\theta_{OLS}(Y_{CV})$,
2. OLS estimation of $\hat{\theta}$ using data generated by model (63) with nonconstant variance observational error: $\theta_{OLS}(Y_{NCV})$,
3. GLS estimation of $\hat{\theta}$ using data generated by model (62) with constant variance observational error: $\theta_{GLS}(Y_{CV})$,
4. GLS estimation of $\hat{\theta}$ using data generated by model (63) with nonconstant variance observational error: $\theta_{GLS}(Y_{NCV})$.

We compare the parameter estimates $\hat{\theta}$ and standard errors $SE(\hat{\theta})$ obtained in each case. Further we discuss how to interpret plots of $r_j = y_j - f(t_j, \hat{\theta})$ versus t_j and $f(t_j, \hat{\theta})$ to assess whether reasonable assumptions have been made in assuming the statistical model for the data.

5.2 Inverse Problem Results: Simulated Data

Data were generated with $n = 60$ time points (equivalent to five years of data), with the set of parameters

$$\vec{\theta}_0 = \begin{pmatrix} \beta \\ \kappa_0 \\ \kappa_1 \end{pmatrix} = \begin{pmatrix} 1.5 \\ 1.4e^{-3} \\ 0.55 \end{pmatrix}.$$

Error was added to the forward solution according to two statistical models, as described in Section 5.1. In the case of constant variance observational error, the error is scaled to the magnitude of the model but not in a time-dependent manner. In this case we generated noisy data by sampling from a $\mathcal{N}(0, 1)$ distribution (we could of course have sampled from any other random variable). Therefore, for constant variance error of about $k\%$ of the average magnitude of the $f(t_j, \vec{\theta}_0)$,

$$\epsilon_j \sim \frac{k}{100} \text{avg}_j f(t_j, \vec{\theta}_0) \mathcal{N}(0, 1).$$

So in this case $\epsilon_j \sim \mathcal{N}(0, [\frac{k}{100}\text{avg}_j f(t_j, \vec{\theta}_0)]^2)$ with ϵ_j (and also R_j) $i.i.d.$ In the second statistical model, the error depends on time and is scaled by the model at each time point, i.e., the error is *relative*. In this case the error is added to the observations by

$$R_j = f(t_j, \vec{\theta}_0)\epsilon_j \sim f(t_j, \vec{\theta}_0) \frac{k}{100} \mathcal{N}(0, 1),$$

with $\epsilon_j \sim \mathcal{N}(0, [\frac{k}{100}f(t_j, \vec{\theta}_0)]^2)$, and again the ϵ_j are $i.i.d.$, but now the R_j are not $i.i.d.$ This enables us to compare different types of error on the same scale: one independent of time and observation magnitude, and one dependent on observation magnitude, and thus time. With the present examples, we have taken $k = 10$.

The results from using an OLS and GLS estimator with data generated with constant variance error are displayed in Table 5, and the fitted model solutions displayed in Fig. 11. Both estimators do an arguably similar job at producing the true values, that is $\hat{\theta}_{OLS}$ and $\hat{\theta}_{GLS}$ are comparably close to θ_0. The standard errors $SE(\hat{\theta}_{GLS})$ for the GLS estimator however, are all smaller, and seem to indicate that the corresponding estimates are more "reliable". This, however, is not true because they are based on incorrect formulae, as we shall see in our examination of the error plots for both of these cases. Note that from Fig. 11 and the residual sum of squares, RSS, in both cases, there is no clear argument from these results as to which estimator is better suited for use with the data.

When OLS and GLS estimation are each used with data with nonconstant variance error, the parameters and standard errors in Table 6 are obtained, and the plot of these model solutions over the generated data is given in Fig. 12. Again, one estimator does not do a clearly better job over the other in terms of predicting parameter values closer to those used to generate the data. However, again, the

Table 5 Parameter estimates from data with constant variance CV error

$\vec{\theta}$	$\vec{\theta}_0$	$\vec{\theta}_{\text{init}}$	$\hat{\theta}_{OLS}$	$SE(\hat{\theta}_{OLS})$	$\hat{\theta}_{GLS}$	$SE(\hat{\theta}_{GLS})$
β	1.5	1.55	1.4845	0.038	1.51186	0.017
κ_0	$1.4e^{-3}$	$1.3e^{-3}$	$1.4188e^{-3}$	$2.1e^{-4}$	$1.3203e^{-3}$	$1.2e^{-4}$
κ_1	0.55	0.65	0.56203	0.050	0.56047	0.019
RSS			$1.6831e^4$		$1.722e^4$	

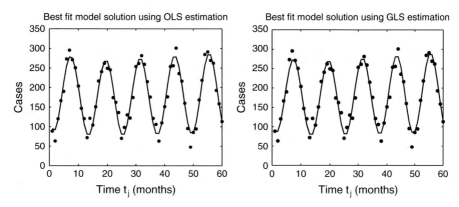

Fig. 11 Best fit model solutions to monthly case notifications with constant variance CV error

Table 6 Parameter estimates from data with nonconstant variance NCV error

$\vec{\theta}$	$\vec{\theta}_0$	$\vec{\theta}_{\text{init}}$	$\hat{\theta}_{OLS}$	$SE(\hat{\theta}_{OLS})$	$\hat{\theta}_{GLS}$	$SE(\hat{\theta}_{GLS})$
β	1.5	1.55	1.4876	0.037	1.4923	0.0079
κ_0	$1.4e^{-3}$	$1.3e^{-3}$	$1.4703e^{-3}$	$2.0e^{-4}$	$1.4301e^{-3}$	$7e^{-5}$
κ_1	0.55	0.65	0.54531	0.047	0.54232	0.012
RSS			$1.6692e^4$		$1.676e^4$	

standard errors from the GLS estimation are smaller as compared to those of the OLS estimation. From this, it would seem that the GLS estimation would always give "better" parameter values, or do a better job at producing reliable results. However, we know that in the case of constant variance error, the GLS estimation makes some incorrect assumptions on the data generation and therefore, the standard errors reported there would give a false sense of confidence in the values (indeed they are based on incorrect asymptotic formulae).

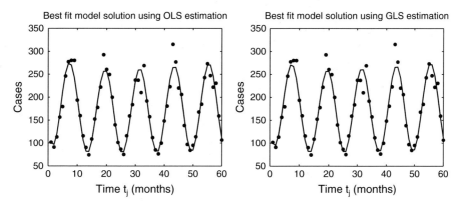

Fig. 12 Best fit model solutions to monthly case notifications with nonconstant variance NCV error

5.2.1 Residual Plots

Here we illustrate use of residual plots to investigate whether our assumptions on the errors incurred in observation of data are correct – that is, whether the ϵ_j are *i.i.d.* for all $j = 1, \ldots, n$, and also are independent of the observation magnitude. As we have already discussed in Section 4, if the errors are *i.i.d.* then a plot of the residuals $r_j = y_j - f(t_j, \hat{\theta})$ versus time t_j should show no discernible pattern. Similarly, a plot of the residual r_j as a function of the model values $f(t_j, \hat{\theta})$ should be random if there is no relationship between these two quantities. While use of the OLS estimation tacitly assumes the statistical model (62), and therefore the residual is a realization of the error random variable, this is not true of the GLS estimation. In that case, the assumed statistical model is shown in (62) with ϵ_j *i.i.d.* but the residual r_j are *not i.i.d.* for all $j = 1, \ldots, n$. Therefore, in the case of GLS we should investigate plots of the residual/model values, $R_j = \frac{Y_j - f(t_j, \theta_0)}{f(t_j, \theta_0)}$ instead of the residuals.

In Fig. 13, we see the relationship between the residuals and time, and that between residuals and the model values when the OLS estimation procedure is applied to data which has been generated with constant variance error. In both the

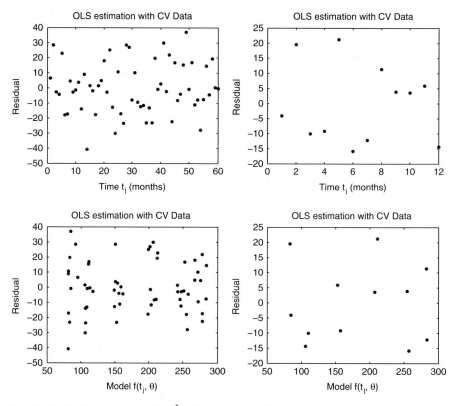

Fig. 13 Residual ($r_j = y_j - f(t_j, \hat{\theta})$) plots of the OLS estimation with CV data ($\epsilon_j = Y_j - f(t_j, \vec{\theta}_0)$); *Left*: nontruncated, *Right*: truncated

top and bottom panels on the left, the full set of $n = 60$ points are used, while on the right hand side, only one year, or $n = 12$ points have been used for the estimation. Both top panels show a random pattern, so the errors are clearly *i.i.d.* But in the bottom left plot, we observe clustering of residuals around certain model values, although there is no clear pattern in the dependent variable, just in the independent variable, $f(t_j, \hat{\theta})$. However, we recognize that this is due to the seasonality of the data and model, so that at regular repeated time points over many periods, there are going to be repeated values of the model. As evidence of this, we see that when only one period is plotted (the bottom right panel), a random pattern is seen, and we confirm that the errors are not dependent on the model values. Thus, if there are vertical bands on a plot such as this, it can be attributed to certain model values repeating and does not indicate any dependence of the error on the model value. To check, one can simply reduce the number of data points used in the estimation so that there are few or no repeated values.

When OLS estimation is carried out with data that has been generated according to the statistical model (63), however, the independence of the error from time is not so clear, as these graphs (Fig. 14) do not show a random pattern. While there

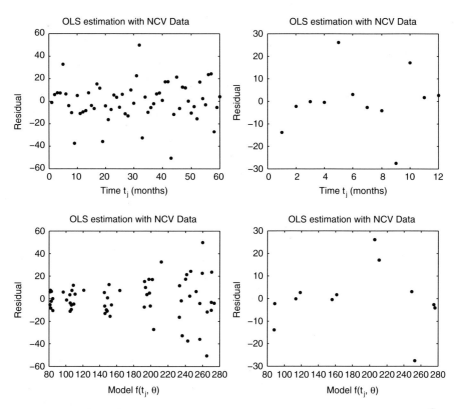

Fig. 14 Residual ($r_j = y_j - f(t_j, \hat{\theta})$) plots of the OLS estimation to NCV data ($\epsilon_j = \frac{Y_j - f(t_j, \vec{\theta}_0)}{f(t_j, \vec{\theta}_0)}$); *Left*: nontruncated, *Right*: truncated

is no clear relationship, there is some randomness in the residuals, and the band of residuals are tighter, not homogeneously distributed across the plot as in Fig. 13. The dependence of the residuals on model value magnitude (seen in the bottom panels) is apparent as the r_j clearly increase with increasing model values, producing a fan shape. In this case the OLS estimation is used incorrectly, and the residual plots exhibit a clear dependence on model values and do not confirm independence from time.

The GLS estimation procedure, however, gave smaller standard errors regardless of the data set used, and therefore, more confidence in the parameter estimates. However, in Fig. 15, we see evidence again of the dependence of the residuals on time and model quantities, thus indicating that our assumptions have been incorrect for GLS estimation. In this case, we would have assumed that the errors are proportional to the observations, thus motivating a GLS estimator. If the variance is constant across time and model values, and the GLS estimator is used, we should expect a systematic behavior in the residual plots. Indeed, the plots in Fig. 15 reveal

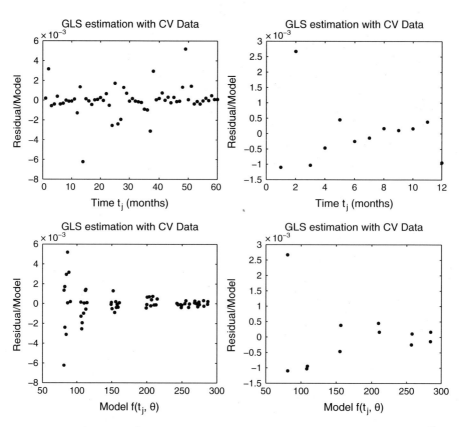

Fig. 15 Residual/Model ($\frac{r_j}{f(t_j,\hat{\theta})}$) plots of the GLS estimation to CV data ($\epsilon_j = Y_j - f(t_j, \vec{\theta}_0)$);
Left: nontruncated, *Right*: truncated

a tight band of points in the $\frac{r_j}{f(t_j,\hat{\theta})}$ versus t_j plots and the reverse fan shape of the plot of the residual/model $\frac{r_j}{f(t_j,\hat{\theta})}$ versus the model values $f(t_j,\hat{\theta})$. This indicates that the relations which give us the parameter estimates and their standard errors no longer hold and we are essentially reporting incorrect values. As we saw in Section 5.2, while the parameter estimates may not necessarily be poor, the reliability provided by the standard errors is incorrect.

When the GLS estimator is used appropriately, however, the randomness of the error plots suggest reasonability of assumptions, as seen in Fig. 16. Here, the error in the data has been generated proportional to the model values, and therefore, not longitudinally constant. So when we plot the ratios $\frac{y_j - f(t_j,\hat{\theta})}{f(t_j,\hat{\theta})}$, we allow for this dependence and see the random patterns we would expect when plotting realizations of a random variable. Again, the vertical bands seen in the bottom left panel indicate repeated model values, as can be seen by the bottom right panel, where the repetitions have been excluded from the data set.

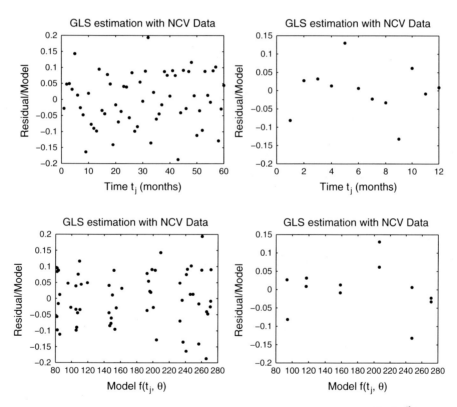

Fig. 16 Residual/Model ($\frac{r_j}{f(t_j,\hat{\theta})}$) plots of the GLS estimation to NCV data ($\epsilon_j = \frac{Y_j - f(t_j,\vec{\theta}_0)}{f(t_j,\vec{\theta}_0)}$); *Left*: nontruncated, *Right*: truncated

5.3 Inverse Problem Results: Australian Surveillance Data

Using the iterative weighted least squares procedure described in Section 2.3.2, we
carried out inverse problem calculations with the model and observations as outlined
in the previous section using Australian IPD data in place of the simulated data. In
this case we assumed constant variance noise in the data and hence used WLS,
e.g., see Equation (27), for our estimation procedure. Details are given in [32]. We
discuss here the case where we used data for the period 2002–2004 (36 months of
monthly data $n_1 = 36$, and $n_2 = 6$ of annual vaccinated or unvaccinated cases) and
estimated $\vec{\theta} = (\beta, \kappa_0, \kappa_1, \delta)^T$ along with σ_1, σ_2 in a weighted least squares (WLS)
functional

$$J_{42}(\vec{\theta}, \sigma_1^2, \sigma_2^2) = \frac{1}{\sigma_1^2} \sum_{j=1}^{36} \left| Y_j^{(1)} - f_j^{(1)} \right|^2 + \frac{9}{\sigma_2^2} \sum_{k=1}^{3} \left\{ \left| Y_k^{(2)} - f_k^{(2)} \right|^2 + \left| Y_k^{(3)} - f_k^{(3)} \right|^2 \right\}.$$
(64)

As usual, we assume there exists a "true" parameter $\vec{\theta}_0$ which generated the data,
and our statistical model is then given by

$$Y_j^{(1)} \equiv f^{(1)}(t_j, \vec{\theta}_0) + \epsilon_j^{(1)} \qquad\qquad j = 1, ..., 36, \tag{65}$$

$$Y_k^{(2)} \equiv f^{(2)}(t_k, \vec{\theta}_0) + \epsilon_k^{(2)} \qquad\qquad k = 1, 2, 3, \tag{66}$$

$$Y_k^{(3)} \equiv f^{(3)}(t_k, \vec{\theta}_0) + \epsilon_k^{(3)} \qquad\qquad k = 1, 2, 3. \tag{67}$$

The errors ($\epsilon_j^{(i)}$ in (65), (66), (67) for $i = 1, 2, 3$) in the above model are assumed
to be random variables with means $E[\epsilon_j^{(i)}] = 0$ and constant variances $var(\epsilon_j^{(i)}) = \sigma_{0,i}^2$, where $\sigma_{0,1} = \sigma_1$, $\sigma_{0,2} = \sigma_{0,3} = \sigma_2$ are unknown. Thus we have assumed that
the size of the errors committed at each time for a given kind of "measurement"
is constant and also does not depend on the magnitude of the measurement itself.
We also assume that $\epsilon_j^{(i)}$ are independent and identically distributed (i.i.d.) random
variables for each fixed i. The observations and the model quantities are related by

- $Y_j^{(1)} \sim f^{(1)}(t_j, \vec{\theta}) = \int_{t_j}^{t_{j+1}} [\kappa(s)E(s) + \delta\kappa(s)E_V(s)] ds$ for $j = 1, 2, .., 36$
  (monthly cases),
- $Y_k^{(2)} \sim f^{(2)}(t_k, \vec{\theta}) = \int_{t_k}^{t_{k+1}} \kappa(s)E(s) ds$ for $k = 1, 2, 3$ (yearly unvaccinated cases),
- $Y_k^{(3)} \sim f^{(3)}(t_k, \vec{\theta}) = \int_{t_k}^{t_{k+1}} \delta\kappa(s)E_V(s) ds$ for $k = 1, 2, 3$ (yearly vaccinated
  cases).

The data fits in Fig. 17 reveal that the model solution with the parameters shown
in Table 7 fits the Australian surveillance data from 2002 to 2004, with the top
panel showing the fit to the monthly case notification data, the bottom left panel the
unvaccinated cases reported annually, and the bottom right the annual vaccinated
cases. The model solution and data agree well, and parameter values are on the
scale of our initial guesses, although their values differ slightly to minimize the cost

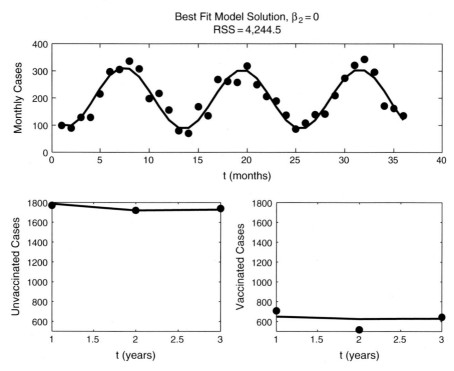

Fig. 17 Best fit solution to Australian IPD data with parameters shown in Table 7. *Top panel*: monthly cases; *bottom left panel*: annual unvaccinated cases; *bottom right panel*: annual vaccinated cases

function in the functional (64). Further, the standard errors are relatively small and suggests that the estimates obtained here are reliable.

To test the assumptions of the statistical model that we have chosen to represent our data, we plotted the residuals between the model and observations as a function of the model, that is, $r_j = y_j^{(1)} - f^{(1)}(t_j, \hat{\theta})$ vs. the model values $f^{(1)}(t_j, \hat{\theta})$ (Fig. 18). The lack of a clear relationship between these two quantities suggests that our assumptions are reasonable and the residuals of each observation do not depend on the model values. However, we see six groups of points, which can be explained

Table 7 Model calibration to Australian IPD data from 2002 to 2004; estimation of $\hat{\psi} = (\hat{\theta}, \hat{\sigma}_1, \hat{\sigma}_2)^T = (\hat{\beta}, \hat{\kappa}_0, \hat{\kappa}_1, \hat{\delta}, \hat{\sigma}_1, \hat{\sigma}_2)^T$

ψ	$\hat{\psi}$	$SE(\hat{\theta})$
β	1.52175	0.02
κ_0	$1.3656e^{-3}$	$1.3e^{-4}$
κ_1	0.56444	0.04
δ	0.7197	0.06
σ_1	28.924	
σ_2	259.158	

Fig. 18 Residuals as a
function of model values. *Top
panel* is over the period
January 2003–June 2003,
middle panel is for January
2003–December 2003, and
bottom panel is for all three
years

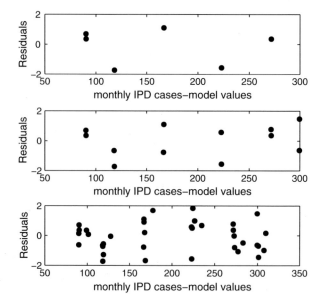

by the oscillatory pattern of the infections. In the top panel we have plotted just
one half of the period of the infection rate and see a completely random pattern,
indicating no relationship among these quantities. When we extend this time period
for another half of a period, thus plotting an entire period in the middle panel, we see
that there are two points in each group of points. Thus, the pattern observed is driven
by the seasonality of the infections and not by any incorrect assumptions. On the
contrary, only a pattern in the dependent variable (the residuals) would suggest that
incorrect assumptions have been made. This analysis suggests that it is reasonable to
assume constant variance among observations of the same type, providing support
for the statistical model underlying the parameter estimation procedure.

6 Sensitivity Functions

The sensitivity matrices $\chi = F_{\vec{\theta}}$ introduced in Section 3 to define covariances
for sampling distributions and associated standard errors are actually well known
in the applied mathematics and engineering literature, where they arise in routine
sensitivity analysis.

In actuality, *sensitivity analysis* is an ensemble of techniques [30] that can
provide information on parameter dependent model behavior, yielding a much better understanding of the underlying mathematical model with a resulting marked
improvement in the estimation results obtained using the models in simulations and
inverse problems. Traditionally, sensitivity analysis referred to a procedure used in
simulation studies (direct problems) where one evaluated the effects of parameter
variations on the time course of model outputs and identified the parameters or the
initial conditions to which the model is most/least sensitive. In recent years however,

investigators' attention has also recently turned to the sensitivity of the solutions to inverse problems with respect to data, in a quest for optimal selection of data measurements in *experimental design*. As part of model validation and verification, one typically needs to estimate model parameters from data measurements, and a related question of paramount interest is related to sampling; specifically, at which time points the measurements are most informative in the estimation of a given parameter. Due to the fact that in practice the components of the parameter estimates are often correlated, *traditional sensitivity functions* (TSF) used alone are not very efficient in answering this question because TSF do not take into account how model output variations affect parameter estimates in inverse problems. Investigators [11, 34] recently proposed a new class of sensitivity functions, called *generalized sensitivity functions* (GSF), which provide information on the relevance of measurements of output variables of a system for the identification of specific parameters. For a given set of time observations, Thomaseth and Cobelli use theoretical information criteria (the Fisher information matrix) to establish a relationship between the monotonicity of the GSF curves with respect to the model parameters and the information content of these observations. Here our interest is in how to use this information content tool along with TSF to improve data collection for estimation of parameters in inverse problems. It is, of course, intuitive that sampling more data points from the region indicated by the GSF to be the "most informative" with respect to a given parameter would result in more information about that parameter, and therefore provide more accurate estimates for it.

To define and discuss these sensitivity functions we consider the general mathematical model (1) with N-vector solutions $\vec{x}$ depending on p-vector parameters $\vec{\theta}$.

6.1 Traditional Sensitivity Functions

Traditional sensitivity functions (TSF) are classical sensitivity functions used in mathematical modeling to investigate variations in the output of a model resulting from variations in the parameters and the initial conditions.

In order to quantify the variation in the state variable $\vec{x}(t)$ with respect to changes in the parameter $\vec{\theta}$ and the initial condition $\vec{x}_0$, we are naturally led to consider *traditional sensitivity functions (TSF)* as defined by the derivatives

$$\vec{s}_{\theta_k}(t) = \frac{\partial \vec{x}}{\partial \theta_k}(t), \qquad k = 1, \ldots, p, \qquad (68)$$

and

$$\vec{r}_{x_{0l}}(t) = \frac{\partial \vec{x}}{\partial x_{0l}}(t), \qquad l = 1, \ldots, N, \qquad (69)$$

where x_{0l} is the l-th component of the initial condition $\vec{x}_0$. If the function $\vec{g}$ is sufficiently regular, the solution $\vec{x}$ is differentiable with respect to θ_k and x_{0l}, and therefore the sensitivity functions $\vec{s}_{\theta_k}$ and $\vec{r}_{x_{0l}}$ are well defined.

In practice, the model under investigation often is sufficiently simple to allow one to compute analytically the sensitivity functions (68) and (69). This is precisely the case (see (55)) with the logistic growth population example of (54) to be discussed below. However, when one deals with a more complex model, as with the epidemiological example of Section 5, it is often preferable to consider these sensitivity functions separately for clarity purposes.

The sensitivity functions are local in nature because they are defined by partial derivatives which have a *local* character. Thus sensitivity and insensitivity (i.e., $\vec{s}_{\theta_k} = \partial \vec{x}/\partial \theta_k$ very close to zero) depend on the time interval, the state values $\vec{x}$, and the values of $\vec{\theta}$ for which they are considered. For example in a certain time subinterval we might find that $\vec{s}_{\theta_k}$ is small so that the state variable $\vec{x}$ is *insensitive* to the parameter θ_k on that particular interval. The same function $\vec{s}_{\theta_k}$ can take large values on a different subinterval, indicating that the state variable $\vec{x}$ is *quite sensitive* to the parameter θ_k on the latter interval. From the sensitivity analysis theory for dynamical systems, one finds (e.g., see (48)) that $s = (\vec{s}_{\theta_1}, \ldots, \vec{s}_{\theta_p})$ is an $N \times p$ vector function that satisfies the matrix ODE system

$$\dot{s}(t) = \vec{g}_{\vec{x}}(t, \vec{x}(t), \vec{\theta})s(t) + \vec{g}_{\vec{\theta}}(t, \vec{x}(t), \vec{\theta}), \qquad (70)$$
$$s(t_0) = 0_{N \times p},$$

so that the dependence of s on $(t, \vec{x}(t))$ as well as $\vec{\theta}$ is readily apparent. Here we have used $\vec{g}_{\vec{x}} = \partial \vec{g}/\partial \vec{x}$ and $\vec{g}_{\vec{\theta}} = \partial \vec{g}/\partial \vec{\theta}$ to denote the derivatives of $\vec{g}$ with respect to $\vec{x}$ and $\vec{\theta}$, respectively.

The sensitivity functions with respect to the components of the initial condition $\vec{x}_0$ define an $N \times N$ vector function $r = (\vec{r}_{x_{01}}, \ldots, \vec{r}_{x_{0N}})$, which satisfies the matrix system

$$\dot{r}(t) = \vec{g}_{\vec{x}}(t, \vec{x}(t), \vec{\theta})r(t), \qquad (71)$$
$$r(t_0) = I_{N \times N}.$$

Equations (70) and (71) can be used in conjunction with Equation (1) to numerically compute the sensitivities s and r for general cases when the function $\vec{g}$ is sufficiently complicated to prohibit an analytical solution.

In many cases the parameters have different units and the state variables may have varying orders of magnitude, and thus in practice it is sometimes more convenient to work with the scaled versions of the TSF, referred to as *relative sensitivity functions* (RSF). However, here we will focus solely on the non-scaled sensitivities, i.e., TSF.

6.2 Generalized Sensitivity Functions

Recently, generalized sensitivity functions were proposed by Thomaseth and Cobelli [34] as a new tool in identification studies to analyze, for a given set of observations, the distribution of the information content of observations relative to its influence on the estimated model parameters. These are formulated in the context of an OLS inverse problem framework in [11, 34] where a rather detailed motivation for defining these "cumulative information" functions is discussed. Roughly speaking, these functions involve sensitivity of estimated parameters with respect to the data collected up to a particular time observation. Recall that the usual sensitivity functions involve influence of the parameters in a model on the model output.

We consider here a scalar observation model with discrete time measurements. When $m = 1$ and C is a $1 \times N$ array in (4)), the *generalized sensitivity functions* (GSF) are defined as

$$\mathbf{gs}(t_l) = \sum_{i=1}^{l} \frac{1}{\sigma^2(t_i)} [F^{-1} \times \nabla_{\vec{\theta}} f(t_i, \vec{\theta}_0)] \bullet \nabla_{\vec{\theta}} f(t_i, \vec{\theta}_0), \tag{72}$$

where $\{t_l\}, l = 1, \ldots, n$ are the times when the measurements are taken,

$$F = \sum_{j=1}^{n} \frac{1}{\sigma^2(t_j)} \nabla_{\vec{\theta}} f(t_j, \vec{\theta}_0) \nabla_{\vec{\theta}} f(t_j, \vec{\theta}_0)^T \tag{73}$$

is the corresponding $p \times p$ *Fisher information matrix* and $\sigma^2(t_j)$ is the observation time dependent variance. The symbol "$\bullet$" represents element-by-element vector multiplication (for motivation and details which lead to the definition above, the interested reader may consult [11, 34]). The Fisher information matrix measures the information content of the data corresponding to the model parameters. In (72) we see that this information is contained in the GSF, making them appropriate tools to indicate the relevance of the measurements to estimation of a parameter in inverse problems.

We observe that the generalized sensitivity functions (72) are vector-valued functions with the same dimension as $\vec{\theta}$. The k-th component gs_k of the vector function **gs** represents the generalized sensitivity function with respect to θ_k. The GSF in (72) are defined only at the discrete time points $\{t_j, j = 1, \ldots, n\}$ and they are cumulative functions involving at time t_l only the contributions of those measurements up to and including t_l; thus gs_k calculates the *influence of measurements up to t_l* on the *parameter estimate* for θ_k.

It is readily seen from the definition that all the components of **gs** are one at the final time point t_n, i.e., $\mathbf{gs}(t_n) = \mathbf{1}$. If one defines $\mathbf{gs}(t) = \mathbf{0}$ for $t < t_1$ (naturally, **gs** is zero when no measurements are collected), then each component of **gs** transitions (not necessarily monotonically) from zero to one. As developed in [11, 34], the time subinterval during which the change in gs_k has the *sharpest increase* corresponds to the *observations which provide the most information in the estimation of θ_k*. That is, regions of sharp increases in gs_k indicate a high concentration of information in the data about θ_k. Thus, the utility of these functions in design of experiments is rather obvious.

The numerical implementation of the generalized sensitivity functions (72) is straightforward, since the gradient of f with respect to $\vec{\theta}$ (or $\vec{x}_0$) is simply the Jacobian of $\vec{x}$ with respect to $\vec{\theta}$ (or $\vec{x}_0$) multiplied by the observation operator $\mathcal{C}$. These Jacobian matrices can be obtained by numerically solving the sensitivity ODE system (70) or (71) coupled with the system (1). One would need to use this approach to compute the GSF for the epidemiological model of Section 5. For the logistic model used below to illustrate ideas, the solution of Equation (54) given by (55) is sufficiently simple to permit an analytical representation of the Jacobians.

6.3 TSF and GSF for the Logistic Equation

The Verhulst-Pearl logistic Equation (54) is a relatively simple example with easily determined dynamics that is useful in demonstrating the utility of the traditional sensitivity functions as well as the generalized sensitivity functions in inverse problems (see [2, 4] for more discussions on TSF and GSF for this example). Unless data are sampled from regions with changing dynamics, it is possible that some of the parameters will be difficult to estimate. Moreover, the parameters that are obtainable may have high standard errors as a result of introducing redundancy in the sampling region (this is illustrated in [2]). In order to investigate sensitivity for the logistic growth example, we will examine varying behavior in the model depending on the region from which t_j is sampled. We consider points τ_1 and τ_2, as depicted in Fig. 19, partitioning the logistic solution curve into three distinct regions: $0 < t_j < \tau_1$, $\tau_1 < t_j < \tau_2$, and $\tau_2 < t_j < T$, with T sufficiently large for our solution to be near its asymptote $x = K$. Based on the changing dynamics of the curve in Fig. 19, we expect differences in the ability to estimate parameters depending on the region in which the solution is observed.

We consider the logistic model with true parameters $\vec{\theta}_0 = (17.5, 0.7, 0.1)$. We analyze the TSF corresponding to each parameter in the initial region of the curve,

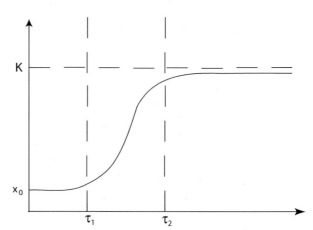

Fig. 19 Regions with different growth in the *Verhulst-Pearl solution curve*

where the solution approaches x_0 as $t \rightarrow 0$. When we consider the initial region of the curve, where $0 < t_j < \tau_1$ for $j = 1, \dots, n$, we have

$$\frac{\partial x(t_j)}{\partial K} \approx 0, \qquad \frac{\partial x(t_j)}{\partial r} \approx 0, \qquad \frac{\partial x(t_j)}{\partial x_0} \approx 1;$$

this follows from considering the limits of the readily computed analytical sensitivity functions as $t \rightarrow 0$. Based on these analytical findings, which indicate low sensitivities with respect to K and r, we expect to have little ability to determine these parameters when we sample data from $[0, \tau_1]$; however we should be able to estimate x_0. This is confirmed by the computational examples in [2, 4].

We next consider the region of the curve which is near the asymptote at $x = K$, in this case for $\tau_2 < t_j < T$, $j = 1, \dots, n$. Here we find that by considering the limits as $t \rightarrow \infty$, we have the approximations

$$\frac{\partial x(t_j)}{\partial K} \approx 1, \qquad \frac{\partial x(t_j)}{\partial r} \approx 0, \qquad \frac{\partial x(t_j)}{\partial x_0} \approx 0.$$

Based on these approximations, we expect to be able to estimate K well when we sample data from $[\tau_2, T]$. However, using data only from this region, we do not expect to be able to estimate very well either x_0 or r. Again these expectations are readily confirmed by the inverse problem calculations presented in [2, 4].

Finally, we consider the part of the solution curve where $\tau_1 < t_j < \tau_2$ for $j = 1, \dots, n$ and where it has nontrivially changing dynamics. We find that the partial derivative values differ greatly from the values in regions $[0, \tau_1]$ and $[\tau_2, T]$. When $[\tau_1, \tau_2]$ is included in the sampling region we expect to recover good estimates for all three parameters (expectations that are met in [2, 4]).

Our analytical observations are fully consistent with information contained in the graphs of the TSF illustrated in Fig. 20(a) for $T = 25$. We note that the curve s_K

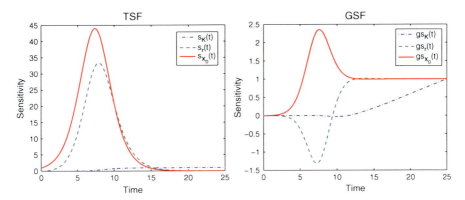

Fig. 20 (a) TSF and (b) GSF corresponding to each parameter for the logistic curve with $\vec{\theta}_0 = (17.5, 0.7, 0.1)$

slowly increases with time and it appears that the solution is insensitive to K until around the flex point of the logistic curve, which occurs shortly after $t = 7$ in this case. The sensitivities s_K and s_r both are close to zero when t is near the origin, and hence we deduce that both K and r will be difficult or impossible to obtain using data in that region. Also, we observe that s_{x_0} and s_r are nearly zero in [15,25], which suggests that we will be unable to estimate x_0 or r using observations in that region.

We numerically computed the GSF using Equation (72) with $\sigma = 1$ and the true value parameters $\vec{\theta}_0 = (17.5, 0.7, 0.1)$. The plots of these functions are shown in Fig. 20(b) where one can observe obvious regions of steep increase in each curve. For the curves $gs_{x_0}(t)$, $gs_r(t)$ and $gs_K(t)$, we find by visual inspection that these regions are approximately [4.5, 7.5], [7, 11] and [12, 25], respectively. By the generalized sensitivity theory, if we increase the number of data points sampled in one of these regions, the estimation of the corresponding parameter is expected to improve. This is precisely what happens in the computational examples found in [2, 4].

While the general algorithms are still under development, the following scenario involving TSF and GSF in design of experiments for data to be used in OLS and GLS formulations are envisioned:

1. One proposes a mechanism, interaction, etc., as represented by a term or terms (such as a nonlinearity, probability distribution, etc.) in a model (ODE, PDE, etc.). One then uses methodology based on the TSF, GSF and the Fisher Information Matrix (FIM) calculations to suggest design of experiments to collect data (duration of experiment, sampling sizes, frequency in time, space, age/size class, etc.) to be used in inverse problem/parameter estimation techniques to investigate the mechanistic based terms.
2. One then designs and carries out the experiments resulting from 1. with guidance in data collection (variables required to be observed, sampling frequency, measurement accuracy needed, etc) being provided for each class of models to be used with the data; questions and models usually will be driven by mechanism based formulation.
3. Finally, one can carry out post experimental modeling analysis (parameter estimation and inverse problems with both OLS and GLS , statistical analysis of variance in data and model fits with residual plots, hypothesis testing and model comparison as described in the next several sections, Kullback-Leibler distance based and information content based model selection techniques such as AIC and recent generalizations [16, 17] and improvements, etc.) to provide a modeling framework and methodology for future investigations of the type proposed here. In the post analysis one can also carry out verification and validation type studies as well as testing predictive capabilities. This can be done in part by comparing the models with data that was not used in the inverse problems for estimation of parameters.

7 Statistically Based Model Comparison Techniques

In previous sections we have discussed techniques (e.g., residual plots) for investigating correctness of the assumed *statistical model* underlying the estimation (OLS or GLS) procedures used in inverse problems. To this point we have not discussed correctness issues related to choice of the *mathematical model*. However there are a number of ways in which questions related to the mathematical model may arise. In general, modeling studies [7, 8] can raise questions as to whether a mathematical model can be improved by *more detail* and/or *further refinement?* For example, one might ask whether one can improve the mathematical model by assuming more *detail* in a given mechanism (constant rate vs. time or spatially dependent rate – e.g., see [1] for questions related to time dependent mortality rates during sub-lethal damage in insect populations exposed to various levels of pesticides). Or one might question whether an *additional mechanism* in the model might produce a better fit to data-see [5–7] for *diffusion alone* or *diffusion plus convection* in cat brain transport in grey vs. white matter considerations.

Before continuing an important point must be made: In model comparison results outlined below, there are really *two models* being compared: the *mathematical model* and the *statistical model*. If one embeds the mathematical model in the *wrong statistical model* (for example, assumes constant variance when this really isn't true), then the mathematical model comparison results using the techniques presented here will be *invalid* (e.g., *worthless*). An important remark in all this is that you must have the mathematical model you want to simplify or improve (e.g., test whether $V = 0$ or not in the example below) embedded in the *correct statistical model* (determined in large part by the observation process), so that the comparison really is *only with regard to the mathematical model*.

To provide specific motivation, we illustrate the formulation of hypothesis testing by considering a mathematical model for a diffusion-convection process. This model was proposed for use with experiments designed to study substance (labeled sucrose) transport in cat brains, which are heterogeneous, containing grey and white matter [7]. In general, the transport of substance in cat's brains can be described by a PDE describing *change in time and space*. This convection/diffusion model, which is widely discussed in the applied mathematics and engineering literature, has the form

$$\frac{\partial u}{\partial t} + V \frac{\partial u}{\partial x} = \mathcal{D} \frac{\partial^2 u}{\partial x^2}. \tag{74}$$

Here, the parameter $\vec{\theta} = (\mathcal{D}, V)$, which belongs to some admissible parameter set Θ, denotes the diffusion coefficient $\mathcal{D}$ and the bulk velocity V of the fluid, respectively. Our problem: test whether the parameter V plays a significant role in the mathematical model. That is, if the model (74) represents a diffusion-convection process, we seek to determine whether diffusion alone or diffusion plus convection best describes transport phenomena represented in cat brain data sets $\{y_{ij}\}$ for

$\{u(t_i, x_j; \vec{\theta})\}$, the concentration of labeled sucrose at times $\{t_i\}$ and location $\{x_j\}$. We then may take $H_0 : \mathcal{V} = 0$ and the alternative $H_A : \mathcal{V} \neq 0$. Consequently, the restricted parameter set $\Theta_H \subset \Theta$ defined by

$$\Theta_H = \{\vec{\theta} \in \Theta : \mathcal{V} = 0\}$$

will be important. To carry out these determinations, we will need some model comparison tests of analysis of variance (ANOVA) type from statistics involving residual sum of squares (RSS).

7.1 RSS Based Statistical Tests

In general, we assume an inverse problem with mathematical model $f(t, \vec{\theta})$ and n observations $\vec{Y} = \{Y_j\}_{j=1}^n$. We define an OLS performance criterion

$$J_n(\vec{\theta}) = J_n(\vec{Y}, \vec{\theta}) = \frac{1}{n} \sum_{j=1}^n [Y_j - f(t_j, \vec{\theta})]^2,$$

where our statistical model again has the form

$$Y_j = f(t_j, \vec{\theta}_0) + \epsilon_j, \quad j = 1, \ldots, n,$$

with $\{\epsilon_j\}_{j=1}^n$ independent and identically distributed, $E(\epsilon_j) = 0$ and constant variance $var(\epsilon_j) = \sigma^2$. As usual $\vec{\theta}_0$ is the "true" value of $\vec{\theta}$ which we assume to exist. As noted above, we use Θ to represent the set of all the admissible parameters $\vec{\theta}$ and assume that Θ is a compact subset of Euclidean space of R^p with $\vec{\theta}_0 \in \Theta$.

Let $\theta^n(\vec{Y}) = \theta_{OLS}^n(\vec{Y})$ be the OLS *estimator* using J_n with corresponding *estimate* $\hat{\theta}^n = \theta_{OLS}^n(\vec{y})$ for a realization $\vec{y} = \{y_j\}$. That is,

$$\theta^n(\vec{Y}) = \arg\min_{\vec{\theta} \in \Theta} J_n(\vec{Y}, \vec{\theta}) \quad \text{and} \quad \hat{\theta}^n = \arg\min_{\vec{\theta} \in \Theta} J_n(\vec{y}, \vec{\theta}).$$

Remark 1. In most calculations, one actually uses an approximation f^N to f, often a numerical solution to the ODE or PDE for modeling the dynamical system. Here we tacitly assume f^N will converge to f as the approximation improves. There are also questions related to approximations of the set Θ when it is infinite dimensional (e.g., in the case of function space parameters such as time or spatially dependent parameters) by finite dimensional discretizations Θ^M. For extensive discussions related to these questions, see [8] as well as [6] where related assumptions on convergences $f^N \to f$ and $\Theta^M \to \Theta$ are given. We shall ignore these issues here, keeping in mind that these approximations will also be of importance in the methodology discussed below in most practical uses.

In many instances, including the motivating example given above, one is interested in using data to address the question whether or not the "true" parameter $\vec{\theta}_0$ can be found in a subset $\Theta_H \subset \Theta$ which we assume for discussions here is defined by

$$\Theta_H = \{\vec{\theta} \in \Theta | H\vec{\theta} = c\} \tag{75}$$

where H is an $r \times p$ matrix of full rank, and c is a known constant.

In this case we want to test the *null hypothesis* H_0: $\vec{\theta}_0 \in \Theta_H$. Define then

$$\theta_H^n(\vec{Y}) = \arg \min_{\vec{\theta} \in \Theta_H} J_n(\vec{Y}, \vec{\theta}) \quad \text{and} \quad \hat{\theta}_H^n = \arg \min_{\vec{\theta} \in \Theta_H} J_n(\vec{y}, \vec{\theta})$$

and observe that $J_n(\vec{Y}, \hat{\theta}_H^n) \geq J_n(\vec{Y}, \hat{\theta}^n)$. We define the related non-negative test statistics and their realizations, respectively, by

$$T_n(\vec{Y}) = n(J_n(\vec{Y}, \theta_H^n) - J_n(\vec{Y}, \theta^n)) \quad \text{and} \quad \hat{T}_n = T_n(\vec{y}) = n(J_n(\vec{y}, \hat{\theta}_H^n) - J_n(\vec{y}, \hat{\theta}^n)).$$

One can establish asymptotic convergence results for the test statistics $T_n(\vec{Y})$, as given in detail in [6]. These results can, in turn, be used to establish a fundamental result about much more useful statistics for model comparison. We define these statistics by

$$U_n(\vec{Y}) = \frac{T_n(\vec{Y})}{J_n(\vec{Y}, \theta_n)}, \tag{76}$$

with corresponding realizations $\hat{U}_n = U_n(\vec{y})$. We then have the asymptotic result that is the basis of our ANOVA–type tests.

Under reasonable assumptions (very similar to those required in the asymptotic sampling distribution theory discussed in previous sections–see [6, 8, 31]) involving regularity and the manner in which samples are taken, one can prove [6]:

(a) We have the estimator convergence $\theta^n \longrightarrow \vec{\theta}_0$ as $n \to \infty$ with probability one;
(b) If H_0 is true, $U_n \overset{D}{\longrightarrow} U(r)$ as $n \to \infty$ where $U \sim \chi^2(r)$, a χ^2 distribution with r degrees of freedom.

An example of the χ^2 density is depicted in Fig. 21 where the density for $\chi^2(4)$ (χ^2 with $r = 4$ degrees of freedom) is graphed.

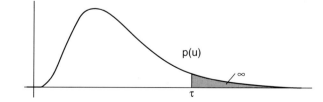

Fig. 21 Example of $U \sim \chi^2(4)$ density

Table 8 $\chi^2(1)$

α	τ	Confidence (%)
.25	1.32	75
.1	2.71	90
.05	3.84	95
.01	6.63	99
.001	10.83	99.9

In this figure two parameters (τ, α) of interest are shown. For a given value τ, the value α is simply the probability that the random variable U will take on a value greater than α. That is, $Prob\{U > \tau\} = \alpha$ where in hypothesis testing, α is the *significance level* and τ is the *threshold*.

We wish to use this distribution to test the null hypothesis, H_0, where we approximate by $U_n \sim \chi^2(r)$. If the test statistic, $\hat{U}_n > \tau$, then we *reject* H_0 as false with confidence level $(1 - \alpha)100\%$. Otherwise, we *do not reject* H_0 as true. For cat brain problem, we use a $\chi^2(1)$ Table 8, which can be found in any elementary statistics text or online and is given here for illustrative purposes.

7.1.1 P-Values

The minimum value α^* of α at which H_0 can be rejected is called the *p-value*. Thus, the smaller the p-value, the stronger the evidence in the data in support of rejecting the null hypothesis and including the term in the model, i.e., the more likely the term should be in the model. We implement this as follows: Once we compute $\hat{U}_n = \bar{\tau}$, then $p = \alpha^*$ is the value that corresponds to $\bar{\tau}$ on a χ^2 graph and so, we reject the null hypothesis at any confidence level, c, such that $c < 1 - \alpha^*$. For example, if for a computed $\bar{\tau}$ we find $p = \alpha^* = .0182$, then we would reject H_0 at confidence level $(1 - \alpha^*)100\% = 98.18\%$ or lower. For more information, the reader can consult ANOVA discussions in any good statistics book.

7.1.2 Alternative Statement

To test the null hypothesis H_0, we choose a significance level α and use χ^2 tables to obtain the corresponding threshold $\tau = \tau(\alpha)$ so that $P(\chi^2(r) > \tau) = \alpha$. We next compute $\hat{U}_n = \bar{\tau}$ and compare it to τ. If $\hat{U}_n > \tau$, then we *reject* H_0 as false; otherwise, we do not reject the null hypothesis H_0.

7.2 Revisiting the Cat-Brain Problem

We summarize use of the above model comparison techniques outlined above by returning to the cat brain example discussed in detail in [7, 8]. There were *3 sets of experimental data* examined, under the null-hypothesis $H_0 : \mathcal{V} = 0$.

For the *Data Set 1*, we found after carrying out the inverse problems over Θ and Θ_H, respectively,

$$J_n(\hat{\theta}^n) = 106.15 \quad \text{and} \quad J_n(\hat{\theta}_H^n) = 180.1,$$

which gives us that $\hat{U}_n = 5.579$ (noting that $n = 8 \neq \infty$), for which $p = \alpha^* = .0182$. Thus, we reject H_0 in this case at *any* confidence level less than 98.18%. Thus, we should *reject* that $V = 0$, which suggests convection is important in describing this data set.

For *Data Set 2*, we found

$$J_n(\hat{\theta}^n) = 14.68 \quad \text{and} \quad J_n(\hat{\theta}_H^n) = 15.35,$$

and thus, in this case, we have $\hat{U}_n = .365$, which implies we *do not reject H_0* with *high degrees of confidence* (p-value very high). This suggests $V = 0$, which is completely opposite to the findings for Data Set 1.

For the final set (*Data Set 3*) we found

$$J_n(\hat{\theta}^n) = 7.8 \quad \text{and} \quad J_n(\hat{\theta}_H^n) = 146.71,$$

which yields in this case, $\hat{U}_n = 15.28$. This, as in the case of the first data set, suggests (with $p < .001$) that $V \neq 0$ is important in modeling the data.

The difference in conclusions between the first and last sets and that of the second set is interesting and perhaps at first puzzling. However, when discussed with the doctors who provided the data, it was discovered that the first and last set were taken from the *white matter* of the brain, while the other was taken from the *grey matter*. This later finding was consistent with observed microscopic tests on the various matter (micro channels in white matter that promote convective "flow"). Thus, it can be suggested with a reasonably high degree of confidence, that white matter exhibits convective transport, while grey matter does not.

8 Epi Model Comparison

We return to the previously introduced epidemiological model as another example of a way in which the model comparison statistic may be used. Here we apply this statistic to determine whether a more sophisticated model is appropriate based on the surveillance data from the Australian NNDS website. Here we introduce the modified model and describe the test statistic for this example. We then present the results from the least squares estimation procedure in both the cases of the simplified and more complex model, and finally, interpret the conclusions indicated by the test statistic.

So far, in our model of invasive pneumococcal disease dynamics, we have considered the progression of individuals from a colonized to an infected state by a constant linear per capita rate. However, this is a gross simplification of more complex physiological processes, many of which occur within the individual and would likely require more sophisticated mathematical representations. But it is also possible that at a population level, this linear term may sufficiently capture the dynamics of the infections when the model solutions are compared with observed data. One specific mechanism that we can explicitly consider is "exogenous reinfection", that is, the establishment of an infection within a colonized individual through repeated exposure to S. pneumoniae via contacts with other individuals harboring the bacteria. The inclusion of this mechanism results in the following modified model equations

$$\frac{dS}{dt} = \lambda - \beta_1 S \frac{E + E_V + I + I_V}{N} + \alpha E + \gamma I - \phi S + \rho S_V - \mu S \qquad (77)$$

$$\frac{dE}{dt} = \beta_1 S \frac{E + E_V + I + I_V}{N} - \alpha E - l\kappa(t)E - \phi E + \rho E_V - \mu E$$

$$- l\beta_2 E \frac{E + E_V + I + I_V}{N} \qquad (78)$$

$$\frac{dS_V}{dt} = \phi S - \epsilon\beta_1 S_V \frac{E + E_V + I + I_V}{N} + \alpha E_V + \gamma I_V - \rho S_V - \mu S_V \qquad (79)$$

$$\frac{dE_V}{dt} = \epsilon\beta_1 S_V \frac{E + E_V + I + I_V}{N} - \alpha E_V + \phi E - \rho E_V - \delta\kappa(t)E_V$$

$$- \mu E_V - \delta\beta_2 \frac{E + E_V + I + I_V}{N} \qquad (80)$$

$$\frac{dI}{dt} = l\kappa(t)E + l\beta_2 E \frac{E + E_V + I + I_V}{N} - (\gamma + \eta + \mu)I \qquad (81)$$

$$\frac{dI_V}{dt} = \delta\kappa(t)E_V + \delta\beta_2 \frac{E + E_V + I + I_V}{N} - (\gamma + \eta + \mu)I_V. \qquad (82)$$

8.1 Surveillance Data

Our interpretation of the case notification data must also be modified to reflect the additional infection mechanism, so that the number of new cases is now

$$Y_j \sim f(t_j, \vec{\theta}) = \int_{t_j}^{t_{j+1}} [l\kappa E + l\beta_2 E \frac{E + E_V + I + I_V}{N} + \delta\kappa E_V$$

$$+ \delta\beta_2 E_V \frac{E + E_V + I + I_V}{N}]ds,$$

where $j = 1, \ldots, 36$. We estimate parameters $\vec{\theta} = (\beta_1, \kappa_0, \kappa_1, \delta, \beta_2)^T$ now from these 36 monthly cases, and from the corresponding annual reports of which of these cases were vaccinated or unvaccinated. These data are represented by

$$Y_i \sim f(t_i, \vec{\theta}) = \int_{t_i}^{t_{i+1}} \left[l\kappa E + l\beta_2 E \frac{E + E_V + I + I_V}{N} \right] ds,$$

and

$$Y_i \sim f(t_i, \vec{\theta}) = \int_{t_i}^{t_{i+1}} \left[\delta \kappa E_V + \delta \beta_2 E_V \frac{E + E_V + I + I_V}{N} \right] ds,$$

for $i = 1, 2, 3$, and $t_i = 1, 13, 25, 37$ months for $i = 1, \ldots, 4$. Again, we assume the statistical model $Y_j = f(t_j, \vec{\theta}_0) + \epsilon_j$ where $E[\epsilon_j] = 0$, $var(\epsilon_j) = \sigma_1^2$ for all $j = 1, \ldots, 36$, and $Y_i = f(t_i, \vec{\theta}_0) + \epsilon_i$ where $E[\epsilon_i] = 0$, $var(\epsilon_i) = \sigma_2^2$ for all $i = 1, 2, 3$. Thus, we have assumed that the variance is constant longitudinally, but not equivalent across types of observations. That is, it is likely that there is more variation in the annually reported observations than those reported on a monthly basis. The least squares estimation procedure is described in more detail in [32].

8.2 Test Statistic

Here we describe the application of a test statistic to this example to compare the modified model to the comparably simpler model. The statistic will provide a basis from which to decide whether the observed data warrants the additional complexity incorporated in the above model.

From the $n = 42$ observations Y_j approximated by the model quantities $f(t_j, \vec{\theta})$, we seek to estimate parameters $\vec{\theta} = (\beta_1, \kappa_0, \kappa_1, \delta, \beta_2)^T$. We obtain these estimates via a least squares estimation process in which our estimate for $\vec{\theta}$ minimizes an objective functional $J_n(\vec{\theta})$. When $f(t_j, \vec{\theta})$ is that for the more sophisticated model above,

$$\hat{\theta} = \arg \min_{\vec{\theta} \in \Theta} J_n(\vec{\theta}),$$

where $\Theta \subset \mathbb{R}_+^5$ is a (compact) feasible parameter set. The constraint operator $H : \mathbb{R}^5 \to \mathbb{R}^1$ of (75) for our example is then the 1×5 vector $H = (0, 0, 0, 0, 1)$ and $c = 0$.

Thus the reduced parameter space (in the case of the reduced model, where $\beta_2 = 0$), is

$$\Theta_H = \{\vec{\theta} \in \Theta : H\vec{\theta} = 0\} = \{\vec{\theta} \in \Theta : \beta_2 = 0\}.$$

The estimate for $\vec{\theta}$ over Θ_H is denoted by $\hat{\theta}_H$, and is found by minimizing the same objective functional over the smaller parameter space Θ_H, i.e.,

$$\hat{\theta}_H = \arg \min_{\vec{\theta} \in \Theta_H} J_n(\vec{\theta}).$$

We use the test statistic

$$U_n = n \frac{J_n(\hat{\theta}_H) - J_n(\hat{\theta})}{J_n(\hat{\theta})}$$

which, under reasonable conditions, converges to a $\chi^2(1)$ distribution. For a significance level α, we would find a threshold τ such that $Pr\{\chi^2(1) > \tau\} = \alpha$. Then if $U_n > \tau$, we reject our null hypothesis as false, otherwise we do not reject. Our null hypothesis in this case is $H_0 : K\vec{\theta}_0 = 0$, or that the true $\beta_2 = 0$.

8.3 Inverse Problem Results

In this section we compare the results of the least squares estimation procedure with and without the "exogenous reinfection" term. The same set of surveillance data, described in Section 8.1, is used in both cases. The parameter estimates and corresponding standard errors are shown in Table 9.

Table 9 Parameter estimates without and with "exogenous reinfection"

$\vec{\theta}$	$\hat{\theta}_H$ ($\beta_2 = 0$)	$SE(\hat{\theta}_H)$	$\hat{\theta}$ ($\beta_2 \neq 0$)	$SE(\hat{\theta})$
β	1.52175	0.02	1.52287	0.0029
κ_0	$1.3656e^{-3}$	$1.3e^{-4}$	$1.3604e^{-3}$	0.0012
κ_1	0.56444	0.04	0.5632	0.52
δ	0.7197	0.06	0.71125	0.38
β_2	N/A	N/A	$2.2209e^{-14}$	0.01

The parameter estimates themselves, $\hat{\theta}_H$ and $\hat{\theta}$, do not differ significantly. Although, the standard errors indicate that our ability to estimate β and $\kappa(t)$ does change drastically depending on whether or not the two mechanisms of infection are considered. When the reinfection term is considered, we see that the standard error for this particular parameter indicates that our data do not provide a significant amount of information on this process. However, the smaller residual, RSS, when the objective functional is minimized over a larger parameter space (when $\beta_2 \neq 0$), might indicate that including the extra term provides a better fit. To resolve these two seemingly contrasting pieces of information, we turn to the test statistic to determine if the difference in residuals is enough to justify the inclusion of this extra infection rate (Fig. 22).

8.4 Model Comparison

The test statistic can be calculated as

$$U_n = n \frac{J_n(\hat{\theta}_H) - J_n(\hat{\theta})}{J_n(\hat{\theta})} = 42 \times \frac{4,244.5 - 4,220.8}{4,220.8} = 0.236.$$

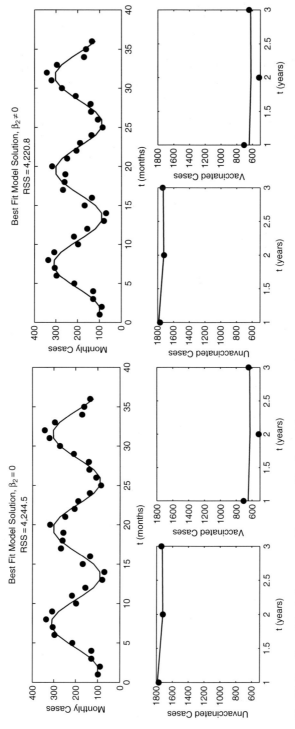

Fig. 22 Best fit model solutions to monthly case notifications with constant variance error

Note that the residual sum of squares is the value of the objective function, so that $RSS = J_n(\hat{\theta})$. We compare this to a $\chi^2(1)$ table (see Table 8) and see that even at a significance level of only 75% we cannot reject our null hypothesis. That is, the difference in residuals, and hence the improvement of the model fits to this data (with $n = 42$), is not sufficient to warrant including the additional infection mechanism. This does not mean that reinfection does not occur, but it does suggest that to accurately capture the dynamics of the population, as evidenced by this surveillance data, it is reasonable to neglect this term. Therefore, we conclude that "reinfection" is not sufficiently present in this data to argue for inclusion of this term in population level models of the infection dynamics.

9 Concluding Remarks

As might be expected, mathematical and statistical models cannot fully represent reality in most scientific situations. The best that one can hope is that models can approximate reality as presented by data from experiments sufficiently well to be useful in promoting basic understanding as well as prediction. We have in this presentation outlined some techniques for evaluation of assumptions regarding statistical models as well as comparison techniques for mathematical models under the assumption that the statistical model assumed is correct. The RSS based techniques discussed represent just one (which happens to enjoy a rigorous theoretical foundation!) of many model comparison/selection techniques available in a large literature. For example, among a wide class of so-called "model selection" methods (some of which are heuristic in nature) are those based on Kullbeck-Leibler information loss. Among the best known of these is the Akaike's Information Criterion (AIC) selection procedure and its numerous variations (AIC_c, TIC, etc.) [13–17, 28] as well as Bayesian model selection (e.g., BIC) procedures. While these are important modeling tools, space limitations prohibit their discussion here.

Finally, we have also limited our discussions to estimation problems based on OLS and GLS with appropriate corresponding data noise assumptions of constant variance and nonconstant variance (relative error), respectively. There are many other important approaches (e.g., regularization, asymptotic embedding, perturbation, equation error, adaptive filtering and identification, and numerous Bayesian based techniques – see [8, 12, 20, 23, 27, 33, 35] and the references therein) which again we ignore because of space limitations.

Acknowledgments This research was supported in part by the National Institute of Allergy and Infectious Disease under grant 9R01AI071915-05, in part by the U.S. Air Force Office of Scientific Research under grant AFOSR-FA9550-04-1-0220, and in part by the Statistical and Applied Mathematical Sciences Institute, which is funded by NSF under grant DMS-0112069.

References

1. Banks HT, Banks JE, Dick LK, Stark JD (2007) Estimation of dynamic rate parameters in insect populations undergoing sublethal exposure to pesticides, CRSC-TR05-22, May, 2005. Bull. Math. Biol. 69:2139–2180.
2. Banks HT, Dediu S, Ernstberger SE (2007) Sensitivity functions and their uses in inverse problems, CRSC-TR07-12, July, 2007. J. Inv. Ill-Posed Probl. 15:683–708.
3. Banks HT, Dediu S, Nguyen HK (2007) Sensitivity of dynamical systems to parameters in a convex subset of a topological vector space, CRSC-TR06-25, September, 2006. Math. Biosci. Eng. 4:403–430.
4. Banks HT, Ernstberger SL, Grove SL (2006) Standard errors and confidence intervals in inverse problems: sensitivity and associated pitfalls, CRSC-TR06-10, March, 2006. J. Inv. Ill-Posed Probl. 15:1–18.
5. Banks HT, Fitzpatrick BG (1989) Inverse problems for distributed systems: statistical tests and ANOVA, LCDS/CCS Rep. 88-16, July, 1988, Brown University; Proc. International Symposium on Math. Approaches Envir. Ecol. Probl. Springer Lecture Note Biomath. 81:262–273.
6. Banks HT, Fitzpatrick BG (1990) Statistical methods for model comparison in parameter estimation problems for distributed systems, CAMS Tech. Rep. 89-4, September, 1989, University of Southern California. J. Math. Biol. 28:501–527.
7. Banks HT, Kareiva P (1983) Parameter estimation techniques for transport equations with application to population dispersal and tissue bulk flow models, LCDS Report #82-13, July 1982, Brown University; J. Math. Biol. 17:253–273.
8. Banks HT, Kunsich K (1989) Estimation Techniques for Distributed Parameter Systems. Birkhauser, Boston.
9. Banks HT, Nguyen HK (2006) Sensitivity of dynamical system to Banach space parameters, CRSC-TR05-13, February, 2005. J. Math. Anal. Appl. 323:146–161.
10. Bai P, Banks HT, Dediu S, Govan AY, Last M, Loyd A, Nguyen HK, Olufsen MS, Rempala G, Slenning BD (2007) Stochastic and deterministic models for agricultural production networks, CRSC-TR07-06, February, 2007. Math. Biosci. and Engineering 4:373–402.
11. Batzel JJ, Kappel F, Schneditz D, Tran HT (2006) Cardiovascular and Respiratory Systems: Modeling, Analysis and Control. SIAM, Philadelphia.
12. Baumeister J (1987) Stable Solution of Inverse Problems. Vieweg, Braunschweig.
13. Bedrick EJ, Tsai CL (1994) Model selection for multivariate regression in small samples. Biometrics 50:226–231.
14. Bozdogan H (1987) Model selection and Akaike's Information Criterion (AIC): The general theory and its analytical extensions. Psychometrika 52:345–370.
15. Bozdogan H (2000) Akaike's Information Criterion and recent developments in information complexity. J. Math. Psychol. 44:62–91.
16. Burnham KP, Anderson DR (2002) Model Selection and Multimodel Inference: A Practical Information-Theoretic Approach. Springer, Berlin Heidelberg New York.
17. Burnham KP, Anderson DR (2004) Multimodel inference: Understanding AIC and BIC in model selection. Sociological Methods and Research 33:261–304.
18. Carroll RJ, Ruppert D (1988) Transformation and Weighting in Regression. Chapman & Hall, New York.
19. Casella G, Berger RL (2002) Statistical Inference. Duxbury, California.
20. Chalmond B (2003) Modeling and Inverse Problems in Image Analysis. Springer, Berlin Heidelberg New York.
21. Cruz JB (ed) (1973) System Sensitivity Analysis. Dowden, Hutchinson & Ross, Stroudsberg, PA.
22. Davidian M, Giltinan D (1998) Nonlinear Models for Repeated Measurement Data. Chapman & Hall, London.
23. Engl HW, Hanke M, Neubauer A (1996) Regularization of Inverse Problems.Kluwer, Dordrecht.

24. Eslami M (1994) Theory of Sensitivity in Dynamic Systems: An Introduction. Springer, Berlin Heidelberg New York.
25. Frank PM (1978) Introduction to System Sensitivity Theory. Academic, New York.
26. Gallant AR (1987) Nonlinear Statistical Models. Wiley, New York.
27. Gelb A (ed) (1979) Applied Optimal Estimation. MIT Press, Cambridge.
28. Hurvich CM, Tsai CL (1989) Regression and time series model selection in small samples. Biometrika 76: 297–307.
29. Jennrich RI (1969) Asymptotic properties of non-linear least squares estimators. Ann. Math. Statist. 40:633–643.
30. Saltelli A, Chan K, Scott EM (eds) (2000) Sensitivity Analysis. Wiley, New York.
31. Seber GAF, Wild CJ (1989) Nonlinear Regression. Wiley, New York.
32. Sutton KL, Banks HT, Castillo-Chávez C (2008) Estimation of invasive pneumococcal disease dynamic parameters and the impact of conjugate vaccination in Australia, CRSC-TR07-15, August, 2007. Math. Biosci. Eng. 5:175–204.
33. Tarantola A (2004) Inverse Problem Theory and Methods for Model Parameter Estimation. SIAM, Philadelphia.
34. Thomaseth K, Cobelli C (1999) Generalized sensitivity functions in physiological system identification. Ann. Biomed. Eng. 27(5):607–616.
35. Vogel CR (2002) Computational Methods for Inverse Problems. SIAM, Philadelphia.
36. Wackerly DD, Mendenhall III W, Scheaffer RL (2002) Mathematical Statistics with Applications. Duxbury Thompson Learning, USA.

The Epidemiological Impact of Rotavirus Vaccination Programs in the United States and Mexico

Eunha Shim and Carlos Castillo-Chavez

Abstract Rotavirus, the most common cause of gastroenteritis among children worldwide, is responsible for approximately 600,000 deaths every year worldwide. Clinical trials of RotaTeq and Rotarix, two commercially generated approved vaccines, have shown a high degree of effectiveness in protecting the most vulnerable individuals against rotavirus infections. RotaTeq and Rotarix are now incorporated into the portfolio of vaccines recommended for regular use by infants in the US and Mexico, respectively. The focus here is to evaluate the impact of vaccine-generated herd immunity, a function of the implementation regimes and coverage policies, on rotavirus transmission dynamics at the population level. In order to evaluate the overall impact of vaccine regimes in the US and Mexico, we develop an age-structured epidemiological model of rotavirus transmission that includes age-specific vaccination rates. This model is parameterized using available epidemiological and vaccine data. Numerical simulations of the parameterized model support the conclusion that reasonable rotavirus vaccination programs can prevent a significant fraction of primary (severe) rotavirus infections in the US and Mexico. Vaccination is likely to have stronger positive impact in Mexico than in the US, because the prevalence of rotavirus infections is higher in Mexico and demographics are distinct in two countries. It is shown that the age distribution of rotavirus cases will shift as a result of vaccination. This shift will be accompanied with decreases in the proportion of primary infections and the change in the distribution of subsequent infections. Effective vaccination regimes tend to increase the average age of both primary and subsequent infections. The observed shifts reduce the average population risk because severity tends to decrease with age.

Keywords Age-structured model · Rotarix · RotaTeq · Rotavirus · Vaccination

E. Shim (✉)
Department of Epidemiology and Public Health, Yale School of Medicine, New Haven, CT
e-mail: eunha.shim@yale.edu

G. Chowell et al. (eds.), *Mathematical and Statistical Estimation Approaches
in Epidemiology*, DOI 10.1007/978-90-481-2313-1_12,
© Springer Science+Business Media B.V. 2009

1 Introduction

Rotavirus infections lead to severe diarrhea requiring hospitalization in approximately one in 50 first-infection cases and results in the death of over 600,000 children annually worldwide. Rotavirus infection accounts for about 5% of all deaths in children under age five [17]. In fact, by the age of five, nearly every child will have experienced a rotavirus infection, one in five will have visited a clinic, and approximately one in 205 will have died from rotavirus induced diarrhea [6].

The primary mode of rotavirus transmission is fecal-oral, although low titers of virus have been reported in respiratory tract secretions and other body fluids. The virus is stable in regular environmental conditions. Transmission occurs through multiple routes including the ingestion of contaminated water or food, or via contacts with contaminated surfaces. Rotavirus infections are especially severe in infants and young children. Infected individuals experience fever, abdominal pain, vomiting, and diarrhea for three to eight days [6]. Treatment of rotavirus infection involves oral rehydration therapy to prevent dehydration. The immunity acquired after infection is partial, that is, prior infections while providing some degree of cross-immunity to rotavirus strains do not provide full protection. However, cross-immunity does play a role, thus recurrent infections tend to be less severe than the first infection. As a result, rotavirus infections among adults tend to be mild.

Previous studies have found that improving hygiene and supplying clean water do not contribute to significant reductions in rotavirus transmission [6]. Consequently, the development of safe and effective rotavirus vaccines has been considered the most promising route towards the development of strategies that reduce rotavirus' prevalence and morbidity [18, 25]. There are currently two live, oral, attenuated rotavirus vaccines in the market: RotaTeq, manufactured by Merck & Co., Inc., and licensed by the US Food and Drug Administration in 2006 and Rotarix, manufactured by GlaxoSmithKline, and licensed by the European Medicines Agency. RotaTeq has been recommended by the Centers for Disease Control and Prevention (CDC) for routine use in the US while Rotarix was approved for the use in Mexico by Mexico's Board of Health in 2004. The use of these rotavirus vaccines may dramatically reduce rotavirus transmission and in the process, it may also reduce rotavirus-induced morbidity and mortality.

RotaTeq and Rotarix differ in their antigenic coverage and cross-reactivity characteristics [15]. RotaTeq is a pentavalent vaccine based on five human-bovine reassortant viruses. The recommended RotaTeq policy includes three doses (once every two months), beginning when the infant reaches the age of two months. Rotarix is a monovalent vaccine derived from the most common human rotavirus strain, G1P [8], and it is given in two doses before the age of six months with a minimum interval of four weeks between doses [9]. Recovery from natural rotavirus infection protects children against the possibility of severe symptoms on re-infection.

Similarly, Rotarix mimics natural infection by generating immunological responses that protect against severe infections from homotypic or heterotypic strains [8, 10]. RotaTeq requires one more dose than Rotarix, partially because the bovine virus grows less well in the human intestine [9]. Regardless of the difference in vaccine formulation, both have proved to be safe and effective in their extensive clinical trials. RotaTeq provides 74% protection against rotavirus infection and 98% protection against severe rotavirus gastroenteritis [15]. Studies have shown that Rotarix confers 73% protection against all rotavirus infection and 85% protection against severe rotavirus gastroenteritis [15, 24]. It is expected that Rotarix and RotaTeq will be given to infants at the same time as the standard childhood vaccination against diphtheria, pertussis, and tetanus (DTaP) [9].

Vaccines offer the best individual protection against rotavirus but the impact of a rotavirus vaccination program at the population level has yet to be assessed. The focus of this study is to evaluate the impact of vaccine-generated levels of herd immunity, a function of the implementation regimes and coverage levels, on the overall transmission dynamics of rotavirus at the population level. The objective here is to explore the impact that the implementation of various rotavirus vaccine regimes may have at the national level (i.e. RotaTeq in the US and Rotarix in Mexico). The simulations are carried out in context, that is, with consideration of the US and Mexico's populations. Age-structured models are used to evaluate changes in age-specific incidence and average age of primary (i.e. first) rotavirus infection in populations where a vaccine program has been implemented.

Rotavirus vaccination regimes provide direct protection to the vaccinated and, in the process they are expected to provide indirect protection to the unvaccinated. The country-specific demographic model is developed to evaluate the possibility of such herd immunity that may be resulted from the implementation of a large-scale vaccination effort. We aim to examine if reasonable rotavirus vaccine coverage levels in the US and Mexico are likely to achieve sufficient levels of herd-immunity. Such levels of coverage will translate into benefits that go beyond the protection of vaccinated individuals. Simulation results are used to evaluate the impact of age-specific vaccine-programs on the prevalence of severe cases of rotavirus infection among young children, the most vulnerable group [2]. However, vaccine-induced immunity wanes with time, thus vaccinated children may experience rotavirus infection after the vaccine effect is gone. That is, rotavirus vaccination can at best delay the timing and lessen the severity of symptoms of rotavirus infection. It is known that vaccination programs often result in changes in the age distribution of disease cases, associated with an increase in the average age of the first infection [11]. In fact, rotavirus vaccine regimes' impact comes from their ability to alter the age distribution of primary and subsequent rotavirus infections. Complications and mortality rates associated with rotavirus infections are significantly lower among adults than children. Hence, the resulting vaccine-generated increases in the average age of the first infection are not necessarily harmful.

2 Method

2.1 Age-Structured Model for Rotavirus Transmission and Its Vaccination

A model with seven distinct epidemiological classes that incorporates the age-specific rotavirus transmission and the aging process via births and deaths is constructed to assess the impact of age-specific rotavirus vaccination regimes (Fig. 1). The model considers primary (severe) and subsequent (mild) rotavirus infections, and assumes current rotavirus vaccine schedules (completed by the age of six months) as well as vaccine-induced temporary immunity. The population is classified according to their immunological status. We consider the following state-densities of epidemiological classes (a and t denote age and time, respectively): susceptible ($S(t, a)$); severely or mildly infected ($I(t, a)$ or $I_m(t, a)$); temporarily recovered with high or low immunity ($R_2(t, a)$ or $R_1(t, a)$); and vaccinated having received a partial or complete vaccine course ($V_1(t, a)$ or $V_2(t, a)$). The number of individuals in epidemiological classes can be obtained by integrating state densities over age group. For instance, the number of individuals in the susceptible class S with ages in the interval $[a_i, a_{i+1}]$ at time t, are given by $\int_{a_i}^{a_{i+1}} S(a, t)da$.

We assume that the population has reached its demographic steady-state age distribution. The demographics of the model are parameterized using fertility and mortality data from the US and Mexico. The total population size in the US is

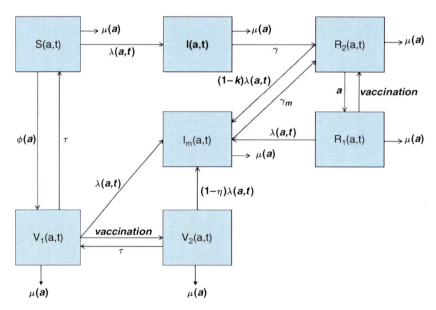

Fig. 1 Transfer diagram for the rotavirus model with vaccination

Table 1 Age groups

Age groups	Range
Group 1	Age 0–4 months
Group 2	Age 5–6 months
Group 3	Age 7–12 months
Group 4	Age 12–23 months
Group 5	Age 24–35 months
Group 6	Age 36–47 months
Group 7	Age 48–59 month
Group 8	Age 5–15 years
Group 9	Age 16–25 years
Group 10	Age 26–60 years
Group 11	Age 60 years and over

assumed to be constant but increasing for Mexico at an annual rate of 1.142%. This framework is used in order to evaluate the impact of rotavirus vaccination at the population level in the US and Mexico, and to predict how the incidence of primary and subsequent infections will change in two countries following the mass vaccination. The overall effectiveness of a vaccination program is dependent on population structure, vaccine efficacy, its coverage level, and the average duration of protection. Vaccine efficacy data for both countries are available and these data are used to test the outcomes of vaccine regimes. Age groupings are chosen based on the availability of age-dependent rotavirus incidence data (Table 1). In US' simulations, age-specific fertility and death rates are modified slightly from those published for 2008 in order to maintain a net growth rate of zero ("International Data Base, Table 028," 2008). In Mexico's simulations, age-specific fertility and death rates are used to match their 2008 reported rates.

All newborns enter the susceptible class, $S(t, a)$, and susceptible individuals who become infected through effective contacts with infectious individuals enter the class, $I(t, a)$, as illustrated in the flow diagram (Fig. 1). Infants (passively immune to rotavirus) are implicitly included in the susceptible class, however, the impact of maternal antibodies on the reduced susceptibility of infants is captured in age-specific reductions in the estimated force of infection (Fig. 2).

Susceptible individuals are vaccinated at the per-capita age-specific rate $\phi(a)$ moving either into the vaccinated V_1 or V_2 classes. Partially vaccinated susceptibles, that is, susceptible individuals who have received the first two doses of RotaTeq (or the first dose of Rotarix) enter the V_1 class. Vaccinated individuals in the class V_1, receiving the last dose, enter the V_2 class. Individuals start immunization at age $a = a_1$ and complete it at age $a = a_2$, with $a_1 < a_2$. The aim here is to follow the actual dose schedules of the rotavirus vaccine, hence, we set $a_1 = 4$ and $a_2 = 6$ months of age. Individuals in the class V_1 who become infected are assumed to get only a mild form of the disease and, consequently, they are moved to the I_m class where they recover after the average infection period, $1/\gamma_m$. Completion of the vaccination scheduled is assumed to reduce the infection incidence rate by the factor, η ($\eta = 0.74$) [6]. Vaccinated individuals will eventually move back to the

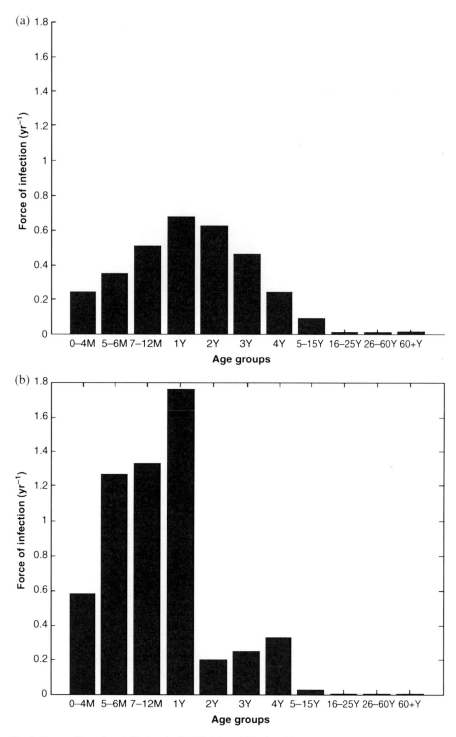

Fig. 2 Force of rotavirus infection in the US (**a**) and Mexico (**b**)

susceptible class or to the mildly infected class since the immunity gained through vaccination is temporary. Immunity wanes after vaccination but explicit data on the length of time this takes are not available. Thus, we assume that immunity, whether from infection or from the vaccine, wanes after three years ($1/\tau = 3$ years) in order to roughly estimate and incorporate the waning effect of the rotavirus immunity.

The force of infection $\lambda(t, a)$, the age-specific rotavirus transmission rate among susceptible individuals of age a at time t, is estimated from age-specific incidence data under some assumptions. Individuals acquire rotavirus infections at the rate $\lambda(t, a)$ from contacts with infectious individuals. A reduced rate of transmissibility for the mild diseases relative to severe ones is assumed, and the factor, ρ_m, that accounts for this reduction in transmissibility, is taken to be 0.5. This value is consistent with epidemiological data [22]. We also assume mean infectious period of $1/\gamma = 5$ days and $1/\gamma_m = 3$ days for primary and subsequent infections, respectively. Following recovery from infection, individuals enter the recovery class with highest immunity, R_2. The process of waning protection is incorporated via the movement of individuals from R_2 to the R_1 class at a fixed per capita rate, $\alpha = 1/3$ year^{-1}. The level of immunity in the class R_1 is lower than in R_2. In fact, it is assumed that the infection rate of mild diseases among individuals in class R_2 is assumed to be reduced by κ compared to the ones in R_1, which is set to be 0.38 [23]. Individuals that have acquired a subsequent infection are first moved to the class $I_m(a, t)$ and sent back to the R_2 class after recovery. The age-specific per capita mortality rate is $\mu(a)$.

The rotavirus infection model is given by the following system of partial differential equations:

$$\left(\frac{\partial}{\partial t} + \frac{\partial}{\partial a}\right) S(t, a) = \tau V_1(t, a) - \{\lambda(t, a) + \phi(a) + \mu(a)\}S(t, a),$$

$$\left(\frac{\partial}{\partial t} + \frac{\partial}{\partial a}\right) I(t, a) = \lambda(t, a)S(t, a) - \{\gamma + \mu(a)\}I(t, a),$$

$$\left(\frac{\partial}{\partial t} + \frac{\partial}{\partial a}\right) I_m(t, a) = \lambda(t, a)\{R_1(t, a) + (1 - \kappa)R_2(t, a) + V_1(t, a)$$

$$+ (1 - \eta)V_2(t, a)\} - \{\gamma_m + \mu(a)\}I_m(t, a),$$

$$\left(\frac{\partial}{\partial t} + \frac{\partial}{\partial a}\right) R_1(t, a) = \alpha R_2(t, a) - \{\lambda(t, a) + \phi(a) + \mu(a)\}R_1(t, a), \qquad (1)$$

$$\left(\frac{\partial}{\partial t} + \frac{\partial}{\partial a}\right) R_2(t, a) = \gamma I(t, a) + \gamma_m I_m(t, a) + \phi(a)R_1(t, a)$$

$$- \{\alpha + (1 - \kappa)\lambda(t, a) + \mu(a)\}R_2(t, a),$$

$$\left(\frac{\partial}{\partial t} + \frac{\partial}{\partial a}\right) V_1(t, a) = \tau V_2(t, a) + \phi(a)S(t, a)$$

$$- \{\tau + \lambda(t, a) + \phi(a) + \mu(a)\}V_1(t, a),$$

$$\left(\frac{\partial}{\partial t} + \frac{\partial}{\partial a}\right) V_2(t, a) = \phi(a)V_1(t, a) - \{\tau + (1 - \eta)\lambda(t, a) + \mu(a)\}V_2(t, a)$$

where

$$\lambda(t, a) = \frac{\int\limits_0^\infty \omega(a, a')[I(t, a') + \rho_m I_m(t, a')]da'}{\int\limits_0^\infty N(t, a)da}$$

and $f(a)$ is the age specific fertility rate.

The boundary conditions at age 0 are given by $S(t, 0) = \int\limits_0^\infty f(a)N(t, a)da$ and $I(t, 0) = I_m(t, 0) = R_1(t, 0) = R_2(t, 0) = V_1(t, 0) = V_2(t, 0) = 0$.

The age specific population density is $N(t, a)$ where $N(t, a) = S(t, a) + I(t, a) + I_m(t, a) + R(t, a) + V(t, a)$. We define $w(a, a')$ as the effective contact rate between the susceptible individuals of age a and infective individuals of age a' [11]. We assume that age-specific contacts are proportional to the age-specific activity levels (a relative measure of the number of age-specific contacts per unit of time) and to the sizes of the age groups [11]. Adding the equations in System (1) leads to the following equations for $N(t, a)$:

$$\left(\frac{\partial}{\partial t} + \frac{\partial}{\partial a}\right) N(t, a) = -\mu(a)N(t, a), \tag{2}$$

$$N(t, 0) = \int\limits_0^\infty f(a)N(t, a)da, \tag{3}$$

where $f(a)$ denotes the per capita age specific fertility rate.

Implementing our vaccination schedule using the above system of partial differential equations is somewhat constraining given data availability and the uncertainties associated with the estimation of the parameters for all ages. As a result, we introduce a rigorously derived model that is tailored to the constraints put by data availability. The age-structured differential equations of this new model include 11 variable age intervals, $[a_{k-1}, a_k]$ $(k = 1 \ldots 11)$ where $0 = a_0 < a_1 < a_2 < \ldots < a_{10} < a_{11}$ (Table 1). These intervals correspond to the age-specific rotavirus incidence data from which this model is parameterized [7, 16]. The age-specific force of infection is estimated from available data on the distributions of rotavirus cases in the above age groups [11]. In the simulations, we use narrow age classes for younger age groups to capture age-specific severe rotavirus infections because they are more likely to occur among children than adults. The process of aging is modeled via movement from one age grouping to the next, at the age-specific per capita rate d_i (per year), given by $d_i = A(a_i)/P_i$ where $A(a_i)$ and P_i denote the population density at age a_i and the size of the ith age group, respectively. We divide our discretized model by the size of the age groups, P_i, in order to normalize our model. We also assume that the population has reached its stable age-distribution (i.e. $N(t, a) = e^{qt}A(a)$) so that we can incorporate relevant demographic effects. By using the approach in [11], we arrive at the system of ordinary differential equations

(Appendix). This system is used to obtain our simulated results. The simulations start from the known pre-vaccination age-specific epidemiological steady state, and the simulations are run over a 100 years of time horizon.

In this study, we do not consider strain-specific vaccine efficacy, thus we do not focus or track strain-specific infections. We assume that both multivalent and monovalent rotavirus vaccines generate about the same levels of immunity against severe clinical infections regardless of the circulating human rotavirus strains. Starting from this rather simple symptomatic immunological perspective, it is assumed that all primary infections generate "equivalent" immunological responses regardless of the strains, that is, they all reduce the severity of subsequent rotavirus infections. These assumptions are based on observations and data that have concluded that an overwhelming proportion of subsequent infections are mild regardless of the strain. In summary, the vaccine is assumed to provide equivalent temporary protection against all circulating strains.

2.2 Parameterization

2.2.1 Force of Infection

The force of infection in the ith age group is the total effective contact rate between the ith age susceptible group and infective individuals of all ages. We use age-specific rotavirus case reports and age-specific serological profiles to parameterize the pre-vaccination force of infection [7, 16]. Similar approaches as our seropositivity data-based estimation procedure of the force of infection have been used to estimate the age-specific force of infection for diseases like measles and pertussis [11–13].

We assume that all individuals have experienced a rotavirus infection during their lifetime, and that the overall incidence, across all age groups, equals the cumulative incidence experienced by a cohort over its lifetime. This indicates that available horizontal information, that is, case reports over a short period of time, is representative of observed longitudinal trends [1]. It is also assumed that all individuals have experienced a rotavirus infection at least once over their lifetimes – an acceptable assumption given the high morbidity of rotavirus infections. Finally, this force of infection (λ_i) estimation approach assumes that the population is unvaccinated and that the disease has reached an equilibrium (endemic) state.

We let p_i denote the proportion of individuals of age a_i who have experienced the infection by age a_i or equivalently we let $(1 - p_i)$ denote the proportion still susceptible at age a_i. The ratio given by the accumulated sum of cases from age 0 to a_i divided by the total number of reported cases over all age classes is used to approximate the proportion of individuals of age a_i, who have experienced a rotavirus infection at least once in their a_i years of life, that is, p_i. Only in the *unrealistic* situation of "equally likely age-specific reporting" of infected individuals, such methods provide a precise approximation. We know, of course, that this is not the case because rotavirus infections are more likely to be reported when experienced by the young. Nevertheless, we chose to use this crude estimate given by equation below since it suffices for our purposes. The fact that rotavirus induced mortality and severity of symptoms are higher among young children than among adults makes our choice less arbitrary.

Under all the above limitations and assumptions, it follows that the pre-vaccination per capita force of infection linked to the age interval a_i to a_{i+1} can be estimated by $\lambda_i = -\ln\left(\frac{1-p_{i+1}}{1-p_i}\right)$[1] (Fig. 2). This estimated force of infections and the steady state age distribution are used to estimate the age-specific rate at which susceptible individuals in each specific age grouping become infected through contacts with infectious individuals from different age groupings. That is, these estimates are used to construct the age-specific matrix "who acquires the infection from whom" (WAIFW). The entries of the WAIFW matrix implicitly involve the effective contact rates between individuals of age a, and individuals of age a', that is, $\omega(a, a')$. The approach used here also assumes that the number of contacts between members of two age groupings is proportional to their corresponding activity levels as well as to the sizes of the two age groupings involved. In conclusion, the force of infection $\lambda(a, t)$ at age a and time t is taken as the sum over all ages a' of the contact rate $\omega(a, a')$ times the number of infectious individuals, divided by the total population size at time t (Fig. 2).

2.2.2 Vaccination Coverage and Efficacy

The first or second dose of RotaTeq are incorporated in the model through the movement of the vaccinated fraction of susceptible individuals in class (S) of age zero to four months, into the vaccinated class (V_1) with ages in the five to six month range, in the aggregated version of our model (Appendix), that transfers vaccinated individuals while keeping track of the aging process. Similar transfers of individuals getting the first dose of Rotarix are made from the susceptible class (S), ages from zero to four months, into the vaccinated class (V_1), ages from five to six month. Partially vaccinated individuals in the V_1 class are moved to the V_2 class at seven months of age if they receive the last dose of RotaTeq or Rotarix.

We evaluate the impact of putting in place a mature vaccine program on disease burden using expected national vaccine coverage in place for the US and Mexico. The rotavirus vaccine will be administered simultaneously with the DTaP immunizations. Hence, we approximate rotavirus vaccine coverage from existing DTaP vaccination coverage data for the US and Mexico. DTaP coverage at seven months of age is in the range of 56.4 to 80.7% with a US national average of 69.5%. These estimates are based on data from the 2006–2007 US National Vaccination Survey [3]. We assume a rotavirus vaccination national coverage level similar to those achieved with DTaP. Hence, we set $\phi_2 = 70\%$, the coverage on completed DTaP immunization in our RotaTeq and Rotarix vaccine program simulations (Fig. 3). We assume that partial vaccination (individuals who do not take all the required doses) gives temporary protection but only against severe infection (no protection against

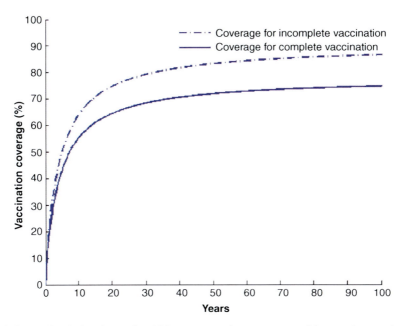

Fig. 3 Incomplete (ϕ_1) and complete (ϕ_2) coverage estimates per year of the rotavirus vaccination program

mild ones). We make this conservative assumption because efficacy data in the presence of incomplete vaccination are not available for RotaTeq and Rotarix. We use the value of 90% as our baseline coverage estimate of the proportion (among the appropriate age groups) that have taken the first dose of Rotarix or the first/second doses of RotaTeq. This value, $\phi_1 = 90\%$, is base on the fact that coverage levels with at least one dose of DTaP by the age of three months of age have been estimated to be around 89.2% [3].

Coverage is assumed to increase from zero to its highest value after some period of time from the start of a vaccination campaign. Thus, we assume that rotavirus vaccine coverage will increase over time until it reaches the baseline levels (Fig. 3). We also assume that coverage decreases as the number of doses increase (Fig. 3). As of May 2007, vaccination coverage for one-dose rotavirus among US infants aged three months was in the range of 40.1–65.4% (mean: 49.1%). These rotavirus vaccination coverage estimates are relatively low when compared with the coverage estimates that have been reported for other infant vaccines ("Rotavirus vaccination coverage and adherence to the Advisory Committee on Immunization Practices (ACIP)-recommended vaccination schedule – United States, February 2006–May 2007," 2008). For instance, the reported coverage levels for pneumococcal conjugate vaccine (PCV7) 1-dose at age three months range from 69.3 to 90.4% (mean: 84.1%) and for the diphtheria, tetanus, and a cellular pertussis (DTaP) they range from 69.5 to 92.3% (mean: 85.7%).

Furthermore, the rotavirus vaccine is assumed to have the efficacy given by the ratio of the prevalence among vaccinated infants and unvaccinated. In general, rotavirus vaccine efficacy increases with disease severity [19]. In the phase three Rotavirus Efficacy and Safety Trial (REST), RotaTeq exhibited an efficacy of 74% (95% CI 67–80%) against G1-G4 rotavirus gastroenteritis of any severity and 98% (95% CI 88–100%) against severe G1–G4 rotavirus gastroenteritis [4]. Rotarix confers 73% protection against any and 85% protection against severe rotavirus gastroenteritis [24]. We use reported data to set the baseline parameters in our simulations, thus we set a vaccine efficacy against primary infections at 74 and 73% (i.e. $\eta = 0.74$ or 0.73) for RotaTeq and Rotarix, respectively.

3 Results

We collect the results of the numerical simulation of the age-structured model of rotavirus transmission and vaccination in the context of the US and Mexico. The simulation results are used to compare the consequences of adopting rotavirus vaccine specific regimes in the US and Mexico over a 100 year time period. We assume the use of the pentavalent vaccine, RotaTeq, in the US in a population at its stable age distribution with zero net population growth. We assume the use of the monovalent vaccine, Rotarix, in Mexico in a population at its stable age distribution that increases its size at 1.142% per year. All the simulations are carried out under the assumption that vaccination starts immediately, that is, in year zero.

As vaccination coverage increases the total incidence of each country decreases. The simulation model is run until a pre-vaccination steady-state epidemiological age distribution is reached using the baseline parameters. A typical individual in each US cohort experiences an average of 0.012 and 0.034 cases of primary and subsequent rotavirus infections per year, respectively (Figs. 4 and 5). The total incidence in Mexico is higher than in the US, thus, a typical individual in this population

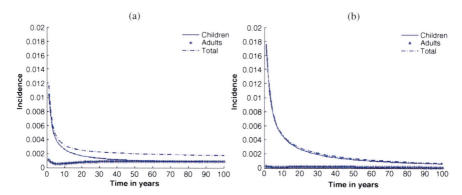

Fig. 4 Primary rotavirus incidences in the simulation model with the baseline parameter values in US (**a**) and Mexico (**b**)

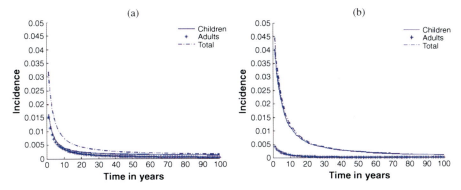

Fig. 5 Subsequent rotavirus incidences in the simulation model with the baseline parameter values in US (**a**) and Mexico (**b**)

experiences an average of 0.018 and 0.045 cases of primary and subsequent infections per year, respectively (Figs 4 and 5). We see that after 50 years, the incidences of primary infections in the US and Mexico become 0.002 and 0.001 per person, respectively. The observed reduction in the incidence of severe cases after vaccination is greater in Mexico than in the US. This may be so, because the relative incidence among adults in the US was initially higher than in Mexico. The impact of vaccination on severe infections among adults may have been therefore reduced.

Figure 6 shows the distribution of primary rotavirus infections among all age groups in the US and Mexico before a program of mass immunization against rotavirus infections was put in place. We observe that among children under the age of five, the incidence is higher in Mexico than in the US. For instance, among infants under age one, the incidence in Mexico is more than three times higher than that in the US. However, among individuals, 6–25 years of age, the incidence in

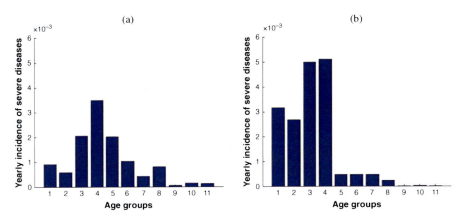

Fig. 6 Age distributions for incidence of primary rotavirus infections before vaccination program is implemented in the US (**a**) and Mexico (**b**)

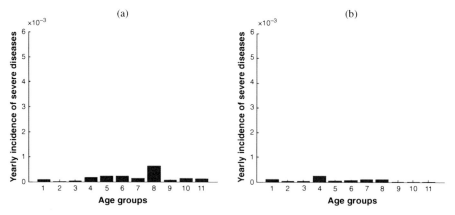

Fig. 7 Age distributions for incidence of primary rotavirus infections after vaccination program is implemented in the US (**a**) and Mexico (**b**)

the US is relatively higher than in Mexico, during the pre-vaccination era. Simulation results suggest that the largest decrease in age-specific incidence following the implementation of a vaccination program occurs among children less than five years of age (that is, among children who have completed rotavirus immunization schedule), because these groups are directly protected by vaccination (Fig. 7). The incidence in the youngest age group is also reduced even though the vaccine has not been administered at this age. These results highlight the impact of herd immunity generated by mass vaccination. On the other hand, the incidences among individuals five years of age or older do not change much, because vaccine-induced immunity wanes for many vaccinated individuals before they enter these age groups.

Figures 8 and 9 portray the distribution of subsequent rotavirus incidences in age groups before and after the introduction of mass vaccination in the US and Mexico.

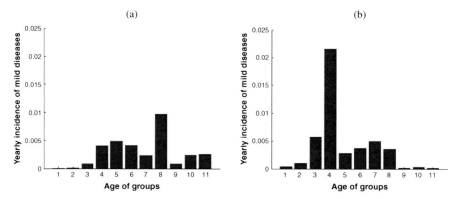

Fig. 8 Age distributions for incidence of mild rotavirus infections before vaccination program is implemented in the US (**a**) and Mexico (**b**)

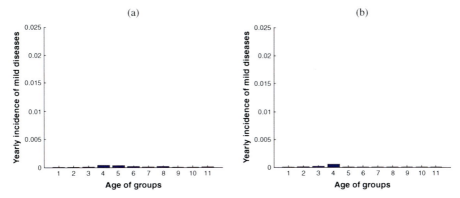

Fig. 9 Age distributions for incidence of mild rotavirus infections after vaccination program is implemented in the US (**a**) and Mexico (**b**)

Simulation results show that mass vaccination can reduce the levels of subsequent infections in the US and Mexico. The largest decrease is observed among Mexican children, 12–23 months of age or among US adolescents, 5–15 years of age. This outcome arises from the fact that incidences in the pre-vaccination era were already relatively high in these age groups. The incidence among the elderly in the US also experiences reductions after vaccination.

The average ages for primary (severe) infections as well as for subsequent (mild) infections are examined (Fig. 10). The average age of primary infections of all age groups in the US increased from four years of age before vaccination to 13 years of age after the introduction of a vaccination program. This result arises from larger decreases in primary infections among young individuals than among older people due to vaccination. The average age of primary infections of all age groups shifted, albeit less dramatically in Mexico than in the US. In Mexico the average age of primary infections among all age groups increased from about two years of age

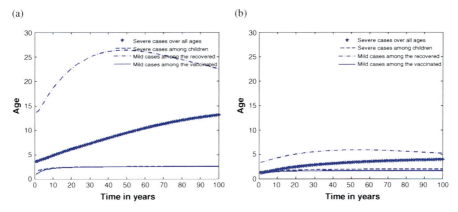

Fig. 10 Average ages of infection in the US (**a**) and Mexico (**b**) with the baseline parameter set

before vaccination to four years of age after vaccination (Fig. 10). This increase is a direct result of the impact of temporary protection of the vaccine at early ages. The population levels of temporary protection among the young translate into significant decreases in the number of primary cases among all age groups while the incidence among unvaccinated infants remain relatively unchanged. It is worth noticing that even slight increases in the average age of full-disease infection in developing countries' scenarios must be considered measures of success since infections among youngsters are linked to severe symptoms in areas where treatment is often unavailable. In Mexico and the US, the average ages of primary infections for individuals under the age of five years increased but only slightly (from about the age of two to the age of three). The average age of mild disease infections in the recovered classes increased significantly, especially among US population. In fact, it increased from 14 years of age to 22 years of age in the US. Or in other words, the planned rotavirus vaccination program is capable of delaying subsequent infections as well as primary ones.

4 Conclusions

Rotavirus, the leading cause of severe acute gastroenteritis among young children, is responsible for high levels of childhood morbidity and mortality worldwide. The withdrawal of Rotashield, an earlier rotavirus vaccine, from the US market in 1998 raised significant concerns regarding the feasibility of developing and implementing effective rotavirus control strategies. It was argued that, for children in some developing nations, the benefits of Rotashield might outweigh its risks, namely, the 1 in 10,000 possible risk of intussusception. The advent of not of one but two safe rotavirus vaccines has brought considerable hope that rotavirus morbidity and mortality in young infants will be reduced. The vaccines RotaTeq and Rotarix have been recommended for routine use among infants in the US and Mexico, respectively. There is uncertainty surrounding the long-term epidemiological impact of massive rotavirus vaccination programs on the populations of developing and developed countries. Mathematical modeling can be used to evaluate and/or predict the potential impact of rotavirus vaccination strategies over various organizational and temporal scales. Here, we evaluate and compare the impact of rotavirus vaccinations at the population level without taking into account potential evolutionary consequences.

A rotavirus transmission model was parameterized with demographic data (i.e., age structure, fertility, and mortality of the population) for the US and Mexico in order to simulate the epidemic-level impact of RotaTeq and Rotarix. We parameterized our model using reported efficacy levels of RotaTeq and Rotarix as well as known rotavirus prevalence levels in the US and Mexico. We used the force of infection and pre-immunization prevalence levels to estimate the entries of the age-specific contact matrix.

The rotavirus incidence generally has been higher in Mexico than in the US and mild and severe cases are most commonly reported among children, prior to initiation of immunization in both countries. In fact, in the pre-vaccination era, nearly all children experienced a rotavirus infection by the age five. The simulations of our age-specific rotavirus transmission model with baseline parameters are used to approximate and explore the effects of rotavirus vaccination programs in the context of the US and Mexico. Yearly rotavirus incidences are simulated before and after implementing a vaccination program. Simulations show rotavirus incidence decreases primarily on those directly protected from infection by the rotavirus vaccine, that is, in children. Decreases in the incidence of unvaccinated susceptible children are also detected, indicating the positive effect of herd immunity. We show that vaccinations reduce mild and severe cases over all age groups but that the impact is greater in Mexico than in the US. We simulate the average age of primary and subsequent infections over time, in order to test the waning effects of vaccine-induced immunity and the overall impact of a rotavirus vaccination program in the long run. We find that vaccination delays the first encounter with the virus, thus increasing the average age of infections in both the US and Mexico.

Epidemiological US data reports significant reduction in the incidence of primary infections among children from vaccination ("Delayed onset and diminished magnitude of rotavirus activity – United States, November 2007–May 2008," 2008) and our simulations support this. Based on the data collected by the National Respiratory and Enteric Virus Surveillance System (NREVSS), the number of individuals who tested positive for rotavirus antigen was substantially lower during the 2007–2008 rotavirus season than during any of the pre-vaccine years. The 2008 data was compared with the total number of positive tests for the seven preceding rotavirus seasons, during the same weeks. The total number of rotavirus positive tests took place during January–May (2008) and had a median 78.5% lower than before. For instance, the percentage of fecal specimens testing positive for rotavirus was reported to be 51% in 2006, 54% in 2007, and 6% in 2008 ("Delayed onset and diminished magnitude of rotavirus activity – United States, November 2007–May 2008," 2008).

The evaluation of the impact of rotavirus vaccination in countries, other than Mexico and the US, should not be extrapolated directly from our results, if nothing else, because the effectiveness of vaccine differs from country to country. In addition, there are further concerns. The bovine virus that is involved in RotaTeq grows less well in the human intestine and therefore whether or not such vaccine will work equally well among children in the developing world where the profiles of maternal antibodies, breast-feeding practice, nutrition status are different from those in developed nations has been raised [9]. Previous studies have shown, for example, that the immune responses of children after the administration of live oral vaccines such as polio or cholera vary in from country to country [20]. In addition, although both vaccines have reported satisfactory levels of efficacy against the full range of serotypes in circulation in the trial population, Rotarix seems to be less efficacious against the G2 strains. Therefore, it remains to be seen how well Rotarix will perform in countries where serotypes, not incorporated into the vaccine, are relatively prevalent.

Our study supports the view that rotavirus vaccination provides the best opportunity to reduce the burden of diarrheal disease in the US and Mexico. Our model can be expanded to include competing/coexisting serotypes of rotavirus and cross-immunity, or to predict vaccine demand in the US or in other countries, where strain diversity is prominent and vaccine effectiveness is in question. The methodologies used here are certainly applicable in the study of the dynamics and control of other infectious diseases.

Two additional points are worth noticing. The first involves the modeling of rotavirus as disease transmitted via age-specific contacts. The fact that rotavirus is so prevalent (in fact, it may be argued that practically everybody is a carrier) means that this disease agent may be best thought of as an environmentally transmitted disease. Hence, whether or not it is relevant or necessary to estimate who had contacts with whom, is quite relevant. Fortunately, indirectly estimated age-specific matrix "who acquires the infection from whom" (WAIFW) can be interpreted as weights that consider the influence of different age classes in the risk of transmission or acquiring an infection. The second point involves the potential evolutionary consequences of massive vaccine use. Such use may alter the competitive landscape where numerous rotavirus strains co-exist. Will dramatic reductions in rotavirus prevalence facilitate the emergence of new strain of rotavirus or other pathogens that can occupy the same niche? Our model only addresses the dynamics of transmission and control over time scales that do not incorporate potential evolutionary changes. The use of mathematical models to address the impact of human interventions on disease evolution poses tough challenges and offers great opportunities.

Acknowledgments Dr. Shim is grateful to NSERC PGS D2 Scholarship (6798-2006-0331613). Dr. Castillo-Chavez was partially supported through National Science Foundation (DMS-0502349), the National Security Agency (DOD-H982300710096), the Sloan Foundation, and Arizona State University grants.

References

1. Anderson, R. M., & May, R. M. (1985). Age-related changes in the rate of disease transmission: implications for the design of vaccination programmes. *J Hygiene 94*: 365–436.
2. Bresee, J. S., Parashar, U. D., Widdowson, M. A., Gentsch, J. R., Steele, A. D., & Glass, R. I. (2005). Update on rotavirus vaccines. *Pediatr Infect Dis J 24*(11):947–952.
3. CDC. (2008). Statistics and Surveillance: July 2006–June 2007 Table Data (Publication. Retrieved May 27, 2008: http://www.cdc.gov/vaccines/stats-surv/nis/data/tables_0607.htm
4. Clark, H. F., Bernstein, D. I., Dennehy, P. H., Offit, P., Pichichero, M., Treanor, J., et al. (2004). Safety, efficacy, and immunogenicity of a live, quadrivalent human-bovine reassortant rotavirus vaccine in healthy infants. *J Pediatr 144*(2):184–190.
5. Delayed onset and diminished magnitude of rotavirus activity – United States, November 2007–May 2008. (2008). *MMWR Morb Mortal Wkly Rep 57*(25):697–700.
6. Dennehy, P. H. (2008). Rotavirus vaccines: An overview. *Clin Microbiol Rev 21*(1), 198–208.

7. Dennehy, P. H., Cortese, M. M., Begue, R. E., Jaeger, J. L., Roberts, N. E., Zhang, R., et al. (2006). A case-control study to determine risk factors for hospitalization for rotavirus gastroenteritis in US children. *Pediatr Infect Dis J 25*(12):1123–1131.
8. Glass, R. I., Bresee, J. S., Turcios, R., Fischer, T. K., Parashar, U. D., & Steele, A. D. (2005). Rotavirus vaccines: Targeting the developing world. *J Infect Dis 192(Suppl 1)*:S160–166.
9. Glass, R. I., & Parashar, U. D. (2006). The promise of new rotavirus vaccines. *N Engl J Med 354*(1), 75–77.
10. Grimwood, K., & Bines, J. E. (2007). Rotavirus vaccines must perform in low-income countries too. *Lancet 370*(9601):1739–1740.
11. Hethcote, H. W. (1997). An age-structured model for pertussis transmission. *Math Biosci 145*(2):89–136.
12. Hethcote, H. W. (1999). Simulations of pertussis epidemiology in the United States: effects of adult booster vaccinations. *Math Biosci 158*(1):47–73.
13. Hethcote, H. W., Horby, P., & McIntyre, P. (2004). Using computer simulations to compare pertussis vaccination strategies in Australia. *Vaccine 22*(17–18):2181–2191.
14. International Data Base, Table 028. (2008). from http://www.census.gov/ipc/www/idb/idbprint.html
15. Nakagomi, O., & Cunliffe, N. A. (2007). Rotavirus vaccines: entering a new stage of deployment. *Curr Opin Infect Dis 20*(5):501–507.
16. Newall, A. T., MacIntyre, R., Wang, H., Hull, B., & Macartney, K. (2006). Burden of severe rotavirus disease in Australia. *J Paediatr Child Health 42*(9):521–527.
17. Parashar, U. D., Bresee, J. S., Gentsch, J. R., & Glass, R. I. (1998). Rotavirus. *Emerg Infect Dis 4*(4):561–570.
18. Podewils, L. J., Antil, L., Hummelman, E., Bresee, J., Parashar, U. D., & Rheingans, R. (2005). Projected cost-effectiveness of rotavirus vaccination for children in Asia. *J Infect Dis 192(Suppl 1)*:S133–145.
19. Rheingans, R. D., Constenla, D., Antil, L., Innis, B. L., & Breuer, T. (2007). Potential cost-effectiveness of vaccination for rotavirus gastroenteritis in eight Latin American and Caribbean countries. *Rev Panam Salud Publica 21*(4):205–216.
20. Roberts, L. (2004). Vaccines. Rotavirus vaccines' second chance. *Science, 305*(5692), 1890–1893.
21. Rotavirus vaccination coverage and adherence to the Advisory Committee on Immunization Practices (ACIP)-recommended vaccination schedule – United States, February 2006–May 2007. (2008). *MMWR Morb Mortal Wkly Rep 57*(15):398–401.
22. Ruuska, T., & Vesikari, T. (1990). Rotavirus disease in Finnish children: use of numerical scores for clinical severity of diarrhoeal episodes. *Scand J Infect Dis 22*(3):259–267.
23. Velazquez, F. R., Matson, D. O., Calva, J. J., Guerrero, L., Morrow, A. L., Carter-Campbell, S., et al. (1996). Rotavirus infections in infants as protection against subsequent infections. *N Engl J Med 335*(14):1022–1028.
24. Vesikari, T., Giaquinto, C., & Huppertz, H. I. (2006). Clinical trials of rotavirus vaccines in Europe. *Pediatr Infect Dis J 25*(1 Suppl):S42–47.
25. Walker, D. G., & Rheingans, R. (2005). The cost–effectiveness of rotavirus vaccines. *Expert Rev. Pharmacoeconomics Outcomes Res 5*(5):593–601.

Appendix

The fractions of the ith group in the epidemiologic classes are used in the simulations in order to present a comprehensive picture of disease progression and aging. The fractions are obtained by dividing the number of individuals in age-specific epidemiological classes by age group size. The differential equations for these fractions are derived from our model and presented below where subscripts indicate age classes.

$$ds_1(t)/dt = \sum_{j=1}^{n} f_j P_j/P_1 + \tau v_{1,1}(t) - (\lambda_1(t) + c_1 + \mu_1 + q)s_1(t),$$

$$ds_2(t)/dt = \tau v_{1,2}(t) + (1 - \phi_1)(c_1 P_1/P_2)s_1(t) - (\lambda_2(t) + c_2 + \mu_2 + q)s_2(t),$$

$$ds_3(t)/dt = \tau v_{1,3}(t) + (1 - \phi_1)(c_2 P_2/P_3)s_2(t) - (\lambda_3(t) + c_3 + \mu_3 + q)s_3(t),$$

$$ds_k(t)/dt = \tau v_{1,k}(t) + (c_{k-1} P_{k-1}/P_k)s_{k-1}(t) - (\lambda_k(t) + c_k + \mu_k + q)s_k(t),$$
$$k = 4, \cdots, 11$$

$$di_1(t)/dt = \lambda_1(t)s_1(t) - (\gamma + c_1 + \mu_1 + q)i_1(t),$$

$$di_k(t)/dt = \lambda_k(t)s_k(t) + (c_{k-1} P_{k-1}/P_k)i_{k-1}(t) - (\gamma + c_k + \mu_k + q)i_k(t),$$
$$k = 2, \cdots, 11$$

$$di_{m,1}(t)/dt = \lambda_1(t)\{r_{1,1}(t) + (1 - \kappa)r_{2,1}(t) + v_{1,1}(t) + (1 - \eta)v_{2,1}(t)\}$$
$$- (\gamma_m + c_1 + \mu_1 + q)i_{m,1}(t),$$

$$di_{m,k}(t)/dt = \lambda_k(t)\{r_{1,k}(t) + (1 - \kappa)r_{2,k}(t) + v_{1,k}(t) + (1 - \eta)v_{2,k}(t)\}$$
$$+ (c_{k-1} P_{k-1}/P_k)i_{m,k-1}(t)$$
$$- (\gamma_m + c_k + \mu_k + q)i_{m,k}(t), \quad k = 2, \cdots, 11$$

$$dr_{1,1}(t)/dt = \alpha r_{2,1}(t) - \lambda_1(t)r_{1,1}(t) - (c_1 + \mu_1 + q)r_{1,1}(t),$$

$$dr_{1,2}(t)/dt = \alpha r_{2,2}(t) - \lambda_2(t)r_{1,2}(t) + (1 - \phi_1)(c_1 P_1/P_2)r_{1,1}(t)$$
$$- (c_2 + \mu_2 + q)r_{1,2}(t),$$

$$dr_{1,3}(t)/dt = \alpha r_{2,3}(t) - \lambda_3(t)r_{1,3}(t) + (1 - \phi_1)(c_2 P_2/P_3)r_{1,2}(t)$$
$$- (c_3 + \mu_3 + q)r_{1,3}(t),$$

$$dr_{1,k}(t)/dt = \alpha r_{2,k}(t) - \lambda_k(t)r_{1,k}(t) + (c_{k-1} P_{k-1}/P_k)r_{1,k-1}(t)$$
$$- (c_k + \mu_k + q)r_{1,k}(t), \quad k = 4, \cdots, 11$$

$$dr_{2,1}(t)/dt = \gamma i_1(t) + \gamma_m i_{m,1}(t) - \{\alpha + (1 - \kappa)\lambda_1(t)\}r_{2,1}(t)$$
$$- (c_1 + \mu_1 + q)r_{2,1}(t),$$

$$dr_{2,2}(t)/dt = \gamma i_2(t) + \gamma_m i_{m,2}(t) - \{\alpha + (1 - \kappa)\lambda_2(t)\}r_{2,2}(t)$$
$$+ (1 - \phi_1)(c_1 P_1/P_2)r_{2,1}(t) - (c_2 + \mu_2 + q)r_{2,2}(t),$$

$$dr_{2,3}(t)/dt = \gamma i_3(t) + \gamma_m i_{m,3}(t) - \{\alpha + (1 - \kappa)\lambda_3(t)\}r_{2,3}(t)$$
$$+ (1 - \phi_1)(c_2 P_2/P_3)r_{2,2}(t) - (c_3 + \mu_3 + q)r_{2,3}(t),$$

$$dr_{2,k}(t)/dt = \gamma i_k(t) + \gamma_m i_{m,k}(t) - \{\alpha + (1 - \kappa)\lambda_k(t)\}r_{2,k}(t)$$
$$+ (c_{k-1}P_{k-1}/P_k)r_{2,k}(t) - (c_k + \mu_k + q)r_{2,k}(t), \quad k = 4, \cdots, 11$$

$$dv_{1,1}(t)/dt = \tau v_{2,1}(t) - \{\tau + \lambda_1(t) + c_1 + \mu_1 + q\}v_{1,1}(t),$$

$$dv_{1,2}(t)/dt = \tau v_{2,2}(t) + \phi_1(c_1 P_1/P_2)\{s_1(t) + r_{1,1}(t) + r_{2,1}(t)\} + (c_1 P_1/P_2)v_{1,1}(t)$$
$$- \{\tau + \lambda_2(t) + c_2 + \mu_2 + q\}v_{1,2}(t),$$

$$dv_{1,3}(t)/dt = \tau v_{2,3}(t) + \phi_1(c_2 P_2/P_3)\{s_2(t) + r_{1,2}(t) + r_{2,2}(t)\}$$
$$+ (1 - \phi_2)(c_2 P_2/P_3)v_{1,2}(t) - \{\tau + \lambda_3(t) + c_3 + \mu_3 + q\}v_{1,3}(t),$$

$$dv_{1,k}(t)/dt = \tau v_{2,k}(t) + (c_{k-1}P_{k-1}/P_k)v_{1,k-1}(t)$$
$$- \{\tau + \lambda_k(t) + c_k + \mu_k + q\}v_{1,k}(t), \quad k = 4, \cdots, 11.$$

$$dv_{2,1}(t)/dt = -\{\tau + (1 - \eta)\lambda_1(t) + c_1 + \mu_1 + q\}v_{2,1}(t),$$

$$dv_{2,2}(t)/dt = (c_1 P_1/P_2)v_{2,1}(t) - \{\tau + (1 - \eta)\lambda_2(t) + c_2 + \mu_2 + q\}v_{2,2}(t),$$

$$dv_{2,3}(t)/dt = (c_2 P_2/P_3)v_{2,2}(t) + \phi_2(c_2 P_2/P_3)v_{1,2}(t) - \{\tau + (1 - \eta)\lambda_3(t)$$
$$+ c_3 + \mu_3 + q\}v_{2,3}(t),$$

$$dv_{2,k}(t)/dt = (c_{k-1}P_{k-1}/P_k)v_{2,k-1}(t) - \{\tau + (1 - \eta)\lambda_k(t) + c_k + \mu_k + q]v_{2,k}(t),$$
$$k = 4, \cdots, 11.$$

Spatial and Temporal Dynamics of Rubella in Peru, 1997–2006: Geographic Patterns, Age at Infection and Estimation of Transmissibility

Daniel Rios-Doria, Gerardo Chowell, Cesar Munayco-Escate, Alvaro Witthembury, and Carlos Castillo-Chavez

Abstract Detailed studies on the spatial and temporal patterns of rubella transmission are scarce particularly in developing countries but could prove useful in improving epidemiological surveillance and intervention strategies such as vaccination. We use highly refined spatial, temporal and age-specific incidence data of Peru, a geographically diverse country, to quantify spatial-temporal patterns of incidence and transmissibility for rubella during the period 1997–2006. We estimate the basic reproduction number (R_0) based on the mean age at infection and the per capita birth rate of the population as well as the reproduction number (accounting for the fraction of the population effectively protected to infection) using the initial intrinsic growth rate of individual outbreaks and estimates of epidemiological parameters for rubella. A wavelet time series analysis is conducted to explore the periodicity of the rubella weekly time series, and the results of our analyses are compared to those carried out for time series of other childhood infectious diseases. We also identify the presence of a critical community size and quantify spatial heterogeneity across geographic regions through the use of Lorenz curves and their corresponding Gini indices. The underlying distributions of rubella outbreak attack rates and epidemic durations across Peru are characterized.

Keywords Rubella · Peru · Epidemic · Periodicity · Reproduction number · Age at infection

1 Introduction

Rubella is a virus that is transmitted via airbone droplets shed from the respiratory secretions of infected persons [1, 2]. In 1814, George Maton characterized rubella as a separate disease from measles and scarlet fever. In 1881, rubella was admitted as an official disease by the international congress of Medicine in London [3]. Rubella

D. Rios-Doria (✉)
School of Human Evolution and Social Change, Arizona State University, Tempe, AZ 85287, USA;
Mathematical, Computational, Modeling Sciences Center, Arizona State University, Tempe, AZ 85287, USA

G. Chowell et al. (eds.), *Mathematical and Statistical Estimation Approaches in Epidemiology*, DOI 10.1007/978-90-481-2313-1_13,
© Springer Science+Business Media B.V. 2009

is most prevalent in children and young adults. The clinical case definition involves three identifiable stages: (i) acute onset of a rash; (ii) temperature higher than 99° F; and (iii) arthralgia or arthritis, lymphadenopathy, or conjunctivitis [4]. Rubella has mean latent and infectious periods of about 10 and 12 days. Recovery from a rubella infection confers life long immunity to the host [5].

Although rubella is a mild disease, the effects of infection during the early stages of pregnancy may cause Congenital Rubella Syndrome (CRS), a disease stage with dangerous birth defects on newborns [4] including deafness and defects in the eyes, heart and brain. More than 100,000 cases of CRS are reported each year world-wide since surveillance began in 1998 [6]. Rubella control via vaccination has been achieved in many countries. Nevertheless, a few developing countries including Peru, are just in the process of eradicating rubella via vaccination.

Soon after the introduction of the first rubella vaccine in 1969 a number of mathematical models have been used to evaluate its impact in the reduction of rubella morbidity and CRS (e.g., [5, 7–13]). The studies are diverse and often specific. For instance, a recent study assessed the impact of the "one child per family" policy on the long term impact of rubella burden in China [5]. Nevertheless, detailed ecological studies on the dynamics of childhood infectious diseases are almost nonexistent for developing countries (e.g., [14–18]). In this paper, we explore the spatial-temporal patterns of incidence and transmissibility for rubella during the period 1997–2006 in the geographically diverse country of Peru using a unique age-specific weekly series of rubella cases stratified by province. The analyses use data stratified by geographic region (e.g., coast, mountain and jungle). The basic reproduction number (R_0) is estimated using estimates of the mean age at infection and the per capita birth rate of the population, respectively, whereas the reproduction number, accounting for the effective fraction of the population effectively protected to rubella, is estimated using the initial intrinsic growth rate of individual outbreaks and rubella epidemiology. A wavelet time series analysis is conducted to test for periodicity of the rubella weekly time series. The results of our analyses are compared to those carried out on childhood infectious diseases. We identify the presence of a critical community size and quantify spatial heterogeneity across geographic regions using the Lorenz curves and corresponding Gini indices. The underlying distributions of rubella outbreak attack rates and epidemic duration across Peru are characterized from these analyses.

2 Materials and Methods

2.1 Demographic and Geographic Data

Peru is a South American country located on the Pacific coast between the latitudes −3 degrees S to −18 degrees S. Peru shares borders with Bolivia, Brazil, Chile, Colombia, and Ecuador (Fig. 1). Peru's estimated total population is 29 million which is heterogeneously distributed throughout a surface area of 1,285,220 km².

Fig. 1 Map of Peru highlighting boundaries of 195 provinces and 25 regions. The geography of Peru covers a range of features, from a western coastal plain (*yellow*), the Andes Mountains in the center (*brown*), and the eastern jungle of the Amazon (*green*). The total population of Peru is about 29 million heterogeneously distributed in an area of 1,285,220 km^2

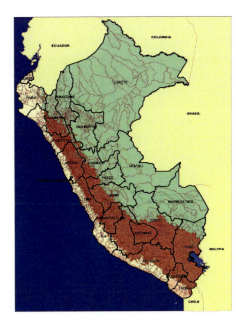

The geography of Peru includes a western coastal plain, the Andes Mountains in the center, and the eastern jungle of the Amazon. Peru is divided in 25 administrative regions further subdivided into 195 provinces. Each province is classified as a member of the coastal, mountain or jungle regions (Fig. 1). Estimates of population size per province (for 1997–2006) are found in the National Institute of Statistics and Informatics of Peru database [19]. Population density (people/km^2) estimates per province are also available. The regional estimates ranged from a mean of 22.3 people/km^2 in the mountain range, 12.38 in the jungle areas, and 172 in the coastal areas [20].

2.2 Rubella Epidemic Data

Rubella data were obtained form the Health Ministry's Department of Epidemiology (1997–2006). The age, gender, classification (probable/confirmed), location (province) and week of onset of symptoms for each rubella case are recorded. Rubella cases are classified following standard WHO guidelines into probable (clinical case) and confirmed (via antibody tests). The identification of probable rubella cases relies on three observations: acute onset of a rash, temperature higher than 99° F and arthralgia or arthritis, lymphadenopathy, or conjunctivitis [4]. The weekly number of cases at onset of symptoms, stratified by province, as recorded by the Health Ministry's Department of Epidemiology are used in this study. We define a local rubella outbreak as the occurrence of five or more recorded rubella cases within at least three consecutive weeks given that the recorded window of time is bounded above and below by the absence of reported rubella cases for at least two consecutive weeks. This approach is selected to minimize the confusion that may result from the diagnosis of imported cases (e.g., symptomatic cases occurring while visiting other provinces). In Peru, a limited vaccination effort that targeted children of one year of age and females of ages 15–19 was carried out in 2003–2005. This effort led to an approximate vaccination coverage of less than 4%. It was not until 2006 (the last year comprising our time series data) that a mass vaccination program resulted in an estimated vaccination coverage of about 68% (Peru's Ministry of Health, Department of Epidemiology). Our statistical analyses confirm that the time series data from 1997 to 2006 are not significantly impacted by the vaccination campaigns.

2.3 Wavelet Time Series Analysis

Wavelet time series analysis [21–23] has been increasingly used to disentangle the spatial and temporal dynamics (time series with non-stationary properties) generated by infectious disease and ecological systems [16, 24]. Here we use the wavelet power spectrum (using the Morlet wavelet) to investigate variations in the dominant periodic cycles across the time series using freely available software [25]. For the Morlet wavelet, the scale is almost equal to the period and consists of a sinusoidal fraction that is damped by a Gaussian function [22]. We logged transformed the time series to manage the variability in the amplitude of the time series.

2.4 Estimation of the Basic Reproduction Number, R_0

The basic reproduction number R_0 is the expected number of secondary cases generated by a typical infectious individual during its period of infectiousness when introduced into a completely susceptible population at a demographic equilibrium [26, 27]. Here we generate rough estimates of the basic reproduction number (R_0) of rubella in Peru using the simple relationships between the mean age at infection and the per capita birth rate of the population [26]. This formula has been used for the estimation of the basic reproduction number for measles and pertussis in rural Senegal where it was then used to assess the impact of vaccination campaigns [28]. Specifically, the mean basic reproduction number, R_0, is estimated by the formula $R_0 \approx G/A$, with the assumption of type I mortality [26]. Here, G is the reciprocal of the per capita birth rate and A is the mean age at infection [26, 28]. This approach requires the availability of age-structured epidemic data.

2.5 Estimation of the Reproduction Number, R

The reproduction number, R, is estimated using the mean initial intrinsic growth rate ("r") and estimates of the latent and infectious periods of rubella [26, 29]. This approach implicitly captures the effective fraction of the population (p) that is protected to infection prior to an epidemic. In a well-mixed population with a constant force of infection, the reproduction number $R \cong (1\text{-}p)\ R_0$. The homogeneous mixing assumption is not always a good assumption. However, the use of homogeneous-mixing models has been successful in assessing the seasonal change in transmissibility for childhood infectious diseases [30, 31]. Bjornstad et al. (2002) [30] used epidemic data from 60 cities in England and Wales during the prevaccination era and concluded that the homogeneous mixing model could not be rejected, which is in agreement with a seasonal well-mixed school population [30]. Here, we generate a lower bound for the reproduction number using the SEIR (susceptible-exposed-infectious-removed) epidemic model with exponentially-distributed latent and infectious periods [32] and an upper bound using a fixed generation interval [29]. From the exponential growth phase of rubella outbreaks, we estimate the intrinsic growth rate, "r". We fit a straight line (with slope "r" and intercept b) to the data on the early reports of weekly cases plotted in a logarithmic scale. The longest epidemic period that is consistent with exponential growth is determined via the goodness-of-fit test statistic [33]. The formula to estimate the reproduction number using the intrinsic growth rate "r" under the assumption of exponential waiting times for the latent and infectious periods of rubella is given by $R = (1 + \frac{r}{k})(1 + \frac{r}{\gamma})$ where $1/k$ and $1/\gamma$ are the mean latent (10 days) and infectious periods (12 days) for rubella, respectively. The mean generation interval between two successive cases is given by $T_c = 1/k + 1/\gamma$. An upper bound for the reproduction number is estimated as $R = e^{rT_c}$ when the generation interval of rubella (mean of 22 days) is assumed to be fixed [29]. The reproduction number is estimated for outbreaks with an initial epidemic phase of at least 5 consecutive weeks.

2.6 Critical Community Size

Various studies dealing with endemic infectious diseases, such as measles, have analyzed disease persistence as a function of community size in isolated and non-isolated communities ([26, 34, 35]). These persistence patterns depend not only on the transmission potential of the infectious agent but also on the characteristics of the host population including migration rates and/or birth that guarantee the replenishing susceptible population [36] and the host mobility patterns that are directly linked to a disease's reintroduction [30]. Here we use the proportion of weeks with no rubella reports for each of the provinces in the time series (1997–2006) to identify possible relationships between community size and rubella persistence in the three geographic regions.

2.7 Scaling Laws in the Distributions of Attack Rates and Duration of Epidemics

Power law distributions, for the final epidemics size and epidemic durations, have been fitted previously to multi-annual measles epidemic data generated from outbreaks in island populations [37, 38]. Here we show that the distribution of attack rates and epidemic durations during 1997–2006 are well characterized by power law (Pareto) distributions, that is, a distribution of the form X^{-b} where b is a positive constant.

2.8 Spatial Heterogeneity of Epidemics

Variations in attack rates across Peru are evaluated using the Lorenz curve and its associated summary Gini index, an approach borrowed from econometrics to quantify the spatial heterogeneity of infectious diseases ([39–42]). The Lorenz curve provides a graphical representation of the cumulative distribution function of a probability distribution. It plots the proportion of cases associated with the bottom y% of the population per region. Equal attack rates (no heterogeneity) result in a first diagonal Lorenz curve. For example, perfectly unbalanced distributions give rise to a vertical line Lorenz curve. Maximum heterogeneity results correspond to the situation when all locations except one had 0 rubella cases. Most empirical attack rate distributions lie somewhere in-between. The Gini index (ranging between 0 and 1) summarizes the statistics generated by the Lorenz curve. A large Gini index close to 1 indicates highly heterogeneous attack rates, that is, when the higher attack rates are concentrated in a small proportion of the population. A Gini index of zero indicates spatial homogeneity, that is, the situation when attack rates are proportional to population size.

3 Results

During the period 1997–2006, one hundred and seventy one provinces reported rubella cases (Fig. 2). Thirty eight percent of the probable rubella cases were confirmed via anti-rubella IgM antibody tests with the support of regional laboratories and the National Reference Laboratory at the National Institute of Health from the Ministry of Health in Peru. Our outbreak definition leads to the identification of 222 rubella outbreaks in 1997–2006. The total number of outbreaks identified decrease to a total of 201 if a threshold of 6 cases is used and to a total of 184 outbreaks using a threshold of 7 cases. In regards to seasonality, we identified seasonal trends in rubella incidence rates that strongly suggest a decay in rubella transmission rates during the winter school holiday (July 15 to August 1), which is consistent with the pattern observed for measles in England and Wales ([43, 44]). We also found the final epidemic size to be strongly correlated with the timing of the epidemic peak (Spearman $\rho = 0.64$ and $P < 0.0001$) and peak size (Spearman $\rho = 0.88$ and $P<0.0001$).

Our wavelet time series analysis at the national level reveals a dominant annual pattern. In addition a biennial pattern also shows strong power during years 2000–2004 (Fig. 2). When the data is stratified by geographic region, the annual pattern is strong across all years in coastal and mountain regions while it only shows

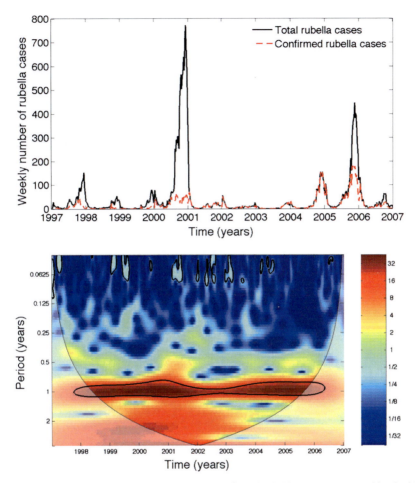

Fig. 2 The total weekly number of probable and confirmed rubella cases as reported by the Ministry of Health of Peru during 1997–2006 (*top panel*) and the wavelet power spectrum for the rubella time series (*bottom panel*), indicating a strong annual pattern across all years. In addition a biennial pattern also shows strong power during years 2000–2004

strong power during 1998–2002 in jungle regions. Biennial cycles show strong power in coastal (1999–2004) and jungle (2000–2003) regions but not in mountain regions (Fig. 3).

3.1 Estimates of the Basic Reproduction Number, R_0

We estimated the overall mean age at infection across provinces and time in Peru to be 8.9 y and the mean per capita birth rate to be 0.0247 (Peru's Health Ministry, Department of Epidemiology). This gives $R_0 \approx G/A = 40.52/8.96 = 4.52$. To

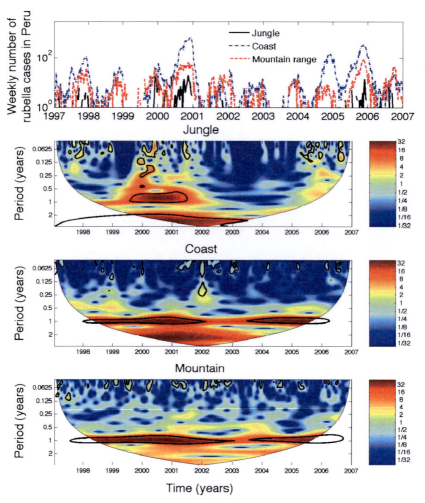

Fig. 3 The *top panel* shows the weekly number of rubella cases stratified by geographic region in Peru during 1997–2006. The *bottom panels* show the wavelet power spectrum for each of the geographic regions, which indicate a strong annual pattern across all years in coastal and mountain regions with only strong power during 1998–2002 in jungle regions. Biennial cycles show strong power in coastal (1999–2004) and jungle (2000–2003) regions but not in mountain regions

explore variations in the basic reproduction number across geographic regions in Peru, we also estimated the mean basic reproduction number by geographic region to be $47.40/8.49 = 5.58$, $36.67/8.77 = 4.18$ and $37.74/11.10 = 3.40$ in coastal, mountain, and jungle regions, respectively. However, province level estimates of the reproduction number by geographic region were not found to be statistically significantly different (ANOVA, $P = 0.14$). By contrast, the estimates of the mean age at infection were found to be significantly different across geographic areas (ANOVA, $P = 0.01$) (Fig. 5). Specifically, the mean age at infection in jungle regions (11.1 y) was found to be significantly higher than that in coastal (8.49 y) or mountain (8.77 y) regions. Furthermore, as we expected, no significant differences in the basic reproduction number were detected when comparing R_0 estimates or the mean age at infection from the initial period 1997–2002 with those estimates in the later period (2003–2006) when the initial vaccination efforts started (ANOVA, $P > 0.11$).

3.2 Estimates of the Reproduction Number, R, for Individual Rubella Outbreaks

We obtained 37 estimates of reproduction number, R, for rubella outbreaks with an initial epidemic phase of at least 5 epidemic weeks (the mean generation interval for rubella of 22 days) (Fig. 4). The assumption of an exponential distribution for the rubella generation time gives an estimate for the mean reproduction number (R) of 2.2 (95% CI: 1.9, 2.5) and the assumption of a fixed generation interval gives $R = 3.0$ (95% CI: 2.0, 4.0). In general, the estimated values of R range from $R = 6.14$ (the highest in 2000, the year of the largest rubella outbreak to date), to $R = 1.3$ (for the years 2001–2005). The estimates of the reproduction number were not correlated with population size or density, latitude or longitude coordinates. Estimates of R were not significantly different in the three geographic regions (one-way ANOVA, $P = 0.7$). R estimates were not found to be correlated with latitude or longitude coordinates or to vary across geographic regions.

3.3 Critical Community Size

Rubella was most persistent in coastal regions where 86.4% of the weeks of the study period (1997–2006) had rubella reports, followed by mountain (79.8%) and jungle regions (30.2%). The proportions of weeks with no rubella reports during the entire period (1997–2006) is negatively correlated with population size in coastal areas (Spearman $\rho= -0.64$, P<0.0001), mountain range areas (Spearman $\rho= -0.77$, P<0.0001), and jungle areas (Spearman $\rho= -0.56$, P<0.0001).

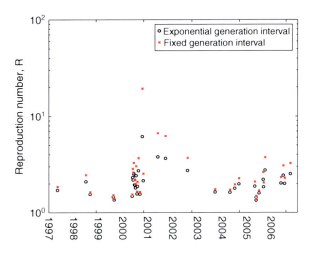

Fig. 4 Estimates of the reproduction number obtained using the initial growth rate (method 1). Lower Bound (assuming exponentially distributed latent and infectious periods) and upper bound (assuming a fixed generation interval) estimates of the reproduction number of individual outbreaks during the period 1997–2006

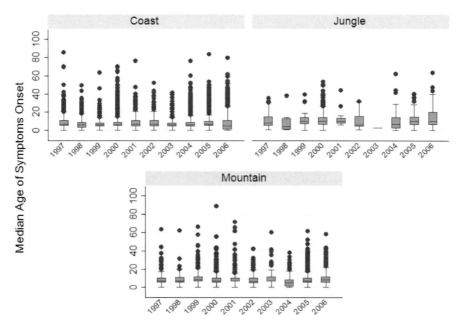

Fig. 5 Boxplots of the mean age at infection for the three geographical regions for 1997–2006. The estimates of the mean age at infection were found to be significantly different across geographic areas (ANOVA, $P = 0.01$). Specifically, the mean age at infection in jungle regions (11.1 y) was found to be significantly higher than that in coastal (8.49 y) or mountain (8.77 y) regions

In coastal regions, less than 40% of the weekly records report zero rubella cases whenever the population is around 1,000,000 or more (Fig. 6).

3.4 Scaling Laws in the Distribution of Attack Rates and Duration of Epidemics

The distribution of attack rates and epidemic durations during 1997–2006 is well characterized by power law (Pareto) distributions. In fact, the distribution of rubella attack rates and epidemic durations (weeks) both follow power-law distributions (coefficient of determination >92%, P<0.0001). Both distributions follow approximately the same power law exponent of −1.8 for epidemics during 1997–2006 (Fig. 7).

3.5 Spatial Heterogeneity

The heterogeneity of rubella incidence, as measured by the Gini index, decreased slightly from the jungle (0.34), to the coastal (0.33) and to the mountain range areas (0.26) (Fig. 8).

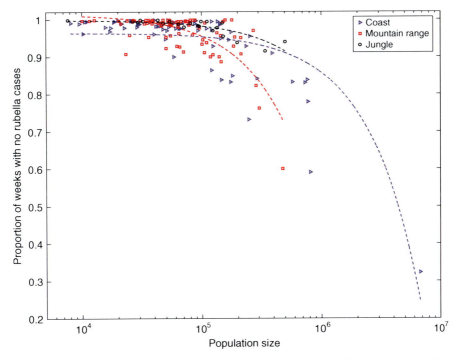

Fig. 6 The proportion of weeks with no rubella reports as a function of population size of the Peruvian provinces classified in coastal, mountain, and jungle areas. The proportion of weeks with no rubella reports during the entire study period were negatively correlated with population size in coastal areas (Spearman $\rho = -0.64$, P<0.0001), mountain range areas (Spearman $\rho = -0.77$, P<0.0001), and jungle areas (Spearman $\rho = -0.56$, P<0.0001). Less than 40% of the weekly records had zero rubella cases in heavily populated areas such as the coastal region, a characteristic not shared by mountain or jungle regions

4 Discussion

To the best of our knowledge this is the first study to evaluate the spatial and temporal dynamics of rubella in a developing country using highly refined temporal, spatial (provinces stratified in three different geographic regions) and age-structured data from Peru. We carried out comprehensive analyses of the transmission dynamics of rubella in Peru, one of the last countries in the world adopting vaccination as a policy. Our analyses include the estimation of the reproduction number using two different approaches and the assessment of periodicity, spatial heterogeneity, and persistence as a function of population size across geographic regions of Peru.

Our results highlight the importance of incorporating the space dimension (e.g., geography) in appropriately disentangling and interpreting the relevant patterns of seasonality and persistence of infectious diseases. That is, data aggregation may

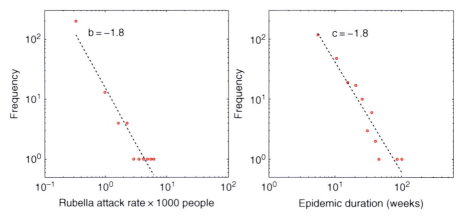

Fig. 7 The distributions of rubella attack rates and epidemic durations follow a power-law distribution with remarkably similar mean scaling exponents of about 1.7. The *dashed lines* are the log–log linear fits to the data (*red circles*)

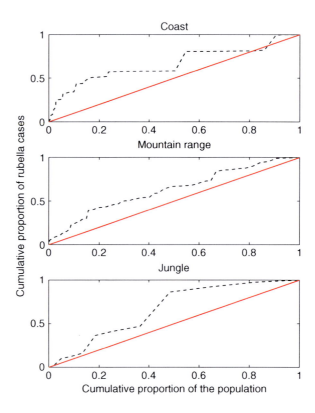

Fig. 8 The Lorenz curves of the distribution of the total number of rubella case notifications as a function of population size across geographic regions in Peru. The *black line* (first diagonal) represents a constant distribution of rubella case notifications (no heterogeneity)

complicate our understanding of the dynamics of rubella in Peru. This complication may be the result of dominant periodic patterns that differ across spatially heterogeneous areas. The results are quite distinct at different scales. At the national level, our wavelet time series analysis identifies strong annual patterns in jungle, coast and mountain regions. By contrast, the wavelet power spectrum showed different patterns by geographic regions with a single strong annual pattern in mountain regions; a dominant annual pattern in coastal regions together with a strong biennial pattern during 2002–2004; and strong annual pattern in jungle regions during 1999–2001 in addition to a strong biennial pattern during approximately 2000–2003. In rural Senegal, both measles and pertusis have a dominant annual pattern before vaccination efforts started (1983–1986) [28] whereas England and Wales experienced a transition from measles biennial cycles until the late 1960s before vaccination to annual cycles after vaccination and then to more irregular patterns [16].

Our estimation approach of the basic reproduction number (R_0) uses values of the mean age at infection and the per capita birth rates of the population [26, 28]. Hence, non-constant reporting rates across age groups can affect our estimates of the mean age at infection. Underreporting of rubella cases cannot be discarded due to the inability for infectious individuals to access medical stations in isolated jungle regions. This hinders the ability to estimate accurate incidence rates and the basic reproduction number in those regions. We observed significantly higher estimates of the mean age at infection in jungle areas compared to coastal and mountain areas. However, we were not able to detect significant differences in R_0 estimates across geographic areas.

We also estimated the reproduction number based on the initial intrinsic growth rates of individual outbreaks across provinces in Peru and the mean generation interval. Consequently, the accuracy of our estimates depends upon generating reliable estimates of these two quantities. The initial growth rate may be affected by underreporting of cases unless reporting remains approximately constant during the initial phase of the outbreaks. Also, R estimates obtained from this method are sensitive to estimates of the mean generation interval. For example, increasing the infectious period from 12 to 16 days (the generation interval increases from 22 to 26 days) increases our mean R estimates from 2.2 to 2.4 (based on exponentially distributed latent and infectious periods [32]) and from 3.0 to 3.9 (based on a fixed generation interval [29]).

Our findings are in agreement with those of Bjornstad et al (2002) [30] and Chowell et al. (2008) [45] who observed an invariant relationship between the reproduction number and population size for measles during the prevaccination era (1944–1966) and the influenza pandemic of 1918–1919, respectively, in England and Wales. This result supports frequency dependent transmission rather than density dependent transmission [46–48]. Moreover, we did not find significant differences in the reproduction number estimates across coastal, mountain and jungle regions of Peru. This suggests a similar effective contact rate for contemporary rubella transmission across geographic regions in Peru. Moreover, as we expected we did not detect significant effects of recent vaccination efforts in Peru as measured by effects on the reproduction number after 2003. Mass vaccination efforts in Peru started in 2006 (the last year considered in our analysis). Properly conducted vaccination efforts against rubella in Peru should lead to eradication of the rubella virus relatively soon. The projected effects of current vaccination campaigns against rubella in Peru are not the focus of our study.

The basic reproduction number for rubella for earlier years has been reported to range between 6–7 in England and Wales and West Germany in 1970, in the range 8–9 in Czechoslovakia in 1970–1977, in the range 11–12 in Poland in 1970–1977 and in the range 15–16 in Gambia in 1976 [26]. For comparison purposes, the basic reproduction number for measles has been reported to range 16–18 in England and Wales during 1950–1968 prior to the introduction of vaccination [26] while lower estimates of 4.6 and 4.5 for measles and pertusis, respectively, have been estimated in rural Senegal before vaccination (1983–1986) [28]. The later study estimated the basic reproduction number using the mean age at infection and the per capita birth rate, the approach that we follow in this study. Our R_0 estimates for rubella in Peru are in good agreement with those of measles and pertussis in rural Senegal [28].

Another research area in the transmission dynamics of infectious diseases is the relation between disease extinction and population size [26, 30, 35, 36]. A population threshold for extinction is the critical community size below which infections like rubella do not persist. The relationship between disease persistence and community size can be explored through the pattern of weeks without reported cases. Our findings suggest that a critical community size of nearly 1,000,000 individuals is needed for sustained epidemics in coastal areas while no clear threshold pattern of population size and rubella persistence could be disentangled in jungle and mountain regions albeit these two quantities were significantly correlated in these geographic regions ($P < 0.05$).

Our analysis reveals the presence of power law scaling relations which can be used for estimating the likelihood of epidemic duration and rubella attack rate [37, 38]. We found that most rubella outbreaks are associated with a small attack rate, although a small number of epidemics are associated with high attack rates. Furthermore, our study suggests that the distribution of rubella attack rates and epidemic durations at the level of provinces in Peru follow power law (Pareto) distributions with similar mean power-law exponents. Power law scaling in duration and size of dengue epidemics have also been reported for Peru during the period 1994–2006 [49].

Our findings indicate that regions with higher population size present higher rubella persistence than regions with lower population size ($P < 0.05$). In all geographical regions, we find low levels of spatial heterogeneity as measured by the Gini index. For comparison, a recent spatial study of dengue in Peru found much higher heterogeneity in coastal areas (Gini ~ 0.59) than the heterogeneity of rubella reported here (Gini ~ 0.34). Higher heterogeneity levels have been reported for various sexually transmitted diseases in King County, Wisconsin (> 0.60), especially for syphilis (= 0.90) [41]. For the study of the 1918–1919 influenza pandemic in England and Wales the heterogeneity was higher in rural areas (Gini ~ 0.23–0.27) than in urban areas with quite low heterogeneity (Gini ~ 0) [45].

The median age at infection in the coastal regions where the rubella incidence rates are highest is low compared to jungle regions where incidence rates have been consistently the lowest during the study period. This is consistent with standard markers that indicate higher population density leading to higher number of outbreaks (more persistence). This also raises the question of whether low incidence rates in jungle areas could be attributed to underreporting issues due to limited health care access. In fact, only one rubella case was reported in the jungle in 2003. Increasing trends in the age at infection during 2004–2006 in jungle areas supports reporting problems. However, protective effects associated to rurality (isolated areas with limited number disease introductions) in jungle areas could be playing an important role [45]. Moreover, it has been observed that with inadequate interventions for eradication, i.e. – introducing vaccination campaigns, may result in an increase of the proportion of pregnant women susceptible to rubella and other childhood infectious diseases [50]. We suggest that the use of age at infection statistics from high resolution spatial data is potentially of great value for real time surveillance of rubella. Steady increases in age at infection could represent the most reliable indicator for CRS risk.

Acknowledgments We thank Karl P. Hadeler for helpful discussions at an early stage of this work and L. Suárez-Ognio at the Health Ministry of Peru for providing rubella incidence data for Peru.

References

1. Benenson AS (1985) Control of Communicable Diseases of Man. vol. 8. 14th ed. American Public Health Association;
2. World Health Organization. Rubella and Congenital Rubella Syndrome (CRS);. http://www.who.int/immunization_monitoring/diseases/rubella/en/ (accessed on September 21, 2008).
3. Pan American Health Organization (1998) Public Health Burden of Rubella and CRS; EPI Newsletter Volume XX, Number 4.
4. Atkinson W, Hamborsky J, McIntyre L, Wolfe S (2007) Centers for Disease Control and Prevention. Epidemiology and Prevention of Vaccine-Preventable Diseases. 10th ed. Washington DC: Public Health Foundation;
5. Gao L, Hethcote HW (2006) Simulations of rubella vaccination strategies in China. Mathematical Biosciences. 202(2):371–385.
6. Robertson SE, Featherstone DA, Gacica-Dobo M, Hersh BS (2003) Rubella and congenital rubella syndrome: global update. Pan American Journal of Public Health. 14(5):306–315.
7. Knox EG (1980) Strategy for rubella vaccination. International Journal of Epidemiology 9(1):13–23.
8. Dietz K (1981) The evaluation of rubella vaccination strategies. In: Hiorns W. Cooke D, eds. The Mathematical Theory of the Dynamics of Biological Populations. vol. 2. New York: Academic Press p. 81–97.
9. Anderson RM, May RM (1983) Vaccination against Rubella and Measles: Quantitative Investigations of Different Policies. The Journal of Hygiene 90(2):259–325.

10. Hethcote HW (1983)   Measles and Rubella in the United States.   American Journal of Epidemiology 117(1):2–13.

11. Edmunds WJ, Gay NJ, Kretzschmar M, Pebody RG (2000) The pre-vaccination epidemiology of measles, mumps and rubella in Europe: Implications for modelling studies. Epidemiology and infection 125(3):635–650.

12. Brisson M, Edmunds WJ. (2003) Economic evaluation of vaccination programs: the impact of herd-immunity. Medical Decision Making 23(1):76–82.

13. Glasser J, Pistol A, Rafila A, Marin M. (2008) Designing interventions to ease an under-ascertained burden via mathematical modeling: Rubella and congenital rubella syndrome in Romania. (Manuscript)

14. Bolker BM, Grenfell BT (1995) Space, persistence and dynamics of measles epidemics. Philosophical Transactions of the Royal Society of London 348(1325):309–320.

15. Rohani P, Earn DJ, Finkenstadt B, Grenfell BT (1998) Population dynamic interference among childhood diseases. Proceedings of the Royal Society B: Biological Sciences 265(1410): 2033–2041.

16. Grenfell BT, Bjornstad ON, Kappey J (2001) Travelling waves and spatial hierarchies in measles epidemics. Nature 414:716–723.

17. Rohani P, Green CJ, Mantilla-Beniers NB, Grenfell BT (2003) Ecological interference between fatal diseases. Nature 422(6934):885–888.

18. Ferrari MJ, Grais RF, Bharti N, Conlan AJK, Bjornstad ON, Wolfson LJ, et al. (2008) The dynamics of measles in sub-Saharan Africa. Nature 451(7179):679–684.

19. Peru Instituto Nacional de Estadistica e Informatica; http://www.inei.gob.pe/ (Accessed 1 February 2008).

20. Wikipedia. Provinces of Peru; http://en.wikipedia.org/wiki/Proveinces_of_Peru (Accessed 1 February 2008).

21. Daubechies I (1992) Ten lectures on wavelets. SIAM

22. Torrence C, Compo G (1998) A practical guide to wavelet analysis. Bullein of the American Meteorological Society. 79(1):61–78.

23. Maraun D, Kurths J (2004) Cross wavelet analysis: Significance testing and pitfalls. Nonlinear Processes in Geophysics. 11:505–514.

24. Cazelles B, Chavez M, Magny GC, Guégan JF, Hales S (2007) Time-dependent spectral analysis of epidemiological time-series with wavelets. Journal of the Royal Society Interface. 4(15):625–636.

25. Grinsted A, Moore JC, Jevrejeva S. Software for Cross Wavelet and Wavelet Coherence; http://www.pol.ac.uk/home/research/waveletcoherence/ (accessed on October 6, 2008).

26. Anderson RM, May RM (1991) Infectious Diseases of Humans: Dynamics and Control. Oxford: Oxford University Press

27. Diekmann O, Heesterbeek JAP (2000) Mathematical Epidemiology of Infectious Diseases: Model Building, Analysis and Interpretation. Wiley.

28. Broutin H, Mantilla-Beniers NB, Simondon F, Aaby P, Grenfell BT, Guegan JF, et al. (2005) Epidemiological impact of vaccination on the dynamics of two childhood diseases in rural Senegal. Microbes and Infection. 7(4):593–999.

29. Wallinga J, Lipsitch M (2007) How generation intervals shape the relationship between growth rates and reproductive numbers. Proceedings of the Royal Society B: Biological Sciences. 274(1609):599.

30. Bjornstad ON, Finkenstadt BF, Grenfell BT (2002) Dynamics of measles epidemics: Estimating scaling of transmission rates using a time series SIR model. Ecological Monographs. 72(2):169–184.

31. Earn DJ, Rohani P, Bolker BM, Grenfell BT (2000) A simple model for complex dynamical transitions in epidemics. Science 287(5453):667–670.

32. Lipsitch M, Cohen T, Cooper B, Robins JM, Ma S, James L, et al. (2003) Transmission dynamics and control of severe acute respiratory syndrome. Science 300(5627).

33. Chowell G, Nishiura H, Bettencourt LM (2007) Comparative estimation of the reproduction number for pandemic influenza from daily case notification data. Journal of The Royal Society Interface 4(12):155–166.

34. Grenfell BT, Bjornstad ON, Kappey J (2001) Travelling waves and spatial hierarchies in measles epidemics. Nature 414:716–723.

35. Grenfell BT, Keeling MJ (1997) Disease extinction and community size: Modeling the presistence of measles. Science 275(5296):65–67.

36. Grenfell B, Harwood J (1997) (Meta)population dynamics of infectious diseases. TRENDS in Ecology and Evolution 12(10):395–399.

37. Rhodes CJ, Anderson RM (1996) Power laws governing epidemics in isolated populations. Nature 381(6583):600–602.

38. Keeling M, Grenfell B (1999) Stochastic dynamics and a power law for measles variability. Philosophical Transactions of the Royal Society of London. 354(1384):769–776.

39. Lee WC (1997) Characterizing exposure-disease association in human populations using the Lorenz curve and Gini index. Statistics in Medicine 16(7):729–739.

40. Woolhouse MEJ, Dye C, Etard JF, Smith T, et al. (1997) Heterogeneities in the transmission of infectious agents: Implications for the design of control programs. In: Proceedings of the National Academy of Sciences of the United States of America. vol. 94; p. 338–342.

41. Kerani RP, Handcock MS, Handsfield HH, Holmes KK (2005) Comparative geographic concentrations of 4 sexually transmitted infections. American Journal of Public Health 95(2):324–330.

42. Green CG, Krause D, Wylie J. (2006) Spatial analysis of Campylobacter infection in the Canadian province of Manitoba. International Journal of Health Geographics 5(1):2.

43. Fine PEM, Clarkson JA (1982) Measles in England and Wales- 1: An analysis of factors underlying seasonal patterns. International Journal of Epidemiology. 11(1):5–14.

44. Grassly NC, Fraser C (2006) Seasonal infectious disease epidemiology. Proceedings of the Royal Society B: Biological Sciences. 273:2541–2550.

45. Chowell G, Bettencourt LM, Johnson N, Alonso WJ, Viboud C (2008) The 1918–1919 influenza pandemic in England and Wales: Spatial patterns in transmissibility and mortality impact. Proceedings of the Royal Society B: Biological Sciences. 275:501–509.

46. Diekmann O, Jong MCMD, Koeijer AAD, Reijnders P (1995) The force of infection in populations of varying size: A modelling problem. Journal of Biological Systems. 3(2):519–529.

47. Jong MCMD, Diekmann O, Heesterbeck H (1995) Epidemic Models: Their Structure and Relation to Data. How does transmission of infection depend on population size. Cambridge University Press

48. McCallum H, Barlow N, Hone J (2001) How should pathogen transmission be modelled? TRENDS in Ecology & Evolution 16(6):295–300.

49. Chowell G, Torre CA, Munayco-Escate C, Suarez-Ognio L, Lopez Cruz RL, Hyman JM, et al. (2008) Spatial and temporal dynamics of dengue fever in Peru: 1994–2006. Epidemiology and Infection 136(12):1667–77.

50. Panagiotopoulos T, Antoniadou I, Valassi-Adam E (1999) Increase in congential rubella occurence after immunisation in Greece: Retrospective survey and systematic review. BMJ. 319:1462–1467.

The Role of Nonlinear Relapse on Contagion Amongst Drinking Communities

Ariel Cintrón-Arias, Fabio Sánchez, Xiaohong Wang,
Carlos Castillo-Chavez, Dennis M. Gorman, and Paul J. Gruenewald

Abstract Relapse, the recurrence of a disorder following a symptomatic remission, is a frequent outcome in substance abuse disorders. Some of our prior results suggested that relapse, in the context of abusive drinking, is likely an "unbeatable" force as long as recovered individuals continue to interact in the environments that lead to and/or reinforce the persistence of abusive drinking behaviors. Our earlier results were obtained via a deterministic model that ignored differences between individuals, that is, in a rather simple "social" setting. In this paper, we address the role of relapse on drinking dynamics but use models that incorporate the role of "chance", or a high degree of "social" heterogeneity, or both. Our focus is primarily on situations where relapse rates are high. We first use a Markov chain model to simulate the effect of relapse on drinking dynamics. These simulations reinforce the conclusions obtained before, with the usual caveats that arise when the outcomes of deterministic and stochastic models are compared. However, the simulation results generated from stochastic realizations of an "equivalent" drinking process in populations "living" in small world networks, parameterized via a disorder parameter p, show that there is no social structure within this family capable of reducing the impact of high relapse rates on drinking prevalence, even if we drastically limit the interactions between individuals ($p \approx 0$). Social structure does not matter when it comes to reducing abusive drinking if treatment and education efforts are ineffective. These results support earlier mathematical work on the dynamics of eating disorders and on the spread of the use of illicit drugs. We conclude that the systematic removal of individuals from high risk environments, or the development of programs that limit access or reduce the residence times in such environments (or both approaches combined) may reduce the levels of alcohol abuse.

Keywords drinking behavior · deterministic model · stochastic model · small-world network · social influence · drinking dynamics.

A. Cintrón-Arias (✉)
Center for Research in Scientific Computation, Box 8212, North Carolina State University, Raleigh, NC 27695-8205, USA

G. Chowell et al. (eds.), *Mathematical and Statistical Estimation Approaches in Epidemiology*, DOI 10.1007/978-90-481-2313-1_14,
© Springer Science+Business Media B.V. 2009

1 Introduction

The mechanisms responsible for observed drinking patterns within and between populations are complex ([25, 42, 56]; and references therein). The development of compartmental and mathematical frameworks geared towards the identification of key "transition" mechanisms that increase the percentage of abusive drinkers must factor in the impact of individuals' socioeconomic characteristics, their propensity to drink (heavy drinking tends to run in families), changes in local environments (going to college), treatment failure, ineffectiveness of educational efforts, cultural norms and community values ([42]; and references therein).

The term drinking (population) dynamics refers to the study and identification of "average" mechanisms, at the individual level, responsible for observed drinking patterns within the organizational and temporal scales of interest. We model drinking dynamics at the population level as the result of individuals' social contacts in pre-specified environments ("drinking contagion"). This modeling approach has proved useful in the identification of the mechanisms behind social patterns that are thought to be, in part, an outcome of intense interactions between individuals in shared social environments. This modeling approach has been applied to the study of the spread of scientific ideas and innovations [5]; in studies that focus on the mechanisms behind the observed increases in prevalence of eating disorders [27]; in studies that address the impact of relapse on the distribution of drinkers [51, 52]; in studies that envision violence as an epidemic [48]; as explanation for the observed growth or decline of crime in cities [26]; and in studies that highlight the explosive increases in the use of illicit drugs, such as ecstasy [37, 53]. Researchers are interested in studying the impact of individual drinking habits and preferences' variability at multiple levels of social organization: from small "isolated" to highly connected communities; and over short or long time horizons. Models have been used to explore the capacity of drinking environments to support communities of drinkers as well as the impact of individuals' movements between drinking venues on the overall distribution of drinking types [42].

The National Institute on Alcohol Abuse and Alcoholism estimates that 18 million Americans suffer from alcohol abuse or dependence. Alcohol-related problems cost the United States (U.S.) nearly $185 billion annually [43] while alcohol abuse was responsible for nearly 80,000 fatalities per year during 2001–05, and it is now the third leading cause of death in the U.S. [17]. Prevention and control efforts that include treatment and education programs that target specific populations including children [35] or adolescents [24] are in need of improvement. Among the many problems confronting these programs are the very high rates of relapse after treatment that are observed. Up to 70% of treated alcohol abusers relapse after treatment (reviewed in [52]). Mathematical studies can be particularly effective as guides to the evaluation, testing and implementation of single or multiple intervention strategies over short or long time scales. This is particularly true in the study of chronic relapsing diseases such as alcohol addiction.

1.1 Social Dynamics, Disease Transmission, and Social Structure

Several aspects linked to disease transmission depend strongly on a population's social dynamics. Disease dynamics can often be driven by factors that include heterogeneity in behavior, frequency of use of mass transportation, travel patterns, and cultural norms and practices. Examples where the use of mathematical models have generated useful insights include studies on the role of behavior on the transmission dynamics of sexually transmitted diseases like gonorrhea or HIV ([3, 16, 29, 30]; and references therein) and studies on the intensity and frequency of travel on the spread of communicable diseases such as SARS [20, 53] and influenza [22, 34]. The most significant study of the role of heterogenous mixing on the transmission dynamics of gonorrhea was carried out by Hethcote and Yorke [29]. These researchers through their introduction of the concept of core group (outliers in the distribution of sexually-active individuals) showed that most secondary cases of gonorrhea infections could be traced to the core (most connected nodes in a network of sexually-active individuals). Furthermore, they showed that focusing surveillance and treatment on core subpopulations resulted in significant reductions in gonorrhea prevalence. The public health policy at that time wrongly focused on the "random" testing of women, a policy derived from data that showed that a large percentage of gonorrhea infected women are indeed asymptomatic ([29]; and references therein).

The systematic study of the role of heterogenous social landscapes on disease dynamics began in direct response to efforts to stop the HIV epidemics. Efforts to compute explicit mixing matrices (who had interactions with whom) and to study the impact of sexual preference in the context of HIV transmission intensified ([3, 6–8, 12–15, 30–33]; and references therein).

Most recently, efforts to explore disease dynamics in the context of heterogenous (fixed) social network structures have proved quite fruitful. The study of epidemics on networks has increased our understanding of the role of "social" heterogeneity on disease dynamics ([45]; and references therein), but the impact of the efforts of the mathematical "network" community goes beyond the study of epidemics on networks, as is evident from the wealth of applications found in the literature (see [4, 45, 46, 55]; and references therein). There is a body of research that contributes to the characterization and validation of some classes of network structures with data [39]; structures whose statistical properties are most often captured via power law distributions [46]. The class of best known or more popular models of this type include small-world [55] and scale-free [4] networks.

Social network analysis is the result (to a great degree) of major contributions by social scientists ([54]; and references therein). Recent mathematical contributions ([45] and references therein; [46, 55]) have increased interactions between social and mathematical scientists. Applications that make use of specialized network structures include studies of the structure of scientific co-authorship networks [45], the organizational structure of committees in the U.S. House of representatives [49], the structure of internet networks [47], the properties of contact tracing networks for SARS [39], and the nature of sexual partnership networks [36]. Efforts to study stochastic epidemic and social processes on networks have also been carried out in the context of homeland security ([21] and references therein) and drinking [11]. Our goal here is "theoretical", that is, we focus on the study of drinking on some networks characterized by scaling laws ([45]; and references therein). Specifically, the primary objective is to explore the role of network structure on the distribution of drinkers in communities (small world type) where relapse rates are high.

This manuscript is organized as follows. Section 2 revisits the results in [51, 52] on the role of relapse on the distribution of drinking types. Section 3 introduces the stochastic analog of the deterministic model to highlight the role of variability in the distribution of drinking types of Section 2. Section 4 simulates *one version* of the stochastic drinking dynamics in a small-world network. Finally, Section 5 discusses the role of relapse in these settings.

2 A Deterministic Contagion Model in Well-Mixed Drinking Communities

In the drinking model formulation proposed in [52], the population is divided in three classes: $S(t)$, moderate and occasional drinkers [18], $D(t)$, problem or heavy drinkers [19, 44], and temporarily recovered, $R(t)$. Table 1 presents the definitions used in [52] where it is assumed that the population is composed of "average" individuals that interact at random with each other. The proportion of contacts of S-individuals with D-individuals per unit of time is therefore proportional to D/N where $N = S + D + R$, denotes the total size of the community. The progression rate from S to D and the relapse rate from R to D depend on frequency-dependent (random) interactions.

Table 1 State variables and parameters of the contagion model in Sánchez et al. [52]

State variable	Description
$S(t)$	Number of occasional and moderate drinkers at time t
$D(t)$	Number of problem drinkers at time t
$R(t)$	Number of recovered individuals at time t
Parameter	Description
β	Effective transmission rate (average number of effective interactions per occasional and problem drinker per unit of time)
ρ	Community-driven relapse rate (average number of effective interactions per problem drinker and recovered individual per unit of time)
ϕ	Per-person treatment rate
μ	Per-person departure rate from the drinking environment
N	Community size (permanent population size)

In [52] the model is given by the following set of nonlinear differential equations:

$$\frac{dS}{dt} = \mu N - \beta S(t)\frac{D(t)}{N} - \mu S(t), \tag{1}$$

$$\frac{dD}{dt} = \beta S(t)\frac{D(t)}{N} + \rho R(t)\frac{D(t)}{N} - (\mu + \phi)D(t), \tag{2}$$

$$\frac{dR}{dt} = \phi D(t) - \rho R(t)\frac{D(t)}{N} - \mu R(t), \tag{3}$$

$$N = S(t) + D(t) + R(t), \tag{4}$$

where β denotes the per-capita effective contact rate (transmission rate), that is, $\beta SD/N$ denotes the rate of transitions from S to D, the result of the frequency-dependent interactions between individuals in the classes S and D; μ denotes the per-capita departure rate from the system; ρ denotes the per-capita effective relapse rate, that is, $\rho RD/N$ denotes the rate of transitions from R to D, the result of the frequency-dependent interactions between R and D; ϕ denotes the per-capita recovery (treatment or education) rate; and μN denotes the total recruitment rate into this homogeneous social mixing community. It is assumed that all "recruits" are S-individuals. Hence, we set the S-recruitment rate equal to μN as it guarantees constant population size. The validity of the analysis is therefore tied to a time horizon where changes in total population size are minimal.

The reproductive number under a treatment/education regime ϕ is given by

$$\mathcal{R}_\phi \equiv \mathcal{R}(\phi) = \frac{\beta}{\mu + \phi}. \tag{5}$$

$\mathcal{R}_\phi$ is a dimensionless quantity (ratio or number) that can be interpreted as the number of D-individuals "generated" in a population of primarily S-individuals sharing a common environment. That is, if we start with $S \approx N$ individuals and introduce a "typical" D-individual then we expect $\mathcal{R}_\phi$ secondary cases generated from the S population per D-individual, but only at the start of the "outbreak". Hence, $\mathcal{R}_\phi > 1$ results in an exponentially growing D-community if N is large enough. We also expect that when $\mathcal{R}_\phi < 1$, the introduction of D-individuals in a population where $S \approx N$ (N large) will not result in the growth and (eventual) establishment of a problem-drinking community (D-individuals). The above observations are on target when the rate of relapse is linear, that is, ρR rather than $\rho RD/N$. However, when the relapse rate is nonlinear, namely, $\rho RD/N$, the outcome is not as "expected". The outcome depends on the ratios

$$\mathcal{R}_\rho = \frac{\rho}{\beta}[1 - \mathcal{R}(\phi)] \tag{6}$$

$$\mathcal{R}_c = \frac{\rho}{\beta}\left[\frac{1}{1 + \frac{1}{\mathcal{R}_0}} - 2\sqrt{\frac{1}{\mathcal{R}_0} - \frac{\mu}{\rho}}\right], \tag{7}$$

where $\mathcal{R}(\phi)$ is defined in Equation (5); $\mathcal{R}_0 \equiv \mathcal{R}(0) = \beta/\mu$.

$\mathcal{R}_\rho$ can be interpreted as the number of problem drinkers (D-individuals) generated from the R-class as a result of the frequency-dependent interactions between the R- and D-classes (R-individuals remain in the same environment). We observe that $\mathcal{R}_\rho > 0$ if and only if $\mathcal{R}(\phi) < 1$. On the other hand $\mathcal{R}_c > 0$ but only as long as

$$\frac{\beta}{\mu + \beta} > 2\sqrt{\frac{1}{\mathcal{R}_0} - \frac{\mu}{\rho}} > 0.$$

We have not been able to interpret the meaning of $\mathcal{R}_c$ in social terms. However, the value of $\mathcal{R}_c$, under some conditions, provides a sharp D-extinction threshold, that is, a threshold that if crossed, would lead to the eventual elimination of the D-class, independent of initial conditions ($D(0)$).

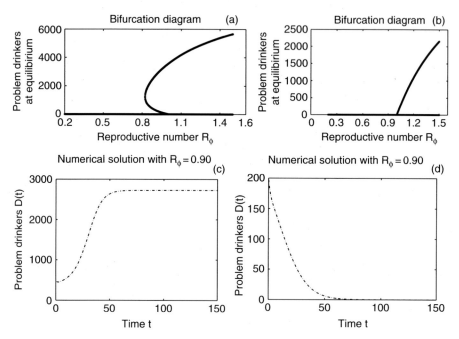

Fig. 1 Numerical simulations of drinking model in a homogeneous drinking community. **Panel (a)** shows a bifurcation diagram that involves the number of problem drinkers at equilibrium versus the reproductive number $\mathcal{R}_\phi$, when $\phi < \rho$. **Panel (b)** displays a bifurcation diagram illustrating the special case when the recovery rate equals the relapse rate ($\phi = \rho = 0.50$). Here, $\mathcal{R}_\phi < 1$ provides a sufficient condition that guarantees the eventual extinction of the population of problem drinkers. **Panels (c) and (d)** display $D(t)$ versus t under different initial conditions. In **Panel (c)** the initial conditions are $S(0) = 0.98N$, $D(0) = 0.02N$ and $R(0) = 0$; in **Panel (d)** they are $S(0) = 0.95N$, $D(0) = 0.05N$ and $R(0) = 0$. The parameter values used are: $N = 10000$, $\mu = 0.50$, $\phi = 0.50$ and $\rho = 7.00$, $0.20 \leq \beta \leq 1.50$ (**Panel (a)**); $N = 10000$, $\mu = 0.50$, $\phi = \rho = 0.50$, $0.20 \leq \beta \leq 1.50$ (**Panel (b)**); $N = 10000$, $\mu = 0.50$, $\phi = 0.50$ and $\rho = 7.00$, $\beta = 0.90$ (**Panels (c) and (d)**)

The distribution of drinking types, in the nonlinear relapse rate case, depends not only on the thresholds $\mathcal{R}_\phi$, $\mathcal{R}_\rho$, and $\mathcal{R}_0$ but also on the size of the initial population of problem drinkers, $D(0)$. In [52] the following results were obtained:

1. If $\mathcal{R}(\phi) > 1$ then the D-class becomes established.
2. Whenever $\mathcal{R}_c < \mathcal{R}(\phi) < 1$ and $\mathcal{R}_\rho < 1$ or whenever $\mathcal{R}(\phi) < \mathcal{R}_c < 1$ the D-class becomes (eventually) extinct.
3. Whenever $\mathcal{R}_c < \mathcal{R}(\phi) < 1$ and $\mathcal{R}_\rho > 1$ whether or not the D-class becomes established is a function of the initial size of the class of D-individuals, $D(0)$ (see Fig. 1c, d).

A per-capita relapse rate greater than the per-capita recovery rate, $\rho > \phi$, leads to explosive growth in the D-class as long as $D(0)$ (the initial population of problem drinkers) is "large enough" (see Fig. 1a). The qualitative behavior displayed in Fig. 1a is commonly called a "backward" bifurcation [52]. We further observe that once the population of problem drinkers becomes established ($\mathcal{R}_c < \mathcal{R}(\phi) < 1$) their extinction can only be carried out if ϕ increases to the point where $\mathcal{R}(\phi) < \mathcal{R}_c$ or if ρ decreases to the point where $\mathcal{R}_\rho < 1$. Figure 1c, d, display $D(t)$ versus t to illustrate, with a time series, the effects of initial conditions, $D(0)$. We observe bistability. The size of the initial number of problem drinkers determines whether or not a D-community becomes established even under unfavorable conditions ($\mathcal{R}(\phi) < 1$). When the per-capita relapse rate equals the recovery rate, $\rho = \phi$, we observe (Fig. 1b) that the D-class grows (gradually) with $\mathcal{R}(\phi)$; multiple endemic (non-negative) stable D-equilibria will not co-exist in this case. When $\rho = \phi$, $\mathcal{R}(\phi) < 1$ guarantees the eventual extinction of the problem drinking class.

3 A Stochastic Contagion Model

The stochastic model of this section is built from the deterministic model given by equations (1), (2), (3), (4) and is used to quantify the role of variability on drinking dynamics.

The derivation of the stochastic model (continuous-time Markov chain) is standard (details are provided in an Appendix)—see for instance [1, 2, 50]). We carry out simulations that highlight the differences between stochastic and deterministic outcomes. Simulation outcomes (distributions) are later used to contrast the results of stochastic simulations of the same drinking process in small-world networks.

The average behavior of the stochastic model is described in Table 2. The simulations of this deterministic version and stochastic analog are computed using identical epidemiological and social parameter values. It is not surprising to see overall agreement between the dynamics of the deterministic model (black curve) and the mean (over 50 realizations) dynamics of the stochastic model (grey curves) when $\mathcal{R}_\phi > 1$ (Fig. 2). The mean results are computed under the condition of non-extinction of the D-class before the preselected time horizon. Setting $\mathcal{R}_\phi < \mathcal{R}_c < 1$

Table 2 Collects the transition rates and infinitesimal probabilities of occurrence of the events linked to a single drinking model outbreak. The dependence on t is omitted, writing S, D, and R, instead of $S(t)$, $D(t)$, and $R(t)$, respectively

Event	Transition	Rate at which event occurs	Probability of transition in time interval $[t, t + dt]$
Recruitment	$S \rightarrow S + 1$	μN	$\mu N dt$
Moderate drinker removal	$S \rightarrow S - 1$	μS	$\mu S dt$
Problem drinker removal	$D \rightarrow D - 1$	μD	$\mu D dt$
Sober removal	$R \rightarrow R - 1$	μR	$\mu R dt$
Drinking contagion	$S \rightarrow S - 1, D \rightarrow D + 1$	$\beta S \frac{D}{N}$	$\beta S \frac{D}{N} dt$
Recovery	$D \rightarrow D - 1, R \rightarrow R + 1$	ϕD	$\phi D dt$
Relapse	$D \rightarrow D + 1, R \rightarrow R - 1$	$\rho R \frac{D}{N}$	$\rho R \frac{D}{N} dt$

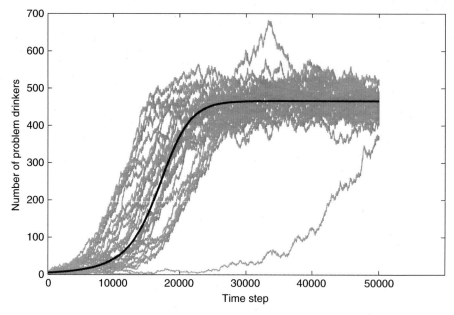

Fig. 2 Results from numerical simulations. 50 stochastic realizations (*grey curves*) and numerical solutions of the deterministic (*black curve*) problem drinker class $D(t)$ versus time t. For these simulations the following values of parameters were used: $N = 1000$, $\beta = 1.20$, $\rho = 7.00$, $\phi = 0.50$ and $\mu = 0.50$ with $\mathcal{R}_\phi = 1.20$ and the initial number of problem drinkers $D(0) = 5$

leads invariably to the eventual extinction of the D-class in the deterministic formulation but not always (as expected) in the stochastic formulation [1, 2].

In well-established drinking communities (including college students) estimates clearly show that $\mathcal{R}_\phi > 1$. Thus, one may ask whether the existence of backward bifurcations (bi-stability) is just of theoretical value? If the goal is to prevent the formation of a drinking community then the above question "makes" sense. However, most often the goal is to reduce or eliminate the D-class and the existence of a backward bifurcation makes this much harder.

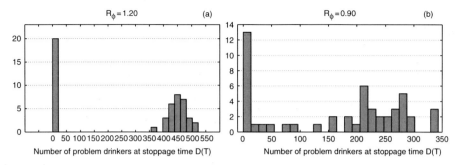

Fig. 3 Histograms of $D(T)$, number of problem drinkers at stoppage time $T = 50000$, resulting from 50 stochastic realizations with $\mathcal{R}_\phi > 1$ (**Panel (a)**) and $\mathcal{R}_\phi < 1$ (**Panel (b)**)

Relapse rates among problem drinkers are high [25, 40]. Hence, the existence of a relapse driven backward bifurcation suggests that efforts to "eliminate" problem drinkers or reduce problem drinking may be futile as long as "R-individuals" remain in the same social environment. Substantial reductions in the relapse parameter—with the ultimate goal of having $\mathcal{R}_\phi < 1$—may be extremely difficult to achieve. Furthermore, treatment and prevention measures even if effective are likely to be insufficient if the goal is to eliminate the D-class (see bifurcation diagram in Fig. 1a).

Histograms (based on 50 stochastic realizations) of the number of problem drinkers at a stoppage time T, denoted by $D(T)$, are examined when $\mathcal{R}_\phi > 1$ (Fig. 3a) and when $\mathcal{R}_\phi < 1$ (Fig. 3b). Figure 3a shows that when $\mathcal{R}_\phi > 1$ most samples of $D(T)$ lie in [350, 550), while for $\mathcal{R}_\phi < 1$ Fig. 3b shows that the problem drinker class may not go extinct. When $\mathcal{R}_\phi < 1$ more than half of the $D(T)$ samples have values between 150 and 350. These results are consistent with those of [52], that is, when the relapse rate is larger than the treatment rate ($\rho > \phi$). In other words, it is possible for a population of problem drinkers to become established even if $\mathcal{R}_\phi < 1$ in a stochastic setting.

4 Drinking Dynamics in Small-World Communities with High Relapse Rates

A network (graph) is a set of nodes with connections (edges) between them. Graphs provide visual representations of the contact structure of individuals in a population [45]. The fact that all social processes (including drinking) depend on contacts between distinct individuals has, in part, motivated the study of epidemics on networks [28, 38, 39, 47].

Watts and Strogatz [55] introduced a one-parameter, p, family of networks. As the disorder parameter p is varied in [0,1], the graph moves from a regular lattice to a random graph. The model can be formulated algorithmically as follows: the initial network is initialized via a one-dimensional periodic ring lattice of N nodes, each connected to its closest $\langle k \rangle$ neighbors (two nodes are neighbors if there is an edge connecting them). The network is updated by re-wiring each edge with probability p (the disorder parameter) to a randomly selected node until it reaches "fixed" statistical properties. When $p \to 0$ the algorithm recovers the initial lattice but when $p \to 1$, most edges are rewired, the resulting network is a random graph [9]. Watts and Strogratz showed that the use of just a few random long-range connections (p small) drastically reduced the *average* distance between any pair of nodes [55]—the kind of property that enhances "transmission", the "small-world effect". The effect was postulated based on the result of a series of letter-forwarding experiments carried out by Milgram [41]. The statistical properties of small-world and "similar" networks have been studied ([46, 55]; and references therein).

Here we model community structure as a small-world network. The terms network and community are used interchangeably, with nodes representing individuals and edges denoting the social connections or interactions, the kind of "social mixing" that may lead to node "transition" (from the moderate drinker into the problem drinker state). Nodes can be in one of three distinct states: moderate drinker, problem drinker, and recovered drinker. The stochastic transitions between nodes' states are modeled as functions of time and the number of "neighbors" in particular states (transition rates). If one starts with a community with N nodes where Node i ($1 \leq i \leq N$) has $\delta(i, t)$ neighbors who, at time t, are in the state "problem drinker", then the probabilities that Node i changes its state given that it alters its state, at each time step are: from moderate to problem drinker, $1 - \exp(-\beta\delta(i, t))$; from problem to recovered, $1 - \exp(-\phi)$; and from recovered to problem drinker, $1 - \exp(-\rho_\tau(t)\delta(i, t))$. This formulation (see Table 3) defines a stochastic process

Table 3 State variables, parameters, events, and transition probabilities of the drinking dynamics model in small-world communities

State variable	Description
$\delta(i, t)$	Number of problem drinker neighbors of node i at time t
$S_p(t)$	Total number of moderate drinkers at time t in a small-world community parameterized by p
$D_p(t)$	Total number of problem drinkers at time t in a small-world community parameterized by p
$R_p(t)$	Total number of recovered individuals at time t in a small-world community parameterized by p

Parameter	Description
β	Transmission rate
ϕ	Per-person treatment rate
$\rho_\tau(t)$	Time-dependent relapse rate

Event	Probability of transition
Node i changes from *moderate* into *problem* drinker	$1 - e^{-\beta\delta(i,t)}$
Node i switches from *problem drinker* into *recovered*	$1 - e^{-\phi}$
Node i changes from *recovered* into *problem drinker*	$1 - e^{-\rho_\tau(t)\delta(i,t)}$

Table 4 Parameter values utilized in simulations of drinking dynamics in small-world communities

Parameter	Description	Baseline value
$\langle k \rangle$	Average connectivity per node	6
N	Community size	1000
β	Transmission rate	0.12
ϕ	Per-person treatment rate	0.7
$\rho_\tau(t)$	Time-dependent relapse rate	$\rho_\tau(t) = 0.90$ whenever $t < \tau$
		$\rho_\tau(t) = 0.12$ if $t \geq \tau$
T	Stoppage time	4000
$D_p(0)$	Initial number of problem drinkers chosen uniformly at random in every community	5
	Number of stochastic realizations	20

on the random variables $S_p(t)$, $D_p(t)$, and $R_p(t)$. These random variables can also be thought of as parameterized by the disorder parameter $p \in [0, 1]$.

Drinking as a "contagious" process is simulated as follows: the stochastic generation of a small-world network [55] is followed by multiple stochastic realizations of the drinking process defined in Table 3 on the selected small-world network. The parameter baseline values are summarized in Table 4. Histograms of $D_p(T)$ and $R_p(T)$, where T denotes the stoppage time in the simulations (see Table 4), are computed for each value of p (see Fig. 4). Figures 5 and 6 highlight the mean and variance (over 20 realizations) of $D_p(T)$ and $R_p(T)$ as a function of p [21, 23].

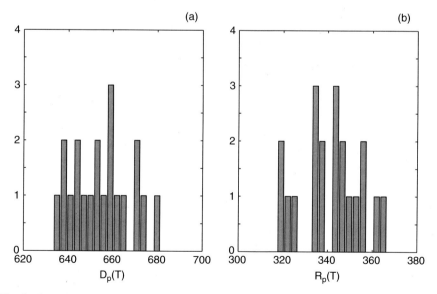

Fig. 4 Histograms of the total number of problem drinkers and recovered individuals, $D_p(T)$ and $R_p(T)$, respectively, at a stoppage time T. Samples obtained from 20 stochastic realizations in simulated communities with $p = 3.02 \times 10^{-4}$ in community size 1000 (nodes)

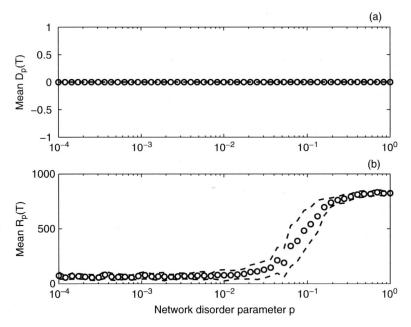

Fig. 5 Average and variance of $D_p(T)$ and $R_p(T)$ as functions of the simulated community architecture parameterized by p (*logarithmic scale*). The mean (*circles*) and mean plus and minus one standard deviation (*dash curves*) are computed from 20 stochastic realizations for each fixed value of p. **Panels (a) and (b)** display results of simulated contagion in small-world communities in the absence of relapse, $\rho \equiv 0$

A drinking wave is detected even as the size of the problem drinking class goes to zero for the case $\rho = 0$ (no relapse) with $\mathcal{R}_\phi > 1$. This feature agrees with deterministic [10] and stochastic "theories" [1] on single-outbreak SIR models. Figure 5a shows that variations on the network structure (modeled by p) have no effect on the mean size of the problem drinker class $D_p(T)$. However, the mean size of the recovered class $R_p(T)$ exhibits a phase transition as $p \to 10^{-1}$ (Fig. 5b). Hence, in the absence of vital dynamics (births and deaths) and relapse, we conclude that community structure does affect the average size of the problem drinking class during the drinking wave. Small values of "p" lead to a phase transition [45], a "small world" effect.

Figure 6 illustrates a worst case scenario in which the average relapse probability is near one for the majority of the time. To see the impact of high, nearly stationary relapse rates, we let $\langle k \rangle$ denote the average number of connections per node in a one-dimensional lattice when $p = 0$ and carry out simulations on this network with the average relapse probability $(1 - e^{-\rho_\tau(t)\langle k \rangle}) \approx 1$. The relapse rate $\rho_\tau(t)$ (defined in Table 4) is modeled as a stepwise constant function that drops its value at precisely $t = \tau$. The worst case scenario here corresponds to the case where $\tau = \infty$. In general, when relapse rates are high for too long, small-world structures (any value of p) have no effect on the mean sizes of the problem and recovered drinking classes. In fact, the size of the problem drinking community is above 60%

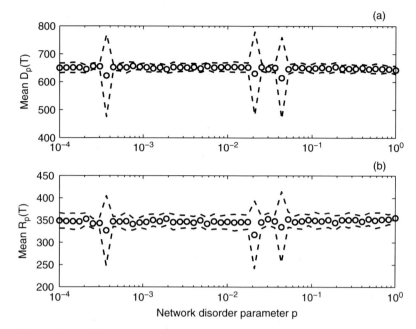

Fig. 6 Dependence of the average and variance of $D_p(T)$ and $R_p(T)$ as a function of community structure p *(logarithmic scale)*. Average *(circles)* and one standard deviation added to and subtracted from the average *(dash curves)* are calculated from 20 stochastic realizations for each fixed value of p. The results shown in **Panels (a) and (b)** assess a "worst case scenario" of having on average every recovered node going into relapse with probability nearly one, in symbols $1 - e^{-\rho_\tau(t)\langle k \rangle} \approx 1$

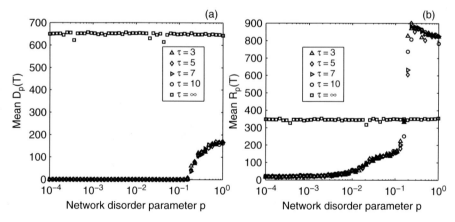

Fig. 7 Average $D_p(T)$ and $R_p(T)$ as functions of the community structure, p. **Panels (a) and (b)** display the results obtained from using a time-dependent relapse rate $\rho_\tau(t)$. The relapse rate jumps from 0.90 to 0.12 at time $t = \tau$, that is, every node diminishes its probability of transition from the recovered into the problem drinker state by half (probabilities go from $1 - e^{-0.90\langle k \rangle} \approx 1$ to $1 - e^{-0.12\langle k \rangle} \approx 0.5$) **Panels (a) and (b)** show the changes in averages as a function of the timing in the jump (τ). The relapse reduction at times, $\tau = 3$ *(upward triangles)*, $\tau = 5$ *(diamonds)*, $\tau = 7$ *(right triangles)*, $\tau = 10$ *(circles)* are highlighted. The averages displayed in Fig. 6 are for the case $\tau = \infty$ *(squares)*

regardless of the value of p (other parameters kept fixed). Furthermore, we see that on average $D_p(T) + R_p(T) = N$ when relapse rates are high. That is, every member of this closed population becomes a problem drinker at least once regardless of the value of p.

Reducing the relapse rate from 0.90 to 0.12 at precisely the time τ reduces the average relapse probability from $1 - e^{-0.90\langle k \rangle} \approx 1.00$ to $1 - e^{-0.12\langle k \rangle} \approx 0.50$ at time τ. Figure 7 shows the impact of increasing the values of $\tau = 3,\ 5,\ 7,\ 10$. We do not observe a lot of differences in the average values of $D_p(T)$ and $R_p(T)$ as a function of τ. However, these averages "improve" in the "right" direction as τ reduces its value from $\tau = \infty$ towards $\tau = 0$.

5 Discussion

Relapse has a significant impact on the dynamics of addictive behavior ([27, 52, 53]; and references therein). The use of a simple system of differential equations [52] shows that for socially-intense processes like drinking, the reproductive number, $\mathcal{R}_\phi$ is not always the key. Frequency dependent relapse rates play a significant role. Frequency dependent relapse rates do increase the possibility of severe outbreaks within "well-behaved" communities, but more importantly they also increase the likelihood of failure of programs aimed at eliminating drinking. Sánchez et al. [52] clearly delineated the possibilities from their mathematical analysis of a simple model where all the mixing takes place in the same drinking environment. Mubayi et al. [42] recently explore the impact of individuals' movement between heterogeneous drinking environments. They showed that frequent movement between *distinct* environments can have a significant (negative) effect on the distribution of drinking types. Here, we only focused on exploring the predictions of [52] in two stochastic settings. The stochastic analog (continuous time Markov chain) of Sánchez et al.'s deterministic model was used to highlight the role of variability. The results were consistent with those of Sanchez et al. with the usual caveats [1]. A small-world network was used to highlight the very strong role played by relapse.

In fact, our study of drinking in a small-world network parameterized by the disorder parameter p leads to the following results: When there is no relapse ($\rho = 0$), we recovered the well understood phase transition effect previously identified from SIR simulations on small-world networks [45], as p crosses a critical value; the introduction of high relapse rates "eliminates" the role of "p". In other words, the form of social connections (who interacts with whom) in populations experiencing strong patterns of relapse has no impact on the prevalence of addictive behaviors. Hence, if relapse rates are high then emphasis on programs that generate substantial and sustained reductions in "mixing" will not be effective. Reducing residence times in risky environments which promote relapse, reducing recruitment into drinking communities, and reducing movement between drinking venues are more likely to be effective [42].

Appendix

Transitions between drinking classes involve discrete events which change the number of individuals in every class, one at a time. For example, when a drinking "contagion" event occurs, the number of moderate drinkers is decreased by one, while the number of problem drinkers increases by one. The probability that an event takes place during an infinitesimal time interval $[t, t + dt]$ is calculated from the average rates in the deterministic model. In this example, the "conversion" event occurs at the rate of $\beta S(t)D(t)/N$ and the probability that it happens in $[t, t + dt]$ is approximately $(\beta S(t)D(t)/N)\, dt$. All the events, their rates of occurrence, and the probabilities at which they take place are listed in Table 2.

It is assumed that the events are described by independent Poisson processes [1]. The term

$$E = \mu N + \mu S + \mu D + \mu R + \beta SD/N + \phi D + \rho RD/N,$$

denotes the rate at which an event occurs at time t. The time between events is exponentially distributed with mean $1/E$. The time at which the next event happens is found, for each realization, by sampling from an exponential distribution with mean $1/E$.

To decide which event takes place (once it is known that an event occurs), we divide up the interval $(0, E)$ into subintervals that correspond to the relative occurrence probabilities of the various events. For example, given that an event has occurred, the probability that it is a recruitment is $\mu N/E$, the probability of the removal of a moderate drinker is $\mu S/E$, the probability of the removal of a problem drinker is $\mu D/E$, etc. A number U is selected randomly from the uniform distribution on $(0, 1)$ and an event is selected if this value falls within the appropriate subinterval. For instance, the event is a recruitment if U satisfies $0 < U < \mu N/E$, a moderate drinker removal if U lies between $\mu N/E$ and $(\mu N + \mu S)/E$, a problem drinker removal if U lies between $(\mu N + \mu S)/E$ and $(\mu N + \mu S + \mu D)/E$, and so on.

Acknowledgments A.C.-A. was supported in part by the Statistical and Applied Mathematical Sciences Institute which is funded by the National Science Foundation under Agreement No. DMS-0112069. Any opinions, findings, and conclusions or recommendations expressed in this material are those of the authors and do not necessarily reflect the views of the National Science Foundations. A.C.-A. was also supported in part by Grant Number R01AI071915-07 from the National Institute of Allergy and Infectious Diseases. The content is solely the responsibility of the authors and does not necessarily represent the official views of the NIAID or the NIH. X.W. and C.C.-C. were supported by NIAAA grant on "Ecosystem Models of Alcohol-Related Behavior", Contract No. HHSN2S1200410012C, ADM Contract No. No1AA410012 through Prevention Research Center, PIRE, Berkeley, the National Science Foundation (DMS-0502349), the National Security Agency (DOD-H982300710096), the Sloan Foundation, and Arizona State University. P.J.G. was supported by Grant Number R01 AA06282 from the National Institute on Alcohol Abuse and Alcoholism.

References

1. Allen, L. J. S. (2003) An Introduction to Stochastic Processes with Applications to Biology. Pearson, Upper Saddle River.
2. Allen, L. J. S., van den Driessche, P. (2006) Stochastic epidemic models with a backward bifurcation. Math. Biosci. Eng. **3**:445–458.
3. Anderson,R., May, R. (1991) Infectious Diseases of Humans: Dynamics and Control. Oxford University Press, Oxford.
4. Barabasi, A. L., Albert, R. (1999) Emergence of scaling in random networks. Science **286**(5439): 509–512.
5. Bettencourt, L. M. A., Cintrón-Arias, A., Kaiser, D. I., Castillo-Chávez, C. (2006) The power of a good idea: quantitative modeling of the spread of ideas from epidemiological models. Physica A **364**:513–536.
6. Blythe, S., Castillo-Chavez, C. (1990) Scaling law of sexual activity, Nature, **344**:202.
7. Blythe, S., Castillo-Chavez, C. (1991) Palmer, P.,Cheng, M.: Towards a unified theory of mixing and pair formation. Math. Biosci. **107**:379–405.
8. Blythe, S., Busenberg, S., Castillo-Chavez, C. (1995) Affinity and paired-event probability. Math. Biosci. **128**:265–284.
9. Bollobás, B. (2001) Random Graphs. Cambridge University Press, Cambridge.
10. Brauer, F., Castillo-Chávez, C. (2001) Mathematical Models in Population Biology and Epidemiology. Springer-Verlag, New York.
11. Braun, R. J., Wilson, R. A., Pelesko, J. A., Buchanan, J. R. (2006) Applications of small-world network theory in alcohol epidemiology. J. Stud. Alcohol **67**: 591–599.
12. Busenberg, S., Castillo-Chavez, C. (1989) Interaction, pair formation and force of infection terms in sexually transmitted diseases. In: Castillo-Chavez, C. (ed.) Mathematical and Statistical Approaches to AIDS Epidemiology. Lecture Notes Biomathematics, Vol. 83, pp. 280–300. Springer-Verlag, Berlin.
13. Busenberg, S., Castillo-Chavez, C. (1991) A general solution of the problem of mixing of subpopulation, and its application to risk- and age-structured epidemic models. IMA J. Math. Appl. Med. Biol. **8**:1–29.
14. Castillo-Chávez, C. (ed.) (1989) Mathematical and Statistical Approaches to AIDS Epidemiology. Lecture Notes in Biomathematics, Vol. 83. Springer-Verlag, Berlin.
15. Castillo-Chavez, C., Huang, W., Li, J. (1996) Competitive exclusion in gonorrhea models and other sexually-transmitted diseases. SIAM J. Appl. Math. **56**:494–508.
16. Castillo-Chavez, C., Song, B., Zhang, J. (2003) An epidemic model with virtual mass transportation: the case of smallpox in a large city. In: Banks, H.T., Castillo-Chavez, C. (eds.) Bioterrorism: Mathematical Modeling Applications in Homeland Security. Frontiers in Applied Mathematics, Vol. 28, pp. 173–198. Society for Industrial and Applied Mathematics, Philadelphia.
17. Centers for Disease Control and Prevention (2008) Alcohol and Public Health. http://www.cdc.gov/alcohol/index.htm. Cited 29 Apr 2008.
18. Centers for Disease Control and Prevention (2008) Frequently Asked Questions: What does moderate drinking mean? http://www.cdc.gov/alcohol/faqs.htm#6. Cited 11 May 2008.
19. Centers for Disease Control and Prevention (2008) Frequently Asked Questions: What do yo mean by heavy drinking? http://www.cdc.gov/alcohol/faqs.htm#10. Cited 11 May 2008.
20. Chowell, G., Fenimore, P. W., Castillo-Garsow, M. A., Castillo-Chavez, C. (2003) SARS outbreaks in Ontario, Hong Kong and Singapore: the role of diagnosis and isolation as a control mechanism. J. Theor. Biol. **224**:1–8.
21. Chowell, G., Castillo-Chávez, C. (2003) Worst-case scenarios and epidemics. In: Banks, H.T., Castillo-Chavez, C. (eds.) Bioterrorism: Mathematical Modeling Applications in Homeland Security. Frontiers in Applied Mathematics, Vol. 28, pp. 35–53. Society for Industrial and Applied Mathematics, Philadelphia.

22. Chowell, G., Ammon, C. E., Hengartner, N. W., Hyman, J. M. (2006) Transmission dynamics of the great influenza pandemic of 1918 in Geneva, Switzerland: Assessing the effects of hypothetical interventions. J. Theor. Biol. **241**:193–204.

23. Chowell, G., Cintrón-Arias, A., Del Valle, S., Sánchez, F., Song, B., Hyman, J. M., Hethcote, H. W., Castillo-Chávez, C. (2006b) Mathematical applications associated with the deliberate release of infectious agents. In: Gummel, A., Castillo-Chávez, C., Clemence, D.P., Mickens, R.E. (eds.) Modeling the Dynamics of Human Disease: Emerging Paradigms and Challenges. Contemporary Mathematics Series, Vol. 410, pp. 51–72. American Mathematical Society, Providence.

24. College Drinking (2008). http://www.collegedrinkingprevention.gov/. Cited 11 May 2008.

25. Daido, K. (2004) Risk-averse agents with peer pressure. Appl. Econ. Lett. **11**: 383–386.

26. Gladwell, M. (1996) The Tipping Point. New Yorker **72**:32–39.

27. González, B., Huerta-Sánchez, E., Ortiz-Nieves, A., Vázquez-Alvarez, T., Kribs-Zaleta, C. (2003) Am I too fat? Bulimia as an epidemic. J. Math. Psychol. **47**:515–526.

28. Grabowski, A., Kosinski, R. A. (2005) The SIS model of epidemic spreading in a hierarchical social network. Acta Phys. Pol. B **36**:1579–1593.

29. Hethcote, H., Yorke, J. (1984) Gonorrhea Transmission Dynamics and Control. Lecture Notes in Biomathematics, Vol. 56. Springer-Verlag, Berlin.

30. Hethcote, H. (2000) The mathematics of infectious diseases. SIAM Rev. **42**:599–653.

31. Hsu, S. (1993) Some Theories, Estimation Methods and Applications of Marriage Functions in Demography and Epidemiology. Dissertation, Cornell University.

32. Hsu, S., Castillo-Chavez, C. (1994) Parameter estimation in non-closed social networks related to the dynamics of sexually-transmitted diseases. In: Kaplan, E.H., Brandeau, M.L. (eds.) Modeling the AIDS Epidemic: Planning, Policy, and Prediction, pp. 533–559. Raven, New York.

33. Hsu, S., Castillo-Chavez, C. (1996) Completion of mixing matrices for nonclosed social networks. In: Lakshmikantham, V.(ed.) Proceedings of the First World Congress of Nonlinear Analysis, pp. 3163–3173. Verlag Walter de Gruyter, Berlin.

34. Hyman, J. M., LaForce, T. (2003) Modeling spread of inuenza among cities. In: Banks, H.T., Castillo-Chavez, C. (eds.) Bioterrorism: Mathematical Modeling Applications in Homeland Security. Frontiers in Applied Mathematics, Vol. 28, pp. 211–236. Society for Industrial and Applied Mathematics, Philadelphia.

35. Leadership to Keep Children Alcohol Free (2008). http://www.alcoholfreechildren.org/. Cited 11 May 2008.

36. Liljeros, F., Edling, C. R., Nunes Amaral, L. A., Stanley, H. E., Aberg, Y. (2001) The web of human sexual contacts. Nature **411**:907–908.

37. Mackintosh, D. R., Stewart, G. T. (1979) A mathematical model of a heroin epidemic: implications for control policies. J. Epidemiol. Commun. H. **33**:299–304.

38. May, R. M., Lloyd, A. L. (2001) Infection dynamics on scale-free networks. Phys. Rev. E. **64**:066112.

39. Meyers, L. A., Pourbohloul, B., Newman, M. E. J., Skowronski, D. M., Brunham, R. C. (2005) Network theory and SARS: Predicting outbreak diversity. J. Theor. Biol. **232**: 71–78.

40. Miller, W. R., Walters, S. T., Bennett, M. E. (2001) How effective is alcoholism treatment in the United States? J. Stud. Alcohol. **62**:211–220.

41. Milgram, S. (1967) The small world problem. Psychol. Today **1**:60–67.

42. Mubayi, A., Greenwood, P., Castillo-Chavez, C., Gruenewald, P., Gorman, D. M. (2009) The impact of relative residence times on the distribution of heavy drinkers in highly distinct environments. Socio. Econ. Plan. Sci. (in press).

43. National Institute of Alcohol Abuse and Alcoholism (2008) Five Year Strategic Plan. http://pubs.niaaa.nih.gov/publications/StrategicPlan/NIAAASTRATEGICPLAN.htm. Cited 29 Apr 2008.

44. National Institute of Alcohol Abuse and Alcoholism (2008) Frequently Asked Questions for the General Public. http://www.niaaa.nih.gov/FAQs/General-English/default.htm. Cited Apr 29 2008.

45. Newman, M. E. J. (2003) The structure and function of complex networks. SIAM Rev. **45**: 167–256.

46. Newman, M. E. J., Barabasi, A. L., Watts, D. J. (2006) The Structure and Dynamics of Networks. Princeton University Press, Princeton.

47. Pastor-Satorras, R., Vespignani, A. (2001) Epidemic spreading in scale-free networks. Phys. Rev. Lett. **86**:3200.

48. Patten, S. B., Arboleda-Florez, J. A. (2004) Epidemic theory and group violence. Soc. Psych. Psych. Epid. **39**:853–856.

49. Porter, M. A., Mucha, P. J., Newman, M. E. J., Warmbrand, C. M. (2005) A network analysis of committees in the U.S. house of representatives. P. Natl. Acad. Sci. USA, **102**:7057–7062.

50. Renshaw, E. (1991) Modelling Biological Populations in Space and Time. Cambridge University Press, Cambridge.

51. Sánchez, F. (2006) Studies in Epidemiology and Social Dynamics. Dissertation, Cornell University.

52. Sánchez, F., Wang, X., Castillo-Chavez, C., Gorman, D. M., Gruenewald, P. J. (2007) Drinking as an epidemic—a simple mathematical model with recovery and relapse. In: Witkiewitz, K. A., Marlatt, G. A. (eds.) Therapist's Guide to Evidence-Based Relapse Prevention: Practical Resources for the Mental Health Professional. Academic, Burlington, 353–368.

53. Song, B., Castillo-Garsow, M., Castillo-Chávez, C., Ríos Soto, K., Mejran, M., Henso, L. (2006) Raves, Clubs, and Ecstasy: The Impact of Peer Pressure. Math. Biosci. Eng. **3**: 249–266.

54. Wasserman, S., Faust, K. (1994) Social network analysis: methods and applications. Cambridge University Press, Cambridge.

55. Watts, D. J., Strogatz, S. H. (1998) Collective dynamics of 'small-world' networks. Nature **383**:440–442.

56. Weitzman, E. R., Folkman, A., Folkman, K. L., Weschler, H. (2003) The relationship of alcohol outlet density to heavy and frequent drinking and drinking-related problems among college students at eight universities. Health Place **9**:1–6.

Index